Acute Care Handbook
for Physical Therapists

Acute Care Handbook for Physical Therapists

Jaime C. Paz, M.S., P.T.

Academic Coordinator of Clinical Education, Department of Physical Therapy, Northeastern University, Boston; Adjunct Staff Therapist, Massachusetts General Hospital, Boston; Newton-Wellesley Hospital, Newton, Massachusetts; and Mount Auburn Home Care, Belmont, Massachusetts; Adjunct Faculty, Department of Physical Therapy, Simmons College, Boston

Michele Panik, M.S., P.T.

Senior Physical Therapist, Inpatient Physical Therapy Services, Massachusetts General Hospital, Boston

Butterworth–Heinemann

Boston Oxford Johannesburg Melbourne New Delhi Singapore

Butterworth–Heinemann supports the efforts of American Forests and the Global ReLeaf program in its campaign for the betterment of trees, forests, and our environment.

Library of Congress Cataloging-in-Publication Data

Paz, Jaime, 1966-
    Acute care handbook for physical therapists / Jaime Paz, Michele Panik.
        p.   cm.
    Includes bibliographical references and index.
    ISBN 0-7506-9822-5
        1. Medicine—Handbooks, manuals, etc. 2. Hospital care-
    -Handbooks, manuals, etc. 3. Physical therapists—Handbooks,
    manuals, etc. I. Panik, Michele, 1969- . II. Title.
        [DNLM: 1. Acute Disease—therapy—handbooks. 2. Intensive Care-
    -handbooks.   WB 39 P348a 1997]
    RC55.P375 1997
    616—dc21
    DNLM/DLC
    for Library of Congress   97-8765
                                                                  CIP

British Library Cataloguing-in-Publication Data
A catalogue record for this book is available from the British Library.

The publisher offers special discounts on bulk orders of this book.
For information, please contact:
Manager of Special Sales
Butterworth–Heinemann
313 Washington Street
Newton, MA 02158–1626
Tel: 617-928-2500
Fax: 617-928-2620

For information on all Butterworth–Heinemann publications available,
contact our World Wide Web home page at: http://www.bh.com

10 9 8 7 6 5 4 3

Printed in the United States of America

To James and Charito, I could be making slippers right now if you hadn't the courage to come to a new country. I'm forever grateful for your undying love and support

To Maria, I couldn't ask for a better sister

And to Aunt Rose and Jennifer, may you always be in peace

JP

To my parents, thank you for sharing your knowledge, professionalism, and sense of discipline and for your constant love and support
MP

Contents

Contributing Authors

Sean M. Collins, M.S., P.T.
Physical Therapist, Rehabilitation Services, Holy Family Hospital and Medical Center, Methuen, Massachusetts; Adjunct Faculty, Department of Physical Therapy, University of Massachusetts, Lowell

Marie Jarrell-Gracious, P.T.
Director of Rehabilitation Services, St. James Hospital, Chicago Heights, Illinois, for GNA Grand Haven, Michigan; Consultant/President, Rehabilitation Outcomes Consulting, Glenwood, Illinois

Cheryl L. Maurer, P.T.
Senior Physical Therapist, Outpatient Physical Therapy Services, Massachusetts General Hospital, Boston

Michele Panik, M.S., P.T.
Senior Physical Therapist, Inpatient Physical Therapy Services, Massachusetts General Hospital, Boston

Jaime C. Paz, M.S., P.T.
Academic Coordinator of Clinical Education, Department of Physical Therapy, Northeastern University, Boston; Adjunct Staff Therapist, Massachusetts General Hospital, Boston; Newton-Wellesley Hospital, Newton, Massachusetts; and Mount Auburn Home Care, Belmont,

Massachusetts; Adjunct Faculty, Department of Physical Therapy, Simmons College, Boston

Marie R. Reardon, P.T.
Clinical Specialist, Inpatient Physical Therapy Services, Massachusetts General Hospital, Boston

Timothy J. Troiano, P.T.
Senior Physical Therapist, Outpatient Physical Therapy Services, Massachusetts General Hospital, Boston

Preface

Acute Care Handbook for Physical Therapists was developed to provide clinicians with a handy reference for patient care in the hospital setting. It was created primarily for physical therapy students and clinicians unfamiliar with acute care. As a member of the health care team, the physical therapist is often expected to understand hospital protocol, medical-surgical "lingo," and the transition of a patient from the intensive care unit to floor-level care. This handbook is therefore intended to be a resource to aid in the interpretation and understanding of the medical-surgical aspects of acute care.

Each chapter in *Acute Care Handbook for Physical Therapists* discusses a major body system. The chapters include the following:

• A review of basic structure and function

• An overview of the medical-surgical workup of an adult patient admitted to the hospital, including evaluation procedures and diagnostic and laboratory tests

• A review of pathophysiology that emphasizes signs and symptoms of specific diseases and disorders

• Pharmacology

• Guidelines for physical therapy intervention

"Clinical Tips" appear throughout each chapter. These helpful hints are intended to help maximize safety, quality, and efficiency of care. The clinical tips are *suggestions* from the editors and contributors that, from clinical experience, have proved to be helpful in acclimating therapists to the acute care setting.

Appendixes provide information to complement topics presented in the chapters.

It is important to remember that all of the information presented in this book is to serve as a guide and to stimulate independent critical thinking within the spectrum of medical-surgical techniques and trends. Developing and maintaining rapport with the medical-surgical team is highly recommended, as the open exchange of information among professionals is invaluable. We believe *Acute Care Handbook for Physical Therapists* can enhance the clinical experience by providing valuable information while you review charts, prepare for therapy intervention, and make clinical decisions in the acute care setting.

JP
MP

Acknowledgments

We offer sincere gratitude to the following people:

Tim Fagerson for getting this ball rolling.

Barbara Murphy and Jana Friedman for their continuous support and editorial expertise.

Dana Tackett for her attention to detail.

The contributors—we couldn't have completed this project without you.

The reviewers: KC, MC, KL, DM, DS, JW, and those anonymous professionals chosen by Butterworth–Heinemann.

PS for computer assistance.

The many patients whose lives have enriched ours, both clinically and personally.

Personal thanks from Jaime to the following:

My colleagues and mentors who have guided me along this professional path: Nancy Zimny M.S., P.T.; Terry Michel M.S., P.T., C.C.S.; Meryl Cohen M.S., P.T., C.C.S.; and Kathy Lee Bishop M.S., P.T., C.C.S.

The students who continually challenge me to become a better educator.

My extended family, all in a special order: John and Alex, Vic and Karen, Steve and Jennifer, Peter and Sally, Mark and Gina, Joe and Michelle, Rick and Cheryl, John and Jill and Jennifer R.

And to Kiegan for making my life complete.

Personal thanks from Michele to the following:

All of my wonderful friends who offered encouragement throughout the publishing process, especially Tracee, Kelly, Maddy, and Kiegan.

Betsy and Lisa, who continually impress me with their unique professional and personal views of work and life.

Ambika, who made my student experience in acute care a memorable one.

The Joneses—I'm trying to keep up with you.

1

Cardiac System

Sean M. Collins

Introduction

Physical therapists in acute care facilities encounter a wide variety of patients with cardiac system dysfunction as either a primary morbidity or a comorbidity. The cardiac system functions to provide the pumping force necessary to circulate blood through the pulmonary, coronary, and systemic circulation. As the energy demands of the body increase, the force required by the cardiac system to maintain output also increases. Therefore, an understanding of normal and abnormal cardiac function, clinical tests, and medical and surgical management of the cardiac system is necessary to safely design and implement an effective physical therapy program.

The objectives of this chapter are to provide the following:

1. A brief overview of the structure and function of the cardiac system

2. An overview of cardiac assessment, including physical examination and diagnostic testing

3. A description of the purpose, mechanisms of action, and side effects of common cardiac medications

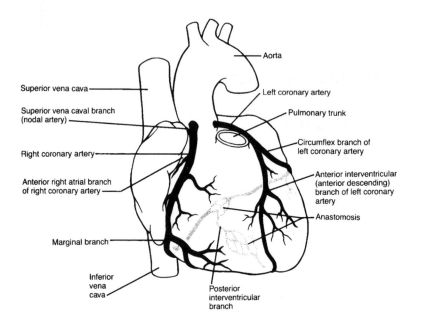

Figure 1-1. *Coronary arteries and cardiac anatomy. (Reprinted with permission from RS Myers. Saunders Manual of Physical Therapy Practice. Philadelphia: Saunders, 1995;199.)*

4.   A description of cardiac diseases and disorders, including clinical findings, medical and surgical management, and physical therapy intervention

Structure

The heart and the roots of the great vessels (Figure 1-1) occupy the pericardium, which is located in the middle of the mediastinum. The mediastinum is bordered anteriorly by the sternum, the costal cartilages, and the medial ends of the third to fifth ribs on the left side. It is bordered inferiorly by the diaphragm; posteriorly by the vertebral column and ribs; and laterally by the pleural cavity (which contains the lungs) [1]. Specific cardiac structures and vessels and their respective functions are outlined in Tables 1-1 and 1-2.

Table 1-1. Primary Structures and Function of the Heart

Structure	Description	Function
Pericardium	Double-walled sac of elastic connective tissue with a strong fibrous outer layer and serous inner layer	Protects against infection and trauma
Epicardium	Outermost layer of cardiac wall, covers surface of heart and great vessels	Protects against infection and trauma
Myocardium	Central layer of thick muscular tissue	Provides major pumping force of the ventricles
Endocardium	Thin layer of endothelium and connective tissue	Lines the inner surface of heart, valves, chordae tendineae, and papillary muscles
Right atrium	Heart chamber	Receives blood from venous system and is a primer pump for the right ventricle
Tricuspid valve	Atrioventricular valve between right atrium and ventricle	Prevents backflow of blood from right ventricle to atrium during ventricular systole
Right ventricle	Heart chamber	Pumps blood to pulmonary circulation
Pulmonic valve	Semilunar valve between right ventricle and pulmonary artery	Prevents backflow of blood from pulmonary artery to right ventricle during ventricle diastole
Left atrium	Heart chamber	Acts as a reservoir for blood and primer pump for left ventricle
Mitral valve	Atrioventricular valve between left atrium and ventricle	Prevents backflow of blood from left ventricle to atrium during ventricular systole
Left ventricle	Heart chamber	Pumps blood to systemic circulation

Table 1-1. *Continued*

Structure	Description	Function
Aortic valve	Semilunar valve between left ventricle and aorta	Prevents backflow of blood from aorta to left ventricle during ventricular diastole
Chordae tendineae	Tendinous attachment of atrioventricular valve cusps to papillary muscle	Prevents valves from everting into atria during ventricular systole
Papillary muscle	Muscle that connects chordae tendineae to floor of ventricular wall	Constricts and pulls on chordae tendineae to prevent eversion of valve cusps during ventricular systole

Table 1-2. Great Vessels of the Heart and Their Function

Structure	Description	Function
Aorta	Major artery from the left ventricle that ascends and then descends after exiting the heart	Ascending aorta delivers blood to neck, head, and arms Descending aorta delivers blood to visceral and lower body tissues
Superior vena cava	Major vein that drains into the right atrium	Drains venous blood from head, neck, and upper body
Inferior vena cava	Major vein that drains into the right atrium	Drains venous blood from viscera and lower body
Pulmonary artery	Major artery from right ventricle	Carries blood to lungs

Note: The mediastinum and the heart can be moved from their normal positions with changes in the lungs secondary to various disorders. For example, a tension pneumothorax will shift the mediastinum away from the side of dysfunction (see Chapter 2 for further description of pneumothorax).

Function

The heart's ability to pump depends on the following [2]:

- Automaticity—the ability to initiate its own electrical impulse
- Excitability—the ability to respond to electrical stimulus
- Conductivity—the ability to transmit electrical impulse from cell to cell within the heart
- Contractility—the ability to stretch as a single unit and recoil
- Rhythmicity—the ability to repeat the cycle in synchrony with regularity

Cardiac Cycle

Blood flow through the cardiac cycle depends on circulatory and cardiac pressure gradients. The right side of the heart is a low-pressure system with little vascular resistance in the pulmonary arteries, whereas the left side of the heart is a high-pressure system with high vascular resistance from the systemic circulation. The cardiac cycle is the period from the beginning of one contraction, which starts with sinoatrial (SA) node depolarization, to the beginning of the next contraction. Systole is the period of contraction, whereas diastole is the period of relaxation. Systole and diastole can also be categorized in the following manner into atrial and ventricular components:

1. *Atrial diastole* is the period of atrial filling. The flow of blood is directed by the higher pressure in the venous circulatory system.

2. *Atrial systole* is the period of atrial emptying and contraction. Initial emptying of 70% of blood occurs as a result of pressure changes from atria to ventricles. Atrial contraction then follows, squeezing out the remaining 30%. This is commonly referred to as the *atrial kick*.

3. *Ventricular diastole* is the period of ventricular filling. It initially occurs with ease, then as the ventricle is filled, atrial contraction is necessary to squeeze the remaining blood volume into the ventricle. The force of contraction is affected by the amount of stretch placed on the ventricular walls during diastole, referred to as *left ventric-*

ular end diastolic pressure (refer to description of preload in "Factors Affecting Cardiac Output").

4. *Ventricular systole* is the period of ventricular contraction. The initial contraction is isovolumic, meaning it does not eject blood, and generates pressure necessary to serve as the catalyst for rapid ejection of ventricular blood.

Cardiac Output

Cardiac output is defined as the amount of blood pumped by the heart in 1 minute. It can also be described in relation to body mass as the *cardiac index*, the amount of blood pumped per minute per square meter of body mass. Systemic circulation competes for tissue perfusion, and total cardiac output adjusts to meet the demands of the body. The heart can adjust cardiac output by changing heart rate (HR) or stroke volume. Changes in heart rate are *chronotropic;* changes in stroke volume are *inotropic* [3].

$$\text{Cardiac output} = \frac{\text{heart rate (beats}}{\text{per minute [bpm])}} \times \frac{\text{stroke volume}}{\text{(liters per minute) [3]}}$$

Factors Affecting Cardiac Output

Preload

Preload is the amount of tension on the ventricular wall before it contracts. It is related to venous return and affects stroke volume by increasing left ventricular end diastolic volume and therefore contraction [4]. This relationship is demonstrated in Figure 1-2.

Frank-Starling Mechanism. The Frank-Starling mechanism defines the relationship between length and tension of the myocardium. In other words, the greater the stretch on the myocardium before systole (preload), the stronger the ventricular contraction. Unlike skeletal muscle, however, relationships between cardiac muscle length and tension consist of the whole heart rather than individual muscle fibers. Length is considered in terms of volume; tension is considered in terms of pressure. A greater volume of blood returning to the heart during diastole means that a greater volume of blood will be ejected during systole. This mechanism can be affected in pathologic situations [5].

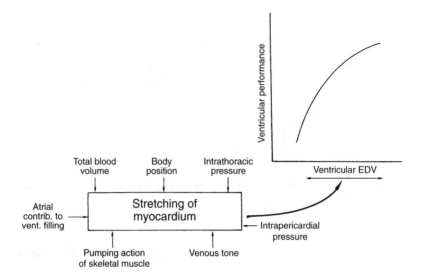

Figure 1-2. *Determinants of myocardial stretch and performance. (EDV = end diastolic volume.) (Reprinted with permission from EA Hillegass, HS Sadowsky. Essentials of Cardiopulmonary Physical Therapy. Philadelphia: Saunders, 1994;139.)*

Afterload

Afterload is the force against which the ventricular wall exerts its contraction. It affects aortic valve opening and is the most obvious measure of load encountered by the ejecting ventricle. An example of afterload is the amount of pressure in the aorta at the time of ventricular systole [4].

Cardiac Conduction System

A schematic of the cardiac conduction system and a normal electrocardiogram (ECG) are presented in Figure 1-3. Normal conduction begins in the SA node and travels through the atria to the atrioventricular (AV) node, where it is delayed momentarily. It then travels to the bundle of His, to the bundle branches, and to Purkinje fibers, resulting in ventricular contraction [6]. Disturbances in conduction can decrease cardiac output [7] (refer to the discussion of rhythm and conduction disturbances in the "Pathophysiology" section).

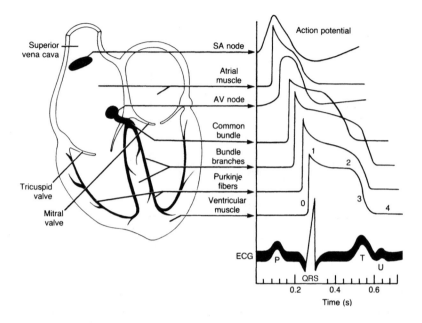

Figure 1-3. *Schematic representation of the sequence of excitation in the heart. (SA = sinoatrial; AV = atrioventricular; ECG = electrocardiogram.) (Reprinted with permission from MD Cheitlin, M Sokolow, MB McIlroy. Clinical Cardiology [6th ed]. East Norwalk, CT: Appleton & Lange, 1993;16.)*

Neural Input

The SA node has its own inherent rate. Neural input can, however, influence heart rate and contractility through the autonomic nervous system [4].

Parasympathetic system neural input generally decelerates cardiac function, thus decreasing heart rate and contractility. Parasympathetic input travels through the vagus nerves. The right vagus nerve primarily stimulates the SA node and affects rate, whereas the left vagus nerve primarily stimulates the AV node and affects contractility [4].

Sympathetic system neural input is through the thoracolumbar sympathetic system and serves mostly to augment ventricular contractility to accelerate cardiac function [4].

Endocrine Input

In response to physical activity or stress, a release in catecholamines influences heart rate, contractility, and peripheral vascular resistance. The net

Table 1-3. Cardiac Effects of Hormones

Hormone	Primary Site	Stimulus	Cardiac Effect
Norepinephrine	Adrenal medulla	Stress and exercise	Vasoconstriction
Epinephrine	Adrenal medulla	Stress and exercise	Coronary artery vasodilation
Angiotensin	Kidney	Decreased arterial pressure	Vasoconstriction, increased blood volume
Vasopressin	Posterior pituitary	Decreased arterial pressure	Vasoconstriction
Bradykinin	Formed by polypeptides in blood when activated	Tissue damage and inflammation	Vasodilation, increased capillary permeability
Histamine	Throughout tissues of body	Tissue damage	Vasodilation, increased capillary permeability

Source: Data from AC Guyton. Textbook of Medical Physiology (8th ed). Philadelphia: Saunders, 1991.

effect of these influences is an increase in cardiac function [4]. For the cardiac effects of hormones produced by the body refer to Table 1-3.

Local Input
Tissue pH, concentration of carbon dioxide (CO_2), concentration of oxygen (O_2), and metabolic products (e.g., lactic acid) can affect vascular tone [3]. During exercise, increased levels of CO_2, decreased levels of O_2, decreased pH, and increased levels of lactic acid at the tissue level dilate local blood vessels and therefore increase cardiac output distribution to that area.

Cardiac Reflexes
Cardiac reflexes influence heart rate and contractility and can be divided into three general categories: baroreflex (or pressure), Bainbridge reflex (or stretch), and chemoreflex (or chemical reflexes).

Baroreflexes are activated through a group of mechanoreceptors located in the heart, great vessels, and intrathoracic and cervical blood vessels. These mechanoreceptors are most plentiful in the walls of the internal carotid arteries [4]. Mechanoreceptors are sensory receptors that are sensitive to mechanical changes such as pressure and stretch. Activation of the mechanoreceptors by high pressures results in an inhibition of the vasomotor center of the medulla that increases vagal stimulation. This chain of events is known as the baroreflex and results in vasodilation, decreased heart rate, and decreased contractility.

Mechanoreceptors located in the right atrial myocardium respond to stretch. With an increased volume in the right atrium, there is an increase in pressure on the atrial wall. This reflex, known as the Bainbridge reflex, stimulates the vasomotor center of the medulla, which in turn increases sympathetic input and increases heart rate and contractility [4].

Chemoreceptors located on the carotid and aortic bodies have a primary effect on increasing rate and depth of ventilation in response to CO_2 levels, but they also have a cardiac effect. Changes in CO_2 during the respiratory cycle can result in a *sinus arrhythmia*, an increased heart rate during inspiration and decreased heart rate during expiration [3].

Coronary Perfusion

For a review of the major coronary arteries, refer to Figure 1-1. Blood is pumped to the large superficial coronary arteries during ventricular systole. At this time, myocardial contraction limits the flow of blood to the myocardium; therefore, myocardial tissue is actually perfused during diastole.

Systemic Circulation

For review of the primary anatomic structures and distribution of the systemic circulation, refer to Figure 1-4. Systemic circulation is affected by total peripheral resistance (TPR), which is the resistance to blood flow by the force created by the aorta and arterial system. Two factors that contribute to resistance are (1) vasomotor tone, in which vessels dilate and constrict, and (2) blood viscosity, in which greater pressure is required to propel thicker blood. Also called *systemic vascular resistance*, TPR along with heart rate (HR) influences

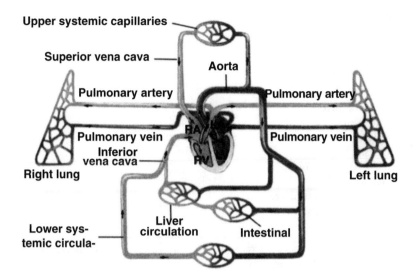

Figure 1-4. *Schematic of systemic circulation. (Reprinted with permission from MM Canobbio. Cardiovascular Disorders. St. Louis: Mosby, 1990;7.)*

blood pressure (BP) [8]. This relationship is illustrated in the following equation:

$$BP = HR \times TPR$$

Assessment

Cardiac assessment consists of patient history, physical examination, laboratory tests, and diagnostic procedures.

Patient History

In addition to the general chart review presented in Appendix I, pertinent information about patients with cardiac dysfunction that should be obtained before physical examination includes the following [2, 5, 9]:

Table 1-4. Cardiac Risk Factors

Major risk factors
    Cigarette smoking
    Hypertension
    Elevated cholesterol
Minor risk factors
    Diabetes
    Sedentary lifestyle
    Obesity
    60 yrs of age or older
    Gender
        Men 35–55 yrs of age
        Postmenopausal women
    Stress

Source: Data from JC Scherer, B Timby. Introductory Medical Surgical Nursing (6th ed). Philadelphia: Lippincott, 1995.

- Presence of chest pain (see Appendix X for an expanded description of characteristics and etiology of chest pain)
  Location, radiation
  Character, quality, and quantity (crushing, burning, numbing, hot)
  Aggravating and alleviating factors
  Precipitating factors
  Accompanying symptoms
  Angina equivalents (what the patient feels as angina such as jaw pain, shortness of breath, diaphoresis, burping, and nausea)
  Treatment sought and its effect

- Family history of heart disease

- Presence of palpitations

- Presence of cardiac risk factors (Table 1-4)

- History of dizziness or syncope

- Previous cardiac studies or procedures

Clinical tip

When discussing angina with a patient, use the patient's terminology. If he or she describes the angina as "crushing" pain, ask the patient if he or she has the crushing feeling during treatment as opposed to asking the patient if he or she has chest pain.

Physical Examination

After obtaining a clinically relevant medical history through chart review, patient interview, or both, the physical examination is performed. The examination consists of observation, palpation, BP measurement, and heart sound auscultation.

Observation

Key components of the observation portion of the physical examination include the following [2, 5]:

1. Inspect extremities for obvious signs of edema.

2. Inspect for signs of trauma (e.g., paddle burns or ecchymosis from cardiopulmonary resuscitation).

3. Inspect for jugular venous distension (JVD), which results from the backing up of fluid into the venous system from right-sided congestive heart failure (Figure 1-5) [5].

    a. Make sure the patient is in a semirecumbent position (45 degrees).

    b. Have the patient turn his or her head away from the side being evaluated.

    c. Observe pulsations in the internal jugular neck region. Pulsations are normally seen 3–5 cm above the sternum. Pulsations higher than this or absent pulsations indicate JVD.

Palpation

Palpation is the second component of the physical examination and is used to evaluate and identify the following:

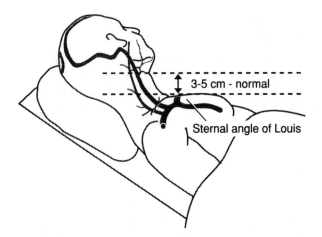

Figure 1-5. *Evaluation of jugular venous distention. (Reprinted with permission from EA Hillegass, HS Sadowsky. Essentials of Cardiopulmonary Physical Therapy. Philadelphia: Saunders, 1994;135.)*

- Pulses for circulation, HR, and rhythm (Figure 1-6)
- Extremities for pitting edema bilaterally (Table 1-5)

Clinical tip

When assessing HR, counting pulses for 15 seconds and multiplying by 4 is sufficient with normal rates and rhythms. If rates are fast (faster than 100 bpm) or slow (slower than 60 bpm), they should be evaluated for 60 seconds. If the rhythm is irregular, auscultation of heart sounds should be performed to identify the HR. In cases of irregular rhythms, the heart may contract without producing a pulse.

Blood Pressure

BP measurement is an indirect measurement of the force exerted against the arterial walls during ventricular systole (systolic force) and during ventricular diastole (diastolic force). Measurement is affected

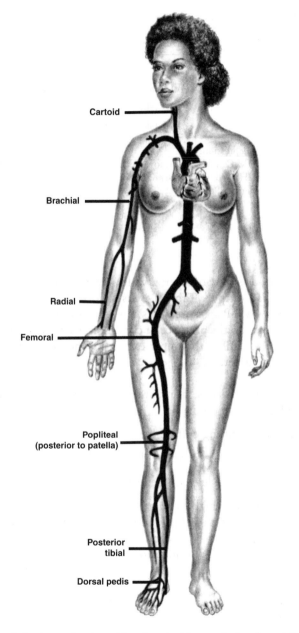

Figure 1-6. *Arterial pulses. (Reprinted with permission from MM Canobbio. Cardiovascular Disorders. St. Louis: Mosby, 1990;26.)*

flow to muscles. In cardiac-compromised or very deconditioned individuals, total cardiac output may not be able to support this increased flow to the muscles and may lead to decreased output to vital areas such as the cerebrum.

• If unable to obtain BP on the arm, the thigh is an appropriate alternative with auscultation at the popliteal artery.

• Falsely high readings will occur if the cuff is too small, applied loosely, or if the brachial artery is lower than the heart level.

• Evaluation of BP and HR in different postures can be used to monitor orthostasis.

Auscultation

Evaluation of heart sounds can yield information about the patient's condition and tolerance to medical treatment and physical therapy through the evaluation of valvular function, rhythm, valvular compliance, and ventricular compliance [5]. To listen to heart sounds, a stethoscope with both a bell and a diaphragm is necessary. For a review of normal and abnormal heart sounds refer to Table 1-8. The examination should follow a systematic pattern using both the bell (for low-pitched sounds) and diaphragm (for high-pitched sounds) and should cover all auscultatory areas as illustrated in Figure 1-7. Abnormal sounds should be noted with a description of the conditions in which they were heard (e.g., after exercise or during exercise).

Clinical tip

• Always ensure proper function of stethoscope by tapping the diaphragm before applying the stethoscope to the patient.

• Rubbing the stethoscope on extraneous objects can add noise and detract from true examination.

• Auscultation of heart sounds over clothing should be avoided because it muffles the intensity of both normal and abnormal sounds.

• If the patient has an irregular cardiac rhythm, HR should be determined through auscultation. To save time, this can

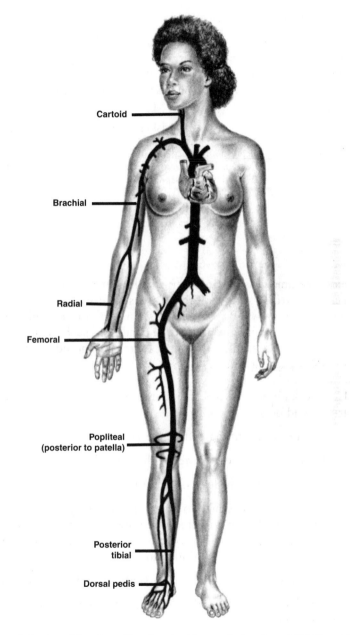

Figure 1-6. *Arterial pulses. (Reprinted with permission from MM Canobbio. Cardiovascular Disorders. St. Louis: Mosby, 1990;26.)*

Table 1-5. Pitting Edema Scale

Scale	Degree (cm)	Description
1+ Trace	Slight	Barely perceptible depression
2+ Mild	0.0–0.6	EID (skin rebounds in <15 secs)
3+ Moderate	0.6–1.3	EID (skin rebounds in 15–30 secs)
4+ Severe	1.3–2.5	EID (skin rebounds in >30 secs)

EID = easily identifiable depression.
Source: Adapted from MM Canobbio. Cardiovascular Disorders. St. Louis: Mosby, 1990; and EA Hillegass, HS Sadowsky. Essentials of Cardiopulmonary Physical Therapy. Philadelphia: Saunders, 1994;134.

by blood volume, elasticity of arterial walls, peripheral vascular resistance, and cardiac output. Table 1-6 lists normal blood pressure ranges. Occasionally, BP measurements can be performed only on certain limbs secondary to the presence of conditions such as intravenous lines, or blood clots. BP of the upper extremity should be measured in the following manner:

1.   Check for posted signs, if any, at the bedside that indicate which arm should be used in taking BP.

2.   Use a properly fitting cuff (Table 1-7).

3.   Position the cuff 2.5 cm above the antecubital crease.

4.   Rest the arm at the level of the heart.

5.   To determine how high to inflate the cuff, palpate radial pulse, inflate until no longer palpable, and note this cuff inflation value. Deflate the cuff, wait 15–30 seconds, and then add 30–40 mm Hg to the previous value for cuff inflation.

6.   Place the bell of the stethoscope gently over the brachial artery.

7.   Reinflate the cuff to the determined value and then slowly deflate the cuff.

8.   Listen for the onset of tapping sounds, which represents blood flow returning to the brachial artery. This is the systolic pressure.

Table 1-6. Blood Pressure Ranges

	Systolic (mm Hg)	Diastolic (mm Hg)
≤8 yrs	85–114	52–85
9–12 yrs	95–135	58–88
Adult (≥13 yrs)	100–140	60–90
Borderline hypertension	140–150	90–100
Hypertension	>150	>100
Normal exercise	Increases during time and with increased load	±10 from baseline

Source: Data from MM Canobbio. Cardiovascular Disorders. St. Louis: Mosby, 1990; and EA Hillegass, HS Sadowsky. Essentials of Cardiopulmonary Physical Therapy. Philadelphia: Saunders, 1994.

Table 1-7. Recommended Sizes of Blood Pressure Cuff Bladders

	Width (cm)	Length (cm)
Child	9.0–10.0	17.0–22.5
Adult, standard	12.0–13.0	22.0–23.5
Adult, large	15.5	30
Adult, thigh	18.0	36

Source: Reprinted with permission from MM Canobbio. Cardiovascular Disorders. Mosby, 1990;32.

9. As the pressure approaches diastolic pressure, the sounds will become muffled and in 5–10 mm Hg will be completely absent. These sounds are referred to as *Korotkoff's sounds* [4].

Clinical tip

• Recording pre- and postexertion BP is important in identifying postactivity hypotensive responses. During recovery from exercise, blood vessels dilate to allow for greater blood

flow to muscles. In cardiac-compromised or very deconditioned individuals, total cardiac output may not be able to
support this increased flow to the muscles and may lead to
decreased output to vital areas such as the cerebrum.

• If unable to obtain BP on the arm, the thigh is an appropriate alternative with auscultation at the popliteal artery.

• Falsely high readings will occur if the cuff is too small,
applied loosely, or if the brachial artery is lower than the
heart level.

• Evaluation of BP and HR in different postures can be
used to monitor orthostasis.

Auscultation

Evaluation of heart sounds can yield information about the patient's
condition and tolerance to medical treatment and physical therapy
through the evaluation of valvular function, rhythm, valvular compliance, and ventricular compliance [5]. To listen to heart sounds, a
stethoscope with both a bell and a diaphragm is necessary. For a review
of normal and abnormal heart sounds refer to Table 1-8. The examination should follow a systematic pattern using both the bell (for low-
pitched sounds) and diaphragm (for high-pitched sounds) and should
cover all auscultatory areas as illustrated in Figure 1-7. Abnormal
sounds should be noted with a description of the conditions in which
they were heard (e.g., after exercise or during exercise).

Clinical tip

• Always ensure proper function of stethoscope by tapping
the diaphragm before applying the stethoscope to the patient.

• Rubbing the stethoscope on extraneous objects can add
noise and detract from true examination.

• Auscultation of heart sounds over clothing should be
avoided because it muffles the intensity of both normal and
abnormal sounds.

• If the patient has an irregular cardiac rhythm, HR should
be determined through auscultation. To save time, this can

Table 1-8. Normal and Abnormal Heart Sounds

Sound	Location	Description
S1 (normal)	All areas	First heart sound; signifies closure of atrioventricular valves and corresponds to onset of ventricular systole
S2 (normal)	All areas	Second heart sound; signifies closure of semilunar valves and corresponds with onset of ventricular diastole
S3 (abnormal)	Best appreciated at apex	Immediately follows S2; occurs early in diastole; represents filling of the ventricle; considered normal in young, healthy individuals (called a *physiologic third sound*); results from decreased ventricular compliance in the presence of heart disease (a classic sign of congestive heart failure)
S4 (abnormal)	Best appreciated at apex	Immediately precedes S1; occurs late in ventricular diastole; is associated with increased resistance to ventricular filling; common in patients with hypertensive heart disease, coronary heart disease, pulmonary disease, myocardial infarction, or after coronary artery bypass grafts
Murmurs (abnormal)	Over respective valves	Indicates regurgitation of blood through valves; can also be classified as systolic or diastolic murmurs; common pathologies resulting in murmurs include mitral regurgitation and aortic stenosis
Pericardial friction rub (abnormal)	Third or fourth intercostal space, anterior axillary line	Sign of pericardial inflammation (pericarditis); associated with each beat of the heart, and sounds like a creak or leather being rubbed together

Source: Data from EA Hillegass, HS Sadowsky. Essentials of Cardiopulmonary Physical Therapy. Philadelphia: Saunders, 1994.

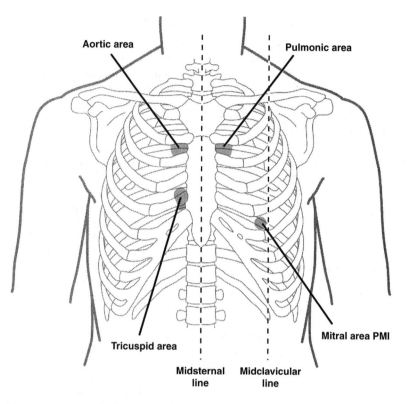

Figure 1-7. *Areas for heart sound auscultation. (PMI = point of maximal impulse.) (Reprinted with permission from EA Hillegass, HS Sadowsky. Essentials of Cardiopulmonary Physical Therapy. Philadelphia: Saunders, 1994;133.)*

be done during a routine auscultatory examination with the stethoscope's bell or diaphragm in any location.

Diagnostic and Laboratory Measures

The diagnostic and laboratory measures discussed in this section provide information that is used to determine diagnosis and prognosis.

Complete Blood Count

Relevant values from the complete blood count are hematocrit, hemoglobin, and white blood cell counts. Elevated levels of hematocrit indicate increased viscosity of blood that can potentially impede blood flow to tissues. Hemoglobin is essential for the adequate oxygen-carrying capacity of the blood. Decreased hemoglobin and hematocrit levels may decrease activity tolerance secondary to decreased oxygen-carrying capacity [9]. Elevated white blood cell counts can indicate that the body is fighting infection, or they can occur with inflammation caused by cell death, such as in myocardial infarction. Sedimentation rate, another hematologic test, is commonly elevated for 2–3 weeks after myocardial infarction secondary to a systemic inflammatory response [10, 11]. Refer to Chapter 6 for more information about these values.

Coagulation Profiles

Coagulation profiles provide information about the clotting time of blood. Patients who undergo treatment with thrombolytic therapy after the initial stages of infarction or who have various cardiac arrhythmias require coagulation profiles to prevent complications of bleeding. The physician determines the patient's therapeutic range of anticoagulation by using the prothrombin time (PT), partial thromboplastin time (PTT), and international normalized ratio (INR) laboratory values [10]. Refer to Chapter 6 for details regarding these values and their significance to treatment.

Patients with low PT and PTT are at higher risk of thrombosis, especially if they have arrhythmias that produce stasis of the blood (e.g., atrial fibrillation). Patients with a PT greater than 2.5 times the reference range should not undergo physical therapy because of the potential for spontaneous bleeding. Likewise, an INR of more than 3 warrants asking the physician if treatment should be withheld [10].

Cholesterol

High cholesterol levels in the blood are thought to be a significant risk factor for atherosclerosis and therefore ischemic heart disease [5]. Measuring blood levels is necessary to determine risk for development of atherosclerosis and to assist in patient education, dietary modification, and medical management. Normal values can be adjusted for age; however, levels of more than 240 mg/dl are generally considered high, and levels of less than 200 mg/dl are considered desirable.

Blood Lipids

A blood lipid analysis categorizes cholesterol into high-density and low-density lipoproteins and provides an analysis of triglycerides.

High-density lipoproteins are formed by the liver and are essentially beneficial. They are considered beneficial because they are readily transportable and do not adhere to the intimal walls of the vascular system. People with higher amounts of high-density lipoproteins are at lower risk for coronary artery disease [10].

Low-density lipoproteins are formed by a diet excessive in fat and are related to a higher incidence of coronary artery disease. Low-density lipoproteins are not as readily transportable because they adhere to intimal walls in the vascular system [10].

Triglycerides are fat cells that are free floating in the blood. When not in use, they are stored in adipose tissue. Their levels increase after eating foods high in fat and decrease with exercise. High levels of triglycerides are associated with a risk of coronary heart disease [10].

Serum Enzymes

After an initial myocardial insult, the presence of tissue necrosis can be determined by increased levels of serum enzymes. Levels of serum enzymes can also be used to determine the extent of myocardial death and the effectiveness of reperfusion therapy. Such analysis typically includes evaluation of isoenzyme levels as well. Isoenzymes are different chemical forms of the same enzyme that are tissue specific and allow differentiation of damaged tissue (e.g., skeletal muscle vs. cardiac muscle) (Table 1-9).

Creatine kinase (CK) (formally called creatine phosphokinase) is released after cell injury or cell death. CK has three isoenzymes. The CK-MB isoenzyme is related to cardiac muscle cell injury or death and constitutes 0–3% of total CK levels. If measured every 2 hours, CK-MB values help physicians estimate the area of infarction and the occurrence of reperfusion. Values peak 33 hours after the initial insult; however, an early peak is a good indication of reperfusion [1]. Values may increase from skeletal muscle trauma, cardiopulmonary resuscitation, defibrillation, and open-heart surgery. Treatment with streptokinase or a tissue plasminogen activator has been shown to falsely elevate the values. CK, with its isoenzyme CK-MB, has emerged as the most useful of all cardiac enzyme tests [9–11].

Lactate dehydrogenase (LDH) is also released after cell injury or death. LDH has five isoenzymes. LDH-1 is specific for cardiac muscle injury. Testing for LDH-1 is valuable for patients admitted a few days after the initial onset of chest pain, because it takes about 3 days to peak and may stay elevated for 5–14 days [9, 10].

Table 1-9. Cardiac Serum Enzymes: Normal Values and Abnormal Trends

Enzyme	Isoenzyme	Normal Value (IU)	Onset of Rise	Time of Peak Rise	Return to Normal
Creatine kinase		55–71	3–4 hrs	33 hrs	3 days
	CK-MB	0–3%	3–4 hrs	33 hrs	3 days
Lactate dehydrogenase		127	12–24 hrs	72 hrs	5–14 days
	LDH-1	14–26%	12–24 hrs	72 hrs	5–14 days

Source: Adapted from AM Smith, JA Therier, SH Huang. Serum enzymes in myocardial infarction. Am J Nurs 1973;73:277; and S Polich, SM Faynor. Interpreting lab test values. PT Magazine 1996;3:110.

Clinical tip

- Active physical therapy should be withheld until CK-MB levels have peaked and begun to fall.
- It is best to await the final diagnosis of location, size, and type (transmural or subendocardial) of myocardial infarction before active physical therapy treatment. This allows for rest and time for the control of possible complications.

Arterial Blood Gas Measurements

Arterial blood gas (ABG) measurements are used to evaluate the oxygenation (PaO_2), ventilation ($PaCO_2$), and pH in patients during acute myocardial infarction and exacerbations of congestive heart failure (CHF). These evaluations can help determine the need for supplemental oxygen therapy and mechanical ventilatory support in these patients [5]. Oxygen is the first drug provided during a suspected myocardial infarction. Refer to Chapter 2 and Appendix III-A for further description of ABG interpretation and supplemental oxygen, respectively.

Oximetry

Oximetry (SaO_2) is used to evaluate the oxygenation in patients on a continuous basis and can be used to titrate supplemental oxygen. Refer to Chapter 2 for a further description of oximetry.

Electrocardiogram

ECG provides a graphic analysis of the heart's electrical activity. The ECG is commonly used to detect arrhythmias, heart blocks, and myocardial perfusion. It can also detect atrial or ventricular enlargement. ECG used for continuous monitoring of patients in the hospital typically involves a two- or three-lead system. A lead represents a particular portion or "view" of the heart. The patient's rhythm is usually displayed in his or her room, in the hall, and at the nurses' station. Lead diagnostic ECG involves a 12-lead analysis, the description of which is beyond the scope of this book. For a review of basic ECG rate and rhythm analysis refer to Table 1-10 and Figure 1-3.

Holter Monitoring

Holter monitoring is 24-hour ECG analysis. This is performed to detect cardiac arrhythmias and corresponding symptoms during a patient's daily activity [2].

Indications for Holter monitoring include the evaluation of the following [2]:

- Syncope

- Dizziness

- Shortness of breath with no other obvious cause

- Palpitations

- Antiarrhythmia therapy

- Pacemaker functioning

- Activity-induced silent ischemia

Clinical tip

Some hospitals use an activity log with Holter monitoring. If this is done, be sure to document physical therapy intervention on the log. If there is no log, be sure to document time of day

Table 1-10. Interpretation of Normal Electrocardiograph Findings

Wave or Segment	Duration (secs)	Amplitude (mm)	Indicates
P wave	<0.10	1–3	Atrial depolarization
PR interval	0.12–0.20	Isoelectric line	Elapsed time between atrial depolarization and ventricular depolarization
QRS complex	0.06–0.10	25–30 (maximum)	Ventricular depolarization and atrial repolarization
ST segment	0.12	–0.5 to 1.0	Elapsed time between ventricular depolarization and repolarization
T wave	0.16	5–10	Ventricular repolarization

Source: Data from RS Meyers. Saunders Manual of Physical Therapy Practice. Philadelphia: Saunders, 1995; B Aehlert. ACLS Quick Review Study Guide. St. Louis: Mosby, 1994; and D Davis. How to Quickly and Accurately Master ECG Interpretation (2nd ed). Philadelphia: Lippincott, 1992.

and intervention during physical therapy in the medical record, as this will help correlate arrhythmias to certain activities.

Echocardiography

Echocardiography is a noninvasive procedure that uses ultrasound to evaluate the function of the heart. Evaluation includes the size of the ventricular cavity, the thickness and integrity of the septum, valve integrity, and motion of individual segments of the ventricular wall. Volumes of the ventricles are quantified, and ejection fraction can be estimated [3].

Transesophageal echocardiography (TEE) is a new technique that provides a better view of the mediastinum in cases of pulmonary disease, chest wall abnormality, and obesity, which make standard echocardiography difficult [2]. For this test, a catheter with an ultrasound head is placed in the esophagus.

Echocardiography is also performed during or immediately after bicycle or treadmill exercise to identify ischemia-induced wall motion abnormalities or during a pharmacologically induced exercise stress test (e.g., a dobutamine stress echocardiograph).

Principal indications for echocardiograph are to assist in the diagnosis of the following [2]:

- Pericardial effusion
- Cardiac tamponade
- Idiopathic congestive cardiomyopathy
- Hypertrophic cardiomyopathy
- Mitral valve regurgitation
- Mitral valve prolapse
- Aortic regurgitation
- Aortic stenosis
- Vegetation of the valves
- Intracardiac masses
- Ischemic cardiac muscle
- Left ventricular aneurysm
- Ventricular thrombi
- Congenital heart disease

Exercise Testing

Exercise testing, or stress testing, is a noninvasive method of assessing cardiovascular responses to increased activity. Exercise testing involves the systematic and progressive increase in intensity of activity. A variety of methods are used to accomplish this task (e.g., treadmill walking, bicycling, stair climbing, arm ergometry). These tests are accompanied by ECG analysis, BP measurements, and subjective reports using the rating of perceived exertion. Occasionally, the use of expired gas analysis can provide useful information about pulmonary function and maximal oxygen consumption [5]. Submaximal tests, such as the 12- and 6-minute walk tests, can be performed to assess a patient's function [5]. For further discussion of the 6-minute walk test, refer to Appendix IX. Submaximal tests differ from maximal tests in that the patient is not pushed to the maximum HR;

instead the test is stopped at a predetermined endpoint, usually at 75% of the patient's predicted maximum HR [5]. For an example of widely used exercise test protocols refer to Table 1-11.

Indications for exercise testing include evaluation of the following:

- Chest pain
- Determination of prognosis and severity of coronary disease
- Effects of medical and surgical treatment
- Arrhythmias
- Hypertension with activity
- Functional capacity
- To provide exercise prescription
- To provide motivation for lifestyle change

Contraindications to exercise testing include the following [5]:

- Recent myocardial infarction (less than 48 hours)
- Acute pericarditis
- Unstable angina
- Ventricular or rapid arrhythmias
- Untreated second- or third-degree heart block
- Overt congestive heart failure
- Acute illness

Exercise test results assist in the formulation of an exercise prescription. Based on the results, the patient's actual or extrapolated maximum HR can be used to determine target HR range to control intensity. Rating of perceived exertion with symptoms during the exercise test can also be used to gauge intensity.

Thallium Stress Testing
Thallium stress testing is an exercise test that involves the injection of a radioactive nuclear marker for detection of myocardial perfusion. The injection is typically given during peak exercise or when symptoms are reported during the stress test. After the test, the subject is passed under

Table 1-11. Comparison of Exercise Test Protocols

Oxygen Requirements (ml O$_2$/kg/min)	Metabolic Equivalents	Treadmill Tests			Bicycle Tests
		Bruce 3-Min Stages (mph/ percentage grade)	Kattus 3-Min Stages (mph/ percentage grade)	Balke (percentage grade at 3.4 mph)	For 70 kg of Body Weight (kgm/min)
56.0	16			26	
52.5	15			24	
49.5	14		4/22	22	
45.5	13	4.2/16		20	1,500
42.0	12		4/18	18	1,350
38.5	11			16	1,200
35.0	10		4/14	14	
31.5	9	3.4/14		12	1,050
28.0	8		4/10	10	900
24.5	7	2.5/12	3/10	8	750
21.0	6			6	600

17.5	5	1.7/10	2/10	4	450
14.0	4			2	300
10.5	3				
					150
7.0	2				
3.5	1				

Source: Adapted from M Cohen, TH Michel. Cardiopulmonary Symptoms in Physical Therapy Practice. New York: Churchill Livingstone, 1988;69.

a nuclear scanner to be evaluated for myocardial perfusion by assessment of the distribution of thallium uptake. The subject then returns 3–4 hours later to be reevaluated for myocardial reperfusion. This test appears to be more sensitive than stress tests without thallium for identifying patients with coronary artery disease [2].

Persantine Thallium Stress Testing
Persantine thallium stress testing is the use of dipyridamole (Persantine) to mimic the cardiac effects of exercise without actually exercising. It is typically used in patients who are very unstable, deconditioned, or unable to ambulate or cycle for the conventional stress testing.

Cardiac Catheterization

Cardiac catheterization, classified as either right or left, is an invasive procedure that involves passing a flexible, radiopaque catheter into the heart to visualize the following [2]:

- Heart chambers
- Coronary arteries
- Great vessels
- Valves
- Cardiac pressures and volumes to evaluate cardiac function (hemodynamic monitoring)

The procedure is also used in the following diagnostic and therapeutic techniques [2]:

- Angiography
- Percutaneous transluminal coronary angioplasty (PTCA) (see "Cardiac Procedures")
- Electrophysiologic studies
- Cardiac muscle biopsy

Right-sided catheterization involves entry through a vein (commonly subclavian) to evaluate right heart pressure readings; calculation of cardiac output; and angiography of the right atrium, right ventricle, tricuspid valve, pulmonic valve, and pulmonary artery [2]. It is also used for continuous hemodynamic monitoring. Indications for right heart catheterization include the following [2]:

- Intracardiac shunt (blood flow between right and left atria or right and left ventricles)
- Myocardial dysfunction
- Pericardial constriction
- Pulmonary vascular disease
- Valvular heart disease
- After heart transplant

Left-sided catheterization involves entry through an artery (commonly femoral) to evaluate the aorta, left atrium, and left ventricle; left ventricular function; mitral and aortic valve function; and angiography of coronary arteries. Indications for left heart catheterization include the following [2]:

- Aortic dissection
- Atypical angina
- Cardiomyopathy
- Congenital heart disease
- Coronary heart disease
- After myocardial infarction complications
- Valvular heart disease
- After heart transplant

Clinical tip

After catheterization, the patient is on bed rest for approximately 4–6 hours when venous access is performed or 6–8 hours when arterial access is performed. The extremity should remain immobile with a sandbag over the access site to provide constant pressure. Physical therapy intervention should be limited to bedside treatment and should work within the limitations of these precautions. During the precautionary period, physical therapy intervention such as bronchopulmonary hygiene or education may be necessary. Bronchopulmonary hygiene is indicated if there are pulmonary complications or if risk of complications exists. Education is warranted when the patient is anxious and needs to have questions answered regarding his or her functional mobility. After the precautionary period, normal mobility can progress to the limit of the patient's cardiopulmonary impairments; however, the catheterization results should be incorporated into the physical therapy treatment plan.

Angiography

Angiography involves the injection of radiopaque contrast material through a catheter to visualize vessels or chambers. Different techniques are used for different assessments [2]:

Aortography is used to assess the aorta and aortic valve.

Coronary arteriography is used to assess coronary arteries.

Pulmonary angiography is used to assess pulmonary circulation.

Ventriculography is used to assess right or left ventricle and AV valves.

Electrophysiologic Studies

Electrophysiologic studies (EPSs) are performed to evaluate the electrical conduction system of the heart. An electrode catheter is inserted through the femoral vein into the right ventricle apex. Continuous ECG monitoring is done both internally and externally. The electrode can deliver programmed electrical stimulation to evaluate conduction pathways, formation of arrhythmias, and the automaticity and refractoriness of cardiac muscle cells. EPSs evaluate the effectiveness of antiarrhythmic medication and can provide specific information about each segment of the conduction system. Indications for EPSs include the following [2]:

- Sinus node disorders
- AV block
- Intraventricular block

- Previous cardiac arrest
- Tachycardia at greater than 200 bpm
- Unexplained syncope

Chest Radiography
Chest x-rays (CXRs) can be ordered for patients to assist in the diagnosis of CHF or cardiomegaly (enlarged heart). Patients in CHF have an increased density in pulmonary vasculature markings, giving the appearance of congestion in the vessels [5]. Refer to Chapter 2 for further description of CXRs.

Hemodynamic Monitoring
For a complete discussion about hemodynamic monitoring, refer to Appendix IV-A.

Pathophysiology

When disease and degenerative changes impair the heart's capacity to perform work, a reduction in cardiac output occurs. If cardiac, renal, or cerebral perfusion is reduced, a vicious circle resulting in heart failure can ensue [3]. Cardiac diseases are generally divided into five major categories: myocardial ischemia and infarction, rhythm and conduction disturbance, valvular heart disease, myocardial and pericardial heart disease, and congestive heart failure [7].

Myocardial Ischemia and Infarction

When myocardial oxygen demand is higher than supply, the myocardium must use anaerobic metabolism to meet energy demands. This system can be maintained for only a short period of time before tissue ischemia will occur, which typically results in angina (chest pain). If the supply and demand are not balanced either by rest, medical management, surgical management, or any combination of these, injury of the myocardial tissue will ensue, followed by infarction (cell death). This balance of supply and demand is achieved in individuals with normal coronary circulation; however, in individuals with compromised coronary circulation, impairment of coronary blood flow can lead to tis-

sue ischemia, infarction (cell death), or both. The following pathologies result in myocardial ischemia and infarction:

- Coronary arterial spasm is a disorder of transient spasm of
coronary vessels that impairs blood flow to the myocardium. It
can occur with or without the presence of atherosclerotic coronary disease. It can result in stable or unstable angina, or myocardial infarction [5].

- Coronary atherosclerotic disease (CAD) is a multistep process
of the deposition of fatty streaks/plaques on artery walls (athero-
sis). The presence of these deposits eventually leads to arterial wall
damage and platelet and macrophage aggregation that then leads
to thrombus formation and hardening of the arterial walls (sclerosis). The net effect is a narrowing of coronary walls. It can result
in stable or unstable angina, or myocardial infarction [5].

Clinical syndromes caused by these pathologies are the following [7]:

- Stable (exertional) angina occurs with increased myocardial
demand, such as during exercise and is relieved by reducing or ter-
minating exercise intensity.

- Unstable angina occurs at rest or with activity below the patient's
usual ischemic baseline. It is not induced by activity or increased
myocardial demand that cannot be met. It can be induced at rest,
when supply is cut down with no change in demand.

- Myocardial infarction occurs with prolonged or unmanaged
ischemia. The location and extent of cell death is determined by the
coronary artery that is compromised. Refer to Table 1-12 for common types of myocardial infarctions and their complications.

Rhythm and Conduction Disturbance

Rhythm and conduction disturbances can range from minor alterations
with no hemodynamic effects to life-threatening episodes with rapid
hemodynamic compromise [7]. Refer to Chapter Appendix 1-A for a
description of atrial, ventricular, and junctional rhythms and atrioventricular blocks. Refer also to Chapter Appendix 1-B for examples of the
most common rhythm disturbances.

Table 1-12. Electrocardiographic Evidence and Complications of Common Types of Myocardial Infarctions

Type of Myocardial Infarction	Wall Affected	Possible Occluded Coronary Artery	Electrocardiographic Evidence	Complication
Anterior MI	Anterior wall of left ventricle	Left coronary artery	Loss of R waves in precordial leads, elevated ST segment and T waves in V1-V4, I, and aVL	Left-sided congestive heart failure Pulmonary edema Bundle branch block Atrioventricular block Ventricular aneurysm (which can lead to congestive heart failure, dysrhythmias, and embolism)
Inferior MI	Inferior wall of left ventricle	Right coronary artery	Elevated ST segment and T wave in leads II, III, and aVF; abnormal Q waves (same leads)	Atrioventricular blocks (which can result in bradycardia) Papillary muscle dysfunction (which can result in valvular insufficiency and eventually congestive heart failure)
Anterolateral MI	Anterolateral wall of left ventricle	LAD, circumflex	Loss of R wave, elevated ST segment and T wave in V4–V6 and aVL	Brady- or tachyarrhythmias Ventricular aneurysm

Table 1-12. *Continued*

Type of Myocardial Infarction	Wall Affected	Possible Occluded Coronary Artery	Electrocardiographic Evidence	Complication
Anteroseptal MI	Septal wall	LAD	Loss of R wave elevated ST and T in leads V1-V3	Brady- or tachyarrhythmias Acute ventricular septal defect
Posterior MI	Posterior wall of left ventricle	RCA, circumflex	Large R wave in V1, elevated ST segment in V4	Bradycardia Heart blocks
Right ventricular MI	Right ventricular wall	RCA	Elevated ST segment and T wave in leads II, III, and aVF	Right ventricular failure (can lead to left ventricular failure and therefore cardiogenic shock) Heart blocks Hepatomegaly Peripheral edema
Transmural MI (Q wave MI)	Full thickness MI at any location	Any artery	Large Q waves	All of the above
Subendocardial MI (non-Q-wave MI)	Partial wall thickness MI at any location	Any artery	ST, T changes for more than 3 days with enzyme changes	All of the above Potential to extend to transmural MI

MI = myocardial infarction; LAD = left anterior descending coronary artery; RCA = right coronary artery.
Source: Data from MD Cheitlin, M Sokolow, MB McIlroy. Clinical Cardiology (6th ed). Norwalk, CT: Appleton & Lange, 1993;1; and LD Hillis, BG Firth, JT Willerson. Manual of Clinical Problems in Cardiology. Boston: Little, Brown, 1984.

Valvular Heart Disease

Valvular hear disease encompasses valvular disorders of one or more of the four valves of the heart [2]. The following three disorders can occur [7]:

1. *Stenosis* involves the narrowing of the valve.

2. *Regurgitation*, the back flow of blood through the valve, occurs with incomplete valve closure.

3. *Prolapse* involves enlarged valve cusps. The cusps can become floppy and bulge backward. This condition may progress to regurgitation

Over time, these disorders can lead to pumping dysfunction and, ultimately, heart failure. The following are common valvular heart diseases:

- Aortic stenosis
- Aortic regurgitation (acute and chronic)
- Mitral stenosis
- Mitral regurgitation (acute and chronic)
- Mitral valve prolapse
- Valvular pulmonic stenosis
- Pulmonic regurgitation
- Tricuspid stenosis

Refer to Table 1-13 for a description of commons signs and symptoms of valvular heart disease.

Myocardial and Pericardial Heart Disease

Myocardial heart disease affects the myocardial muscle tissue; pericardial heart diseases affect the pericardium (the protective layer surrounding the heart). The following is a list of common myocardial and pericardial diseases:

- Cardiomyopathy (Tables 1-14 and 1-15)

Table 1-13. Possible Signs and Symptoms of Valvular Heart Diseases

Disease	Symptoms	Signs
Aortic stenosis	Angina Syncope or near syncope Symptoms of left ventricle failure (i.e., dyspnea, orthopnea, cough)	Elevated left ventricular wall pressure Decreased subendocardial blood flow Systolic murmur Ventricular hypertrophy
Chronic aortic regurgitation	Angina Symptoms of left ventricular failure	Dilated aortic root Dilated left ventricle Diastolic murmur Left ventricular hypertrophy
Acute aortic regurgitation	Rapid progression of symptoms of left ventricular failure, pulmonary edema, or angina	Sinus tachycardia to compensate for decreased stroke volume Loud S3 Diastolic murmur Signs of ventricular failure
Mitral stenosis	Symptoms of pulmonary vascular congestion (i.e., dyspnea, orthopnea) If patient develops pulmonary hypertension (which can cause hypoxia, hypotension), he or she may have angina or syncope	Left atrial hypertrophy Pulmonary hypertension Atrial fibrillation Can have embolus formation (especially if in atrial fibrillation) Long diastolic murmur
Chronic mitral regurgitation	Symptoms of pulmonary vascular congestion Angina Syncope Fatigue	Left atrial enlargement Atrial fibrillation Elevated left atrial pressure
Acute mitral regurgitation	Rapid progression of symptoms of pulmonary vascular congestion	Sinus tachycardia Presence of S3 Presence of S4 Pulmonary edema
Mitral valve prolapse	Most commonly asymptomatic Fatigue Palpitations Syncope	Systolic click May have tachyarrhythmia

Source: Data from LD Hillis, BG Firth, JT Willerson. Manual of Clinical Problems in Cardiology. Boston: Little, Brown, 1984.

Table 1-14. Functional Classifications of Cardiomyopathies

Classification	Dysfunction	Comments
Dilated	Systolic	Dilated ventricle Marked contractile dysfunction of myocardium
Hypertrophic	Diastolic	Thickened ventricular myocardium Less compliant to filling, decreasing filling during diastole
Restrictive	Systolic and diastolic	Endocardial scarring of ventricles Decreased compliance during diastole Decreased contractile force during systole

Source: Adapted from L Cahalin. Cardiac Muscle Dysfunction. In EA Hillegass, HS Sadowsky (eds), Essentials of Cardiopulmonary Physical Therapy. Philadelphia: Saunders, 1994;126.

- Pericarditis (acute and constrictive)
- Pericardial effusion
- Left ventricular hypertrophy
- Ventricular aneurysm
- Pericardial tamponade
- Endocarditis

Refer to Table 1-16 for possible signs and symptoms of myocardial and pericardial heart disease.

Congestive Heart Failure

Congestive heart failure is the term that refers to a lack of pumping of blood. Cardiac output is not maintained and life cannot be sustained if CHF continues without treatment. Etiologies of CHF include the following [5]:

- Myocardial ischemia or infarction
- Arrhythmias

Table 1-15. Etiologic Classifications of Cardiomyopathies

Etiology	Examples
Inflammatory	Viral infection Bacterial infection
Infiltrative	Sarcoidosis Neoplastic disease
Metabolic	Selenium deficiency Diabetes mellitus
Hematologic	Sickle cell anemia
Fibroplastic	Carcinoid fibrosis Endomyocardial fibrosis
Toxic	Alcohol Bleomycin
Hypersensitivity	Cardiac transplant rejection Methyldopa
Physical agents	Heat stroke Hypothermia Radiation
Genetic	Hypertrophic cardiomyopathy Duchenne's muscular dystrophy
Miscellaneous	Postpartum cardiomyopathy Acquired obesity
Idiopathic	Idiopathic hypertrophic cardiomyopathy

Source: Adapted from LP Cahalin. Cardiac Muscle Dysfunction. In EA Hillegass, HS Sadowsky (eds), Essentials of Cardiopulmonary Physical Therapy. Philadelphia: Saunders, 1994;126.

Table 1-16. Possible Signs and Symptoms of Myocardial and Pericardial Heart Diseases

Disease	Symptoms	Signs
Cardiomyopathy	See Table 1-15	See Table 1-15
Acute pericarditis	Retrosternal chest pain (worsened by supine, deep inspiration, or both) Dyspnea, cough, hoarseness, dysphagia, chills,	Pericardial friction rub Diffuse ST segment elevation Decreased QRS voltage in all leads if pericardial effusion also present

Disease	Symptoms	Signs
	and weakness may occur	Fever
Constrictive pericarditis	Fatigue Dyspnea Dizziness, syncope, or both Symptoms of pulmonary venous congestion Vague nonspecific retrosternal chest pain	Jugular venous distention QRS voltage diminished Atrial fibrillation (occasionally) Abdominal swelling Peripheral edema
Chronic pericardial effusion (without tamponade)	May have vague fullness in anterior chest Cough Hoarseness Dysphagia	Muffled heart sounds May have pericardial friction rub QRS voltage diminished Chest x-ray shows cardiomegaly without pulmonary congestion
Pericardial tamponade	Symptoms of low cardiac output (dyspnea, fatigue, dizziness, syncope) May have retrosternal chest pain May have cough, hiccoughs, hoarseness	Jugular venous distention Cardiomegaly Diminished QRS voltage Cardiac effusion becomes tamponade when right heart catheterization shows equal pressures in right atrium, ventricle, and capillary wedge (signifies left atria pressure) and left heart catheterization would show equal pressure on left and right side of the heart
Left ventricular aneurysm	Symptoms of low cardiac output (dyspnea, fatigue, dizziness, syncope)	Persistent ST elevation Can appear on chest x-ray

Source: Data from MD Cheitlin, M Sokolow, MB McIlroy. Clinical Cardiology (6th ed). East Norwalk, CT: Appleton & Lange, 1993;1; and LD Hillis, BG Firth, JT Willerson. Manual of Clinical Problems in Cardiology. Boston: Little, Brown, 1984.

- Renal insufficiency
- Cardiomyopathy
- Pericardial effusion
- Myocarditis
- Pulmonary embolism
- Valvular heart diseases

The following are types of CHF [5]:

Left-sided heart failure refers to failure of the left ventricle resulting in back flow into the lungs.

Right-sided failure refers to failure of the right side of the heart resulting in back flow into the systemic venous system.

High-output failure refers to heart failure that is secondary to renal system failure to filter off excess fluid. The renal system failure places a higher work load on the heart that cannot be maintained.

Low-output failure refers to the condition in which the heart is not able to pump the minimal amount of blood to support circulation.

Systolic dysfunction refers to a problem with systole or the actual strength of myocardial contraction.

Diastolic dysfunction refers to a problem during diastole or the ability of the ventricle to allow the filling of blood.

Possible signs and symptoms of CHF are described in Table 1-17. The New York Heart Association Functional Classification of Heart Disease is described in Table 1-18. Activity guidelines for patients hospitalized with CHF are described in Table 1-19.

Management

Cardiac Procedures

The following section discusses pharmacologic interventions, surgical and nonsurgical procedures, and physical therapy interventions for patients with cardiac dysfunction.

Table 1-17. Signs and Symptoms of Congestive Heart Failure

Symptoms
  Dyspnea
    Paroxysmal nocturnal dyspnea
  Orthopnea
  Cough
  Fatigue
Signs
  Tachypnea
  Cold, pale possibly cyanotic extremities
  Weight gain
  Peripheral edema
  Hepatomegaly
  Jugular venous distention
  Crackles (rales)
  Tubular breath sounds and consolidated S3 heart sound
  Sinus tachycardia
  Decreased exercise tolerance and physical work capacity

Source: Adapted from LP Cahalin. Heart failure. Phys Ther 1996;76:520.

Table 1-18. New York Heart Association's Functional Classification of Heart Disease

Classification	Description
Class I	Patients with cardiac disease but without resulting limitations of physical activity Ordinary physical activity does not cause undue fatigue, palpitation, dyspnea, or anginal pain
Class II	Patients with cardiac disease that results in a slight limitation of physical activity Patients are comfortable at rest, but ordinary physical activity results in fatigue, palpitations, dyspnea, or anginal pain
Class III	Patients with cardiac disease that results in a marked limitation of physical activity Patients are comfortable at rest, but less than ordinary activity causes fatigue, palpitations, dyspnea, or anginal pain
Class IV	Patients with cardiac disease that results in an inability to carry on any physical activity without discomfort Fatigue, palpitations, dyspnea, or anginal pain may be present even at rest If any physical activity is undertaken, symptoms increase

Source: Reprinted with permission from LP Cahalin. Cardiac Muscle Dysfunction. In EA Hillegass, HS Sadowsky (eds), Essentials of Cardiopulmonary Physical Therapy. Philadelphia: Saunders, 1994;137.

Table 1-19. Activity Guidelines for Patients Hospitalized with Congestive Heart Failure*

Day	Standard Activity Regimen	Gradual Activity Regimen
1	Movement from and to commode and chair	Bed rest
2	Room ambulation	Bed rest Gentle, active strengthening exercises
3	Hallway ambulation and cycle ergometry (2 times) (1–5 min) MET level goal = 2.0–3.0	Movement from and to commode Movement from and to chair Movement from and to bathroom Restorator Cycling Room ambulation Gentle strengthening exercises
4	Independent hallway ambulation (3 times) (1–10 min) MET level goal = 3.0–4.0 Patient adequately ascends and descends two flights of stairs and is showering independently Patient adequately understands the home exercise program Outpatient cardiac rehabilitation scheduled Patient discharged	Hallway ambulation/restorator or cycle ergometer (2 times) (1–5 min) MET level goal = 1.0–2.0 Strengthening exercises
5		Hallway ambulation/restorator or cycle ergometer (2 times) (1–8 min) MET level goal = 1.5–2.5 Strengthening exercises Hallway ambulation/restorator or cycle ergometer (2 times) (1–15 min) MET level goal = 2.0–3.0 Strengthening exercises
6		Hallway ambulation (2 times) (1–15 min) MET level goal = 2.0–4.0 Strengthening exercises

Day	Standard Activity Regimen	Gradual Activity Regimen
7		Discharge criteria same as for standard regimen (see day 4)

MET = metabolic equivalent.
*Activity guidelines are based on risk stratification of patients (i.e., degree of ventricular dysfunction and signs and symptoms) and on the cardiopulmonary response (heart rate no greater than 20 would show equal pressure on left and right side of the hypoadaptive blood pressure response [no greater than a 10- to 20-mm Hg decrease] and without dysrhythmias or dyspnea).
Source: Reprinted with permission from LP Cahalin. Heart failure. Phys Ther 1996;76:530.

Percutaneous Revascularization Procedures

Percutaneous revascularization procedures are used to return blood flow through coronary arteries that have become occlusive secondary to atherosclerotic plaques. The following list briefly describes three percutaneous revascularization procedures [2]:

1. PTCA is performed on small atherosclerotic lesions that do not completely occlude the vessel. The distal end of a catheter is equipped with a balloon. The balloon inflates and presses the lesion against the arterial wall.

2. Directional coronary atherectomy can be performed by inserting a catheter with a cutter housed at the distal end on one side of the catheter and a balloon on the other side. The balloon inflates and presses the cutter against the atheroma (plaque). The cutter can then cut the atheroma and remove it from the arterial wall. This can also be performed with a laser on the tip of the catheter.

3. Endoluminal stents are tiny spring-like tubes that can be placed permanently into the coronary artery to increase the intraluminal diameter. Stents are occasionally necessary when initial prevascularization fails.

Coronary Artery Bypass Graft

A coronary artery bypass graft (CABG) is performed when the coronary artery has become completely occluded or when it cannot be corrected by PTCA, directional coronary arthrectomy, or stenting. A vascular graft is used to revascularize the myocardium. The saphenous vein and the left internal mammary artery are commonly used as vascular grafts. The incision required is a median sternotomy, which extends caudally from just inferior to the suprasternal notch to below the xiphoid process and splits the sternum longitudinally. After a CABG, patients are placed on sternal precautions for at least 8 weeks. They should avoid lifting of moderate to heavy weights with the upper extremities (e.g., less than 10 lbs).

Clinical tip

To help patients understand this concept, inform them that a gallon of milk weighs about 8.5 lbs.

Secondary to the sternal incision, patients are at risk of developing pulmonary complications after a CABG. The physical therapist should be aware of postoperative complication risk factors as well as postoperative indicators of poor pulmonary function. Refer to Appendix V for further description of postoperative pulmonary complications.

Cardiac Pacemaker Implantation and Automatic Implantable Cardiac Defibrillator

Cardiac pacemaker implantation involves the placement of a unipolar or bipolar electrode onto the myocardium. This electrode is used to create an action potential in the management of certain arrhythmias. Indications for cardiac pacemaker implantation include the following:

- Sinus node disorders (bradyarrhythmias [HR lower than 60 bpm])

- Atrioventricular disorders (complete heart block, Mobitz type II block)

- Tachyarrhythmias (supraventricular tachycardia, frequent ectopy [HR greater than 100 bpm])

Temporary pacing may be performed after an acute myocardial infarction to help control transient arrhythmias and after a CABG when vagal tone is increased [7]. Table 1-20 classifies the various pacemakers.

Automatic implantable cardiac defibrillator (AICD) is used to manage uncontrollable, life-threatening ventricular arrhythmias by sensing the heart rhythm and defibrillating the myocardium as necessary to return the heart to a normal rhythm. Indications for AICD include the following:

- Ventricular tachycardia
- Ventricular fibrillation

Valve Replacement

Valve replacement is an acceptable method for treatment of valvular disease. Patients with mitral and aortic stenosis, regurgitation, or both are the primary candidates for this surgery. Like the CABG, a median sternotomy is the route of access to the heart.

Cardiac Transplantation

Cardiac transplantation is an acceptable intervention for the treatment of end-stage heart disease. A growing number of facilities are performing heart transplantation, and a greater number of physical therapists are involved in the rehabilitation of pre- and post-transplant recipients. Physical therapy intervention is vital for the success of heart transplantation, as recipients have often survived a long period of convalescence both before and after surgery, rendering them deconditioned. In general, heart transplant patients are immunosuppressed and are without neurologic input to their heart. These patients rely first on the Frank-Starling mechanism to augment stroke volume and then on the catecholamine response to augment both HR and stroke volume. It is beyond the scope of this text to discuss cardiac transplantation; however, several recommended readings for the therapist working with heart transplant patients are listed in the references.

Cardiac Medications

Cardiac medications are classified according to functional indications, drug classes, and mechanism of action. Cardiac drug classes are occasionally indicated for more than one clinical diagnosis. The primary functional indications are listed below. Chapter Appendix 1-C lists the functional indications, mechanisms of action, and side effects of cardiac medications.

Table 1-20. Pacemaker Classifications

First Symbol Pacing Location	Second Symbol Sensing Location	Third Symbol Response to Pacing	Fourth Symbol Programmability/Modulation	Fifth Symbol Antitachyarrhythmia Function
O = None	N = None	O = None	O = None	O = None
A = Atrium	A = Atrium	I = Inhibited	S = Simple programmable	P = Pacing
V = Ventricle	V = Ventricle	T = Triggered	M = Multiprogrammable	S = Shock
D = Dual	D = Dual	D = Dual	C = Communicating	D = Dual
			R = Rate modulation	

Dual = atrium and ventricle can be sensed independently, paced independently, or both; inhibited response = pending stimulus is inhibited when a spontaneous stimulation is detected; triggered response = detection of stimulus produces an immediate stimulus in the same chamber; simple programming = rate adjustment, output adjustment, or both; multiprogrammable = can be programmed more extensively; communicating = has telemetry capabilities; rate modulation = can adjust rate automatically based on one or more other physiologic variables.
Source: Adapted from AD Bernstein, AJ Camm, RD Fletcher, et al. The NASPE/BPEG generic pacemaker code for antibradyarrhythmia and adaptive pacing and antitachyarrhythmia devices. PACE 1987;10:795.

Anti-Ischemic Drugs

Anti-ischemic drugs attempt to reestablish the balance between myocardial oxygen demand and supply [5]. To balance the supply and demand, medications can decrease HR or systemic BP or increase arterial lumen size by decreasing spasm or thrombus.

Medications that are successfully used for this task include the following [5]:

- Beta-blockers (see Chapter Appendix Table 1-C.1)

- Calcium channel blockers (see Chapter Appendix Table 1-C.2)

- Nitrates (smooth muscle cell selective) (see Chapter Appendix Table 1-C.3)

- Thrombolytic agents (see Chapter Appendix Table 1-C.4)

- Antiplatelet and anticoagulation agents (see Chapter Appendix Table 1-C.5)

Congestive Heart Failure Medications

Heart failure treatment may include oral medications for a low-level chronic condition or intravenous medications for an acute and life-threatening condition. Medical management generally attempts to improve the pumping capability of the heart by reducing preload, increasing contractility, reducing afterload, or a combination of these.

Medication classes successful in achieving these goals include the following [5]:

- Diuretics (see Chapter Appendix Table 1-C.6)

- Positive inotropes (see Chapter Appendix Table 1-C.7; see Table 1-21 for signs and symptoms of digitalis toxicity)

- Vasodilators (see Chapter Appendix Table 1-C.8)

- Angiotensin-converting enzyme inhibitors (see Chapter Appendix Table 1-C.9)

Antiarrhythmic Drugs

Antiarrhythmic drugs attempt to normalize conduction of the cardiac electrical system [5]. These drugs are classified in the following manner according to their mechanism of action:

Table 1-21. Signs and Symptoms of Digitalis Toxicity

System Affected	Effects
Central nervous system	Drowsiness
	Fatigue
	Confusion
	Visual disturbances
Cardiac system	Premature atrial contractions, premature ventricular contractions, or both
	Paroxysmal supraventricular tachycardia
	Ventricular tachycardia
	High degrees of atrioventricular block
	Ventricular fibrillation
Gastrointestinal system	Nausea
	Vomiting
	Diarrhea

Source: Data from EA Hillegass, HS Sadowsky. Essentials of Cardiopulmonary Physical Therapy. Philadelphia: Saunders, 1994.

- Class I (sodium channel blockers) (see Chapter Appendix Table 1-C.10)

- Class II (beta-blockers) (see Chapter Appendix Tables 1-C.1 and 1-C.10)

- Class III (refractory period alterations) (see Chapter Appendix Table 1-C.10)

- Class IV (calcium channel blockers) (see Chapter Appendix Tables 1-C.2 and 1-C.10)

Antihypertensive Drugs

Antihypertensive drugs attempt to assist the body in maintenance of normotension by decreasing blood volume, dilating blood vessels, preventing constriction of blood vessels, preventing the retention of sodium, or a combination of these.

Medication classes successful in achieving these goals include the following [5]:

- Diuretics (see Chapter Appendix Table 1-C.6)
- Beta-blockers (see Chapter Appendix Table 1-C.1)
- Alpha-blockers (see Chapter Appendix Table 1-C.1)
- Calcium channel blockers (see Chapter Appendix Table 1-C.2)
- Angiotensin-converting enzyme inhibitors (see Chapter Appendix Table 1-C.9)
- Vasodilators (see Chapter Appendix Table 1-C.8)

Lipid-Lowering Drugs
Lipid-lowering drugs attempt to decrease lipid levels. They are usually prescribed in combination with a change in diet and exercise habits (see Chapter Appendix Table 1-C.11) [5]. Medications successful in lowering lipid levels are the following:

- Anion exchange resin
- Fibric acid derivatives
- HMG-CoA reductase inhibitor
- Nicotinic acid
- Probucol
- Fish oils

Physical Therapy Intervention

This section discusses basic treatment guidelines for physical therapists working with patients who have cardiac impairments.

Goals
The primary goals in treating patients with primary or secondary cardiac pathology are the following [12]:

- Assess hemodynamic response in conjunction with medical or surgical management during self-care activities and functional mobility
- Maximize activity tolerance

- Provide patient and family education regarding behavior modification and risk factor reduction (especially in patients with CAD, status post myocardial infarction, status post PTCA, status post CABG, or status post cardiac transplant)

Basic Concepts for the Treatment of Patients with Cardiac Dysfunction

The status of the patient's medical or surgical course should be considered because it is inappropriate to treat an unstable patient. The following are some general guidelines of when to withhold acute care therapy (i.e., instances in which further medical care should precede physical therapy) [12]:

- Decompensated CHF

- Second-degree heart block coupled with premature ventricular contractions (PVCs) of ventricular tachycardia at rest

- Third-degree heart block

- Hypertensive resting BP (systolic >160 mm Hg, diastolic <80 mm Hg)

- Hypotensive resting BP (systolic <80 mm Hg)

- More than 10 PVCs per minute at rest

- Myocardial infarction or extension of infarction within the previous 2 days

- Unstable angina pectoris with recent changes in symptoms (less than 24 hours)

- Dissecting aortic aneurysm

- Uncontrolled metabolic diseases

- Psychosis or other unstable psychological condition

Activity Level Guidelines

General patient activity levels are provided below. This progression may be accomplished in as little as 3–4 days in a patient with cardiac dysfunction who is medically stable and has no complications. Physical therapy intervention can be initiated at any stage of this progression [12].

1. The patient is on complete bed rest (independent morning care of washing of upper body with arms supported, self-feeding, complete bed bath with assistance, and bedside commode).

2. The patient takes a complete bed bath (self-shaving [males]), uses a bedside commode, and sits up in chair at bedside with feet elevated 20–30 minutes twice a day.

3. In bed, the patient bathes all but his or her back, legs, and feet; he or she may ambulate with assistance. Supine, sitting, and standing BP and pulse are recorded. The patient walks to chair in the room and sits for 30–60 minutes three times a day.

4. The patient bathes as at level 3 and uses the bathroom as desired; he or she sits up in a chair in the room three times a day for 30–60 minutes. Ambulation is monitored.

5. The patient has a sponge bath while sitting in the bathroom, and the nurse bathes his or her back. The patient ambulates in the room, sits in a chair as desired, and ambulates with continuous monitoring in the hallway.

6. The patient has a sit-down shower and walks in the hallway three times a day.

7. The patient walks up and down one flight of stairs.

8. The patient undergoes low-level treadmill test before or after discharge.

Physical therapy intervention may include a warm-up phase of seated or standing exercises; a conditioning phase of walking or stationary cycling; and a cool down, relaxation phase of deep breathing and stretching.

Listed below are various ways to monitor the patient's activity tolerance.

1. HR—HR is the primary means of setting the exercise intensity level in patients who are not taking beta-blockers or on non–rate-responsive pacemakers. There is a normal linear correlation between HR and work. In general, a 20- to 30-beat increase from the resting value during activity is a safe intensity level in which a patient can exercise. If a patient has undergone a stress test during the hospital stay, a percentage (e.g., 60–80%) of the maximum HR achieved during the test can be calculated to determine the exercise intensity [13]. An exam-

ple of a disproportionate HR response to low-level activity (bed or seated exercises or ambulation in room) is an HR of more than 120 bpm or less than 50 bpm [13].

When prescribing activity intensity for a patient taking beta-blockers, the HR should not exceed 20 beats above resting HR. If prescribing activity intensity using HR for patients with an AICD, the exercise target heart rate should be 20–30 beats below the threshold rate on the defibrillator [13].

HR cannot be used to prescribe exercise status post heart transplant secondary to denervation of the heart during transplantation.

Baseline HR and recent changes in medications should always be considered before beginning an exercise session.

2.   BP—Refer to the cardiac assessment section regarding BP measurements and Table 1-6 on BP ranges. Examples of a disproportionate response to exercise is a systolic pressure decrease of 10 mm Hg below the resting value, a hypertensive systolic response of more than 180 mm Hg, or a hypertensive diastolic response of more than 110 mm Hg [13].

3.   Rating of perceived exertion (RPE)—See Table 1-22 for Borg's rating of perceived exertion. Borg's RPE scale was initially proposed in 1962 and has evolved today to be the classic means of objectively documenting subjective feelings of exercise intensity. This scale can be easily used to monitor exercise intensity for the purpose of exercise prescription in a variety of patient populations. It is the preferred method of prescribing exercise intensity for a patient taking beta-blockers. A general guideline for everyone is to exercise to a point no greater than 5 on the 10-point scale and no greater than 13 on the original scale [14].

4.   Rate pressure product (RPP)—RPP = HR × systolic BP and is an indication of myocardial oxygen demand. If a patient undergoes maximal exercise testing and has myocardial ischemia, RPP can be calculated at the point when ischemia is occurring to establish the patient's ischemic threshold. This RPP value can then be used during exercise to provide a guideline of safe intensity.

5.   Heart sounds—See the assessment section on heart sounds and Table 1-8 for normal and abnormal heart sounds. The onset of murmurs, S3 heart sounds, or S4 heart sounds during treatment may be detected and could indicate a decline in cardiac function during

Table 1-22. Borg's Rating of Perceived Exertion

Original Scale	10-Point Scale
6	0 Nothing at all
7 Very, very light	0.5 Very, very slight
8	1 Very slight
9 Very light	2 Slight
10	3 Moderate
11 Fairly light	4 Somewhat severe
12	5 Severe
13 Somewhat hard	6
14	7 Very severe
15 Hard	8
16	9 Very, very severe
17 Very hard	(almost maximal)
18	10 Maximal
19 Very, very hard	
20	

Source: Adapted from American College of Sports Medicine. Guidelines for Exercise Testing and Prescription (4th ed). Philadelphia: Lea & Febiger, 1991;70.

activity. This finding should be brought to the attention of the nurse and physician.

6.   Breath sounds—Refer to Chapter 2 for a discussion on auscultation. The presence of bibasilar crackles during activity that were not present at rest may be indicative of acute CHF. Activity should be terminated and the nurse and physician notified.

7.   ECG rhythm—Refer to the section on ECG and the pathophysiology discussion of rhythm and conduction disturbances. When treating patients that are being continuously monitored by an ECG, it is important to know their baseline rhythm, the most recently observed rhythm, what lead is being monitored, and why they are being monitored.

It is important to recognize their normal rhythm and any deviations from this norm. It is also important to recognize changes that could indicate a decline in cardiac status. Examples include the following:

- Onset of ST changes (elevation or depression of >1 mm) could indicate ischemia
- Increased frequency of PVCs (trigeminy to bigeminy or couplets)
- Unifocal PVCs to multifocal PVCs
- PACs to atrial flutter or atrial fibrillation
- Atrial flutter to atrial fibrillation
- Any progression in heart blocks (first-degree to Mobitz I)
- Loss of pacer spike capturing (pacer spike without resultant QRS)

The physical therapist should also be able to recognize signs and symptoms of cardiac decompensation and immediately notify the physician if any develop.

Common visual signs include diaphoresis (profuse sweating), cyanosis (bluish coloring indicating hypoxia), nasal flaring (indicates difficulty breathing), and increased accessory muscle use (indicates difficulty breathing). It is important to record any signs noted during activity and other objective data at that time.

Common signs and symptoms include weakness, fatigue, dizziness lightheadedness, angina, palpitations, and dyspnea. It is important to record any symptoms reported by the patient and any objective information at that time (ECG readings; BP, HR, and RPP measurements; breath sounds).

References

1. Moore K. Clinically Oriented Anatomy (3rd ed). Baltimore: Williams & Wilkins, 1992;7.
2. Canobbio MM. Cardiovascular Disorders. St. Louis: Mosby, 1990.
3. Cheitlin MD, Sokolow M, McIlroy MB. Clinical Cardiology (6th ed). Norwalk, CT: Appleton & Lange, 1993;1.
4. Guyton AC. Textbook of Medical Physiology (8th ed). Philadelphia: Saunders, 1991;98.
5. Davis D. How to Quickly and Accurately Master ECG Interpretation (2nd ed). Philadelphia: Lippincott, 1992.

6. Hillis LD, Firth BG, Willerson JT. Manual of Clinical Problems in Cardiology. Boston: Little, Brown, 1984.
7. Hillegass EA, Sadowsky HS. Essentials of Cardiopulmonary Physical Therapy. Philadelphia: Saunders, 1994.
8. Urden LD, Davie JK, Thelan LA. Essentials of Critical Care Nursing. St. Louis: Mosby, 1992.
9. Cohen M, Michel TH. Cardiopulmonary Symptoms in Physical Therapy Practice. New York: Churchill Livingstone, 1988.
10. Polich S, Faynor SM. Interpreting lab test values. PT Magazine, 1996;3:110.
11. Goodman CC, Snyder TEK. Differential Diagnosis in Physical Therapy: Musculoskeletal and Systemic Conditions. Philadelphia: Saunders, 1990;43.
12. Cahalin LP, Ice RG, Irwin S. Program Planning and Implementation. In S Irwin, JS Tecklin (eds), Cardiopulmonary Physical Therapy (3rd ed). St Louis: Mosby, 1995;144.
13. Wegener NK. Rehabilitation of the Patient with Coronary Heart Disease. In RC Schlant, RW Alexander (eds), Hurst's The Heart (8th ed). New York: McGraw-Hill, 1994;1227.
14. American Colleges of Sports Medicine. Guidelines for Exercise Testing and Prescription (4th ed). Philadelphia: Lea & Febinger, 1991;26.

Suggested Reading

Braith RW, Limacher MC, Leggett SH, Pollock ML. Skeletal muscle strength in heart transplant recipients. J Heart Lung Transplant 1993;12:1018.

Edinger KE, McKeen S, Bemis-Dougherty A. Physical therapy following heart transplant. Phys Ther Pract 1992;1:25.

O'Connell JB, Bourge RC, Costanzo-Nordin MR, et al. AHA medical/scientific statement. Cardiac transplantation: recipient selection, donor procurement and medical follow-up. Circulation 1992;86:1061.

Sadowsky HS. Cardiac transplantation: a review. Phys Ther 1996;76:498.

Stevenson LW, Steimle AE, Fonarow G, et al. Improvement in exercise capacity of candidates awaiting heart transplantation. J Am Coll Cardiol 1995;25:163.

Appendix 1-A:
Abnormal Heart Rhythms

Table 1-A.1. Electrocardiograph Characteristics and Causes of Atrial Rhythms

Name	Electrocardiograph Characteristics	Common Causes	Physical Therapy Considerations
Supraventricular tachycardia	Regular rhythm Heart rate = 160–250 bpm Can originate from any location above atrioventricular node Can be paroxysmal (comes and goes without reason)	RHD Mitral valve prolapse Cor pulmonale Digitalis toxicity	Can produce palpitations, chest tightness, dizziness, anxiety, apprehension, and weakness Physical therapy would not treat if in SVT until controlled
Atrial flutter	Rhythm can be regular or irregular Atrial rate of 250–350 bpm Ventricular rate is variable and depends on conduction ratio (atrial: ventricular) (e.g., 2:1. Atrial rate = 250, ventricular rate = 125 bpm) Classic sawtooth P waves	Mitral stenosis CAD Hypertension	Signs and symptoms depend on presence or absence of heart disease but can lead to CHF, palpitations, angina, and syncope, if cardiac output decreases far enough to reduce myocardial and cerebral blood flow Physical therapy treatment would depend on patient's tolerance to the rhythm
Atrial fibrillation (one of the most commonly encountered abnormal rhythms)	Irregular rhythm Atrial has no rate (just quivers) Ventricular rate varies	CHF CAD RHD Hypertension Cor pulmonale	Can produce CHF and syncope secondary to no atrial kick If new diagnosis, physical therapy held until medical treatment If chronic and not in CHF, treat with caution

| Premature atrial contractions | Irregular rhythm (can be regularly irregular [e.g., skip every third beat])
Heart rate normal (i.e., 60–100 bpm) | Normal in people affected by caffeine, smoking, or emotional disturbances
Abnormal in people with CAD, CHF, or electrolyte disturbances | Usually asymptomatic but should be considered with other cardiac issues at time of treatment
Can proceed with treatment with close monitoring
If premature atrial contractions are consistent and increasing, they can progress to atrial fibrillations |

RHD = rheumatoid heart disease; SVT = supraventricular tachycardia; CAD = coronary artery disease; CHF = congestive heart failure.
Source: Data from B Aehlert. ACLS Quick Review Study Guide. St. Louis: Mosby, 1994; and EK Chung. Manual of Cardiac Arrhythmias. Boston: Butterworth–Heinemann, 1986.

Table 1-A.2. Electrocardiograph Characteristics and Causes of Ventricular Rhythms

Name	Electrocardiograph Characteristics	Common Causes	Physical Therapy Considerations
Agonal rhythm	Irregular rhythm Heart rate of less than 20 bpm No P wave	Near death	Do not treat
VT	Usually regular rhythm Heart rate greater than 100 bpm No P wave or with retrograde conduction and appears after the QRS	CAD most common after acute MI Can occur in RHD Cardiomyopathy Hypertension	Do not treat Patient needs immediate medical assistance Patient may be stable (maintain CO) for short while, but can progress quickly to unstable condition (no CO) called *pulseless VT*
Multifocal VT (torsades de pointe)	Irregular rhythm Heart rate greater than 150 bpm No P waves	Drug-induced with anti-arrhythmic medications (quinidine, procainamide) Hypokalemia Hypomagnesemia MI Hypothermia	Do not treat Patient needs immediate medical attention
Premature ventricular contractions (focal or multifocal)*	Irregular rhythm (can be regularly irregular [e.g., skip every fourth beat])	In normal individuals, secondary to caffeine consumption, smoking, or	Frequency will dictate affect on CO Need to monitor ECG with

		treatment
Heart rate varies, but is usually normal (i.e., 60–100 bpm) *Couplet* is two premature ventricular contractions in a row. *Bigeminy* is a premature ventricular contraction every other beat. *Trigeminy* is a premature ventricular contraction every third beat.	emotional disturbances CAD MI Cardiomyopathy MVP Digitalis toxicity	Can progress to VT (this is more likely if multifocal in nature or if greater than six premature ventricular contractions per minute) Stop treatment or rest if change in frequency or quality
Ventricular fibrillation Chaotic	Severe heart disease most commonly after acute MI Hypercalcemia Electrocution	Patient needs immediate medical assistance No physical therapy treatment
Idioventricular rhythm Essentially regular rhythm Ventricular rate 20–40 bpm	Advanced heart disease High degree of atrioventricular block Usually a terminal arrhythmia	CHF is common secondary to slow rates Hold treatment unless rhythm is well-tolerated

CAD = coronary artery disease; MI = myocardial infarction; RHD = rheumatoid heart disease; CO = cardiac output; MVP = mitral valve prolapse; ECG = electrocardiograph; VT = ventricular tachycardia; AV = atrioventricular; CHF = congestive heart failure.
*Focal premature ventricular contractions have one ectopic foci, all waveforms look the same; multifocal premature ventricular contractions have more than one ectopic foci and different wave forms.

Source: Data from B Aehlert. ACLS Quick Review Study Guide. St. Louis: Mosby, 1994; and EK Chung. Manual of Cardiac Arrhythmias. Boston: Butterworth–Heinemann, 1986.

Table 1-A.3. Electrocardiograph Characteristics and Causes of Junctional Rhythms

Name	Electrocardiograph Characteristics	Common Causes	Physical Therapy Considerations
Junctional escape rhythm	Regular rhythm Ventricular rate of 20–40 bpm Inverted P wave before or after QRS Starts with ectopic foci in AV junction tissue	Usual cause is physiologic to control the ventricles in AV block, sinus bradycardia, atrial fibrillation, SA block, or drug intoxication	If occasional and intermittent during bradycardia or chronic AF, usually insignificant and can treat (with close watch of possible worsening condition via symptoms and vital signs) If consistent and present secondary to AV block, acute MI, or drug intoxication, can be symptomatic with CHF (see Table 1-17)
Junctional tachycardia	Regular rhythm Ventricular rate of 100–180 bpm P wave as with junctional escape rhythm	Most common with chronic AF Also with CAD, RHD, and cardiomyopathy	Can produce or exacerbate symptoms of CHF or angina secondary to decreased CO Physical therapy treatment depends on patient tolerance In cases of new onset, wait for medical treatment

AV = atrioventricular; SA = sinoatrial; AF = atrial fibrillation; MI = myocardial infarction; CHF = congestive heart failure; CAD = coronary artery disease; RHD = rheumatic heart disease; CO = cardiac output.
Source: Data from B Aehlert. ACLS Quick Review Study Guide. St. Louis: Mosby, 1994; and EK Chung. Manual of Cardiac Arrhythmias. Boston: Butterworth–Heinemann, 1986.

Table 1-A.4. Electrocardiograph Characteristics and Causes of Atrioventricular Blocks

Name	Electrocardiograph Characteristics	Common Causes	Physical Therapy Considerations
First-degree AV block	Regular rhythm Heart rate normal (i.e., 60–100 bpm) Prolonged PR interval greater than 0.20 (constant)	Elderly with heart disease Acute myocarditis Acute MI	If chronic, be more cautious of underlying heart disease If new onset, monitor closely for progression to higher level block
Second-degree AV block			
Type I (Wenckebach, Mobitz I)	Irregular rhythm Atrial rate faster than ventricular rate (both usually 60–100 bpm) PR interval lengthens until P wave appears without a QRS complex	Acute infection Acute MI	Symptoms are uncommon Same as for first-degree AV block
Type II (Mobitz II)	Irregular rhythm Atrial rate greater than ventricular rate PR interval may be normal or prolonged but is constant for each conducted QRS	Anteroseptal MI	CHF is common Can have dizziness, fainting, or complete unconsciousness Patient may need a pacemaker Physical therapy should be held for medical management

Table 1-A.4. *Continued*

Name	Electrocardiograph Characteristics	Common Causes	Physical Therapy Considerations
Third-degree AV block (complete heart block)	Regular rhythm Atrial rate greater than ventricular rate	Anteroseptal MI Drug intoxication Infections Electrolyte imbalances CAD Degenerative sclerotic process of atrioventricular conduction system	Severe CHF Patient will need medical management A pacer (temporary or permanent depending on reversibility of etiology) is almost always necessary

AV = atrioventricular; MI = myocardial infarction; CHF = congestive heart failure; CAD = coronary artery disease.
Source: Data from B Aehlert. ACLS Quick Review Study Guide. St. Louis: Mosby, 1994; and EK Chung. Manual of Cardiac Arrhythmias. Boston: Butterworth–Heinemann, 1986.

Appendix 1-B:
Electrocardiogram Tracings
of Abnormal Heart Rhythms

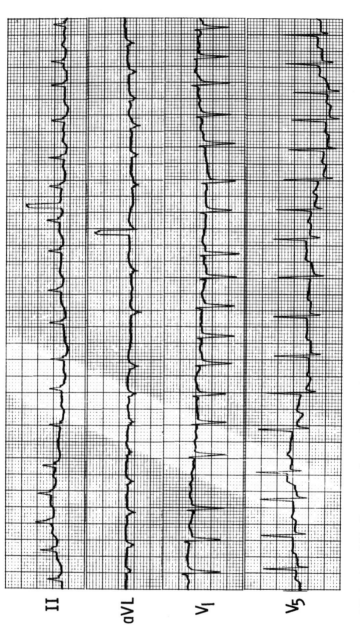

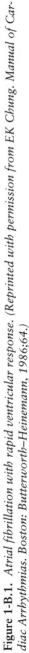

Figure 1-B.1. Atrial fibrillation with rapid ventricular response. (Reprinted with permission from EK Chung. Manual of Cardiac Arrhythmias. Boston: Butterworth–Heinemann, 1986;64.)

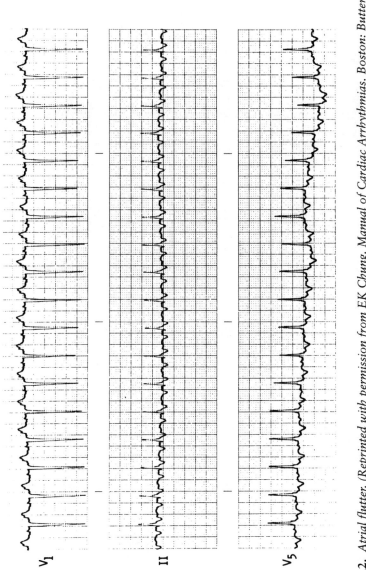

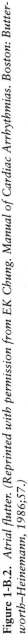

Figure 1-B.2. *Atrial flutter. (Reprinted with permission from EK Chung. Manual of Cardiac Arrhythmias. Boston: Butterworth–Heinemann, 1986;57.)*

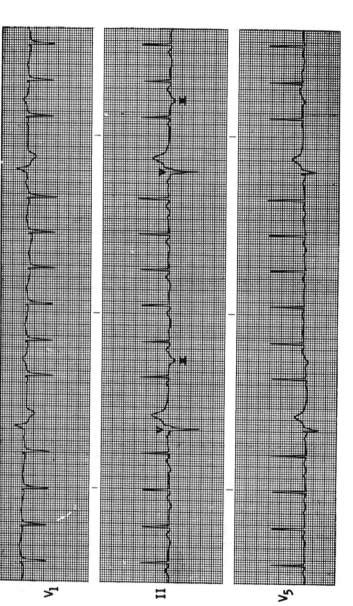
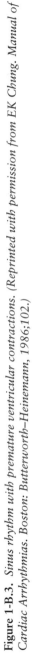

Figure 1-B.3. *Sinus rhythm with premature ventricular contractions. (Reprinted with permission from EK Chung. Manual of Cardiac Arrhythmias. Boston: Butterworth–Heinemann, 1986;102.)*

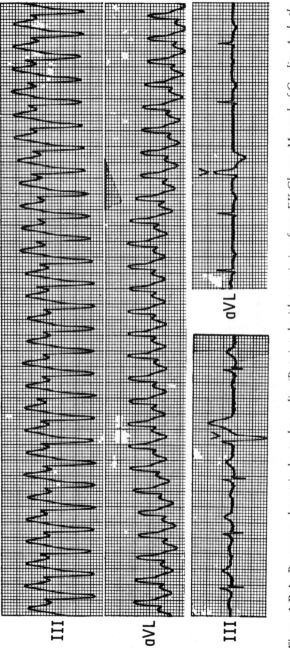
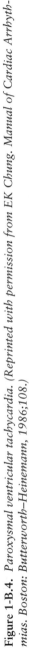

Figure 1-B.4. *Paroxysmal ventricular tachycardia. (Reprinted with permission from EK Chung.* Manual of Cardiac Arrhythmias. *Boston: Butterworth–Heinemann, 1986;108.)*

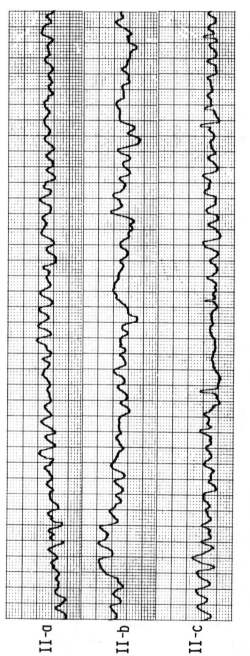

II-a

II-b

II-c

Figure 1-B.5. *Ventricular fibrillation. (Reprinted with permission from EK Chung. Manual of Cardiac Arrhythmias. Boston: Butterworth–Heinemann, 1986;118.)*

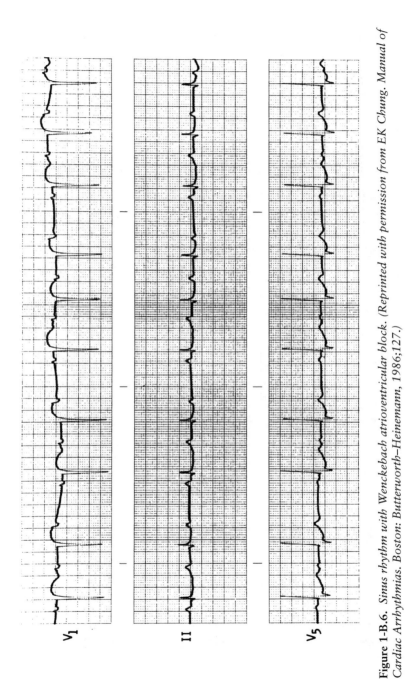

Figure 1-B.6. *Sinus rhythm with Wenckebach atrioventricular block. (Reprinted with permission from EK Chung. Manual of Cardiac Arrhythmias. Boston: Butterworth–Heinemann, 1986;127.)*

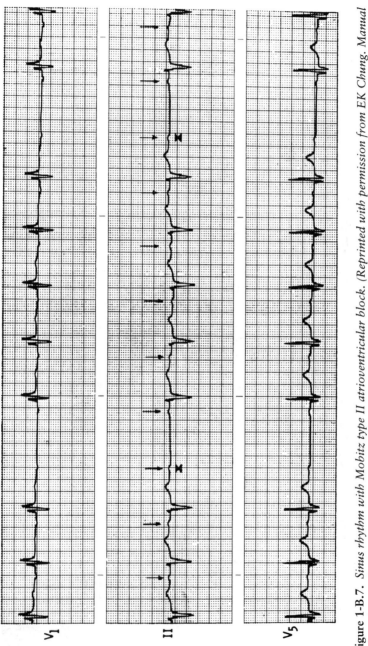

Figure 1-B.7. *Sinus rhythm with Mobitz type II atrioventricular block. (Reprinted with permission from EK Chung. Manual of Cardiac Arrhythmias. Boston: Butterworth–Heinemann, 1986;129.)*

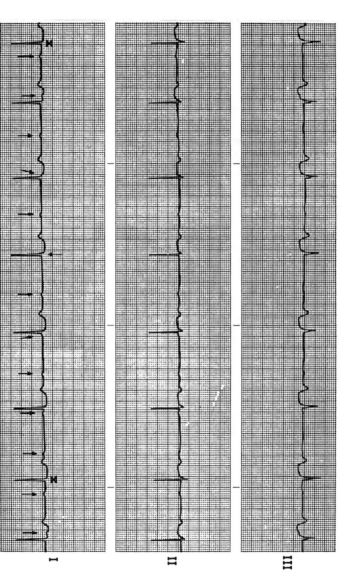

Figure 1-B.8. *Sinus rhythm with advanced atrioventricular block. (Reprinted with permission from EK Chung. Manual of Cardiac Arrhythmias. Boston: Butterworth–Heinemann, 1986;135.)*

Appendix 1-C: Cardiac Medications

Table 1-C.1. Beta Blockers

Indications
  Ischemia
  Hypertension
  Arrhythmia
Selective*
  Beta-1 selective
    Metoprolol (Lopressor)
    Atenolol (Tenormin)
    Acebutolol (Sectral)
    Esmolol (Brevibloc)
    Alprenolol
  Beta-2 selective
    Butoxamine
  Alpha and beta antagonists
    Labetalol (Normodyne, Trandate)
Nonselective*
  Propranolol (Inderal)
  Timolol (Blocadren)
  Nadolol (Corgard)
  Pindolol (Visken)
  Labetalol (Normodyne)
Mechanism of action
  Decreases myocardial oxygen demand by decreasing sympathetic input to
    myocardium, therefore decreasing heart rate and contractility

Table 1-C.1. *Continued*

Side effects
  Smooth muscle spasm (bronchospasm)
  Exaggeration of therapeutic cardiac actions (bradycardia)
  Fatigue
  Insomnia
  Masking of hypoglycemic symptoms in diabetics
  Impaired glucose tolerance
  Decreased high-density lipoproteins cholesterol

*Selective refers to blockade of either beta-1, beta-2, or alpha receptors. Nonselective means not selective in blocking receptors.
Source: Data from EA Hillegass, HS Sadowsky. Essentials of Cardiopulmonary Physical Therapy. Philadelphia: Saunders, 1994; C Peel, KA Mossberg. Effects of cardiovascular medications on exercise responses. Phys Ther 1995;75:387; and CD Ciccone. Current trends in cardiovascular pharmacology. Phys Ther 1996;76:481.

Table 1-C.2. Calcium Channel Blockers

Indications
  Ischemia
  Arrhythmia
  Hypertension
Generic name (brand name)
  Nifedipine (Procardia, Adalat)
  Verapamil (Isoptin, Calan)
  Diltiazem (Cardizem)
  Nicardipine (Cardene)
  Isradipine (DynaCirc)
Mechanism of action
  Decreases myocardial oxygen demand and increases supply of myocardial oxygen by slowing transport of calcium on smooth muscle and myocardial cells, therefore reducing contractility and afterload
Side effects
  Negative inotrope at high doses
  Orthostatic hypotension

Source: Data from EA Hillegass, HS Sadowsky. Essentials of Cardiopulmonary Physical Therapy. Philadelphia: Saunders, 1994; C Peel, KA Mossberg. Effects of cardiovascular medications on exercise responses. Phys Ther 1995;75:387; and CD Ciccone. Current trends in cardiovascular pharmacology. Phys Ther 1996;76:481.

Table 1-C.3. Nitrates

Indications
  Ischemia
  Hypertension
Generic name (brand name; route of entry)
  Amyl nitrate (Aspirol, Vaporole; inhalation)
  Nitroglycerin (Nitro-Bid, Nitrostat; sublingual, spray, percutaneous oint-
    ment, oral [sustained release, intravenous]) (Nitro-Dur, Transdermal-
    NTG, Nitrodisc; transdermal patch)
  Isosorbide dinitrate (Isordil, Sorbitrate; sublingual, oral, chewable)
  Pentaerythritol tetranitrate (Peritrate; sublingual) (Pentrinitrol, Pentafin;
    oral) (Vasitol; sustained release)
  Erythrityl tetranitrate (Tetranitrol, Erythrol tetranitrate; oral) (Cardilate;
    sublingual)
Mechanism of action
  Decreases myocardial oxygen demand and increases myocardial oxygen
    supply
  Venodilates by promoting smooth muscle relaxation on both the venous
    and arterial side, therefore reducing preload and afterload
Side effects
  Headache
  Hypotension

Source: Adapted from K Grimes, M Cohen. Cardiac Medications. In EA Hillegass, HS
Sadowsky (eds), Essentials of Cardiopulmonary Physical Therapy. Philadelphia:
Saunders, 1994;493.

Table 1-C.4. Thrombolytic Agents

Indications
  Ischemia

Generic name (brand name)
  Anistreplase (Eminase)
  Streptokinase (Kabinase, Streptase)
  Tissue-type plasminogen activator (Alteplase)
  Urokinase (Abbokinase)

Mechanism of action
  Increases myocardial oxygen supply by facilitation of the breakdown of
    clots that already have formed in the coronary arteries

Side effects
  Decreases blood clotting
  Cerebral vascular accident
  Genitourinary bleeding
  Gastrointestinal bleeding

Source: Adapted from EA Hillegass, HS Sadowsky. Essentials of Cardiopulmonary
Physical Therapy. Philadelphia: Saunders, 1994;494; and CD Ciccone. Current trends
in cardiovascular pharmacology. Phys Ther 1996;76:481.

Table 1-C.5. Antiplatelet and Anticoagulation Agents

Indications
  Ischemia

Class
  Anticoagulants (generic name [brand name])
    Heparin (Heparin)
    Warfarin (Coumadin)
  Antiplatelets (generic name [brand name])
    Acetyl-salicylic acid (aspirin)
    Dipyridamole (Persantine)

Mechanism of action
  Used prophylactically to prevent thrombus formation

Side effects
  Decreases blood clotting
  Hemorrhage

Source: Adapted from EA Hillegass, HS Sadowsky. Essentials of Cardiopulmonary
Physical Therapy. Philadelphia: Saunders, 1994;497; and CD Ciccone. Current trends
in cardiovascular pharmacology. Phys Ther 1996;76:481.

Table 1-C.6. Diuretics

Indications
  Heart failure
  Hypertension
Category (generic name [brand name])
  Thiazide
    Bendroflumethiazide (Naturetin)
    Benzthiazide (Exna, Hydrex)
    Chlorothiazide (Diuril)
    Chlorthalidone (Hygroton)
    Cyclothiazide (Anhydron)
    Hydrochlorothiazide (Esidrix)
    Hydroflumethiazide (Diucardin, Saluron)
    Methyclothiazide (Enduron)
    Metolazone (Diulo, Zaroxolyn)
    Polythiazide (Renese)
    Quinethazone (Hydromox)
    Trichlormethiazide (Metahydrin, Naqua)
  Loop
    Bumetanide (Bumex)
    Ethacrynic acid (Edecrin)
    Furosemide (Lasix, Furomide)
  Potassium-sparing
    Amiloride (Midamor)
    Spironolactone (Aldactone)
    Triamterene (Dyrenium)
Mechanism of action
  Reduces preload
Side effects
  Volume reduction
  Hypotension
  Arrhythmias
  Hypokalemia

Source: Adapted from EA Hillegass, HS Sadowsky. Essentials of Cardiopulmonary Physical Therapy. Philadelphia: Saunders, 1994;497; and CD Ciccone. Current trends in cardiovascular pharmacology. Phys Ther 1996;76:481.

Table 1-C.7. Positive Inotropes

Category	Generic Name (Brand Name)	Indications	Mechanism of Action	Side Effects
Cardiac glycosides Digitalis	Digitoxin (Crystodigin) Digoxin (Lanoxin) Deslanoside (Cedilanid-DIV)	Heart failure	Increases contractility	Decreases heart rate Conduction delay Digitalis toxicity (see Table 1-21)
Sympathomimetics	Dobutamine (Dobutrex)	Heart failure	Increases contractility	Smooth muscle dilation (bronchodilation and vasodilation) Prolonged use can decrease sensitization of beta receptors (decreased inotropy)
Beta-1 non-selective	Epinephrine (Adrenaline) Isoproterenol (Isuprel)	See Dobutamine (Dobutrex), above	See Dobutamine (Dobutrex), above	See Dobutamine (Dobutrex), above
Dopaminergics	Dopamine (Intropin, Dopastat)	See Dobutamine (Dobutrex), above	See Dobutamine (Dobutrex), above	See Dobutamine (Dobutrex), above
Mixed alpha and beta receptors	Norepinephrine (Levophed)	See Dobutamine (Dobutrex), above	See Dobutamine (Dobutrex), above	See Dobutamine (Dobutrex), above

| Bipyridines | Amrinone (Inocor) | See Dobutamine (Dobutrex), above | See Dobutamine (Dobutrex), above | See Dobutamine (Dobutrex), above | Can exacerbate ischemia and can worsen ectopy |

Source: Adapted from EA Hillegass, HS Sadowsky. Essentials of Cardiopulmonary Physical Therapy. Philadelphia: Saunders, 1994:497; C Peel, KA Mossberg. Effects of cardiovascular medications on exercise responses. Phys Ther 1995;75:387; and CD Ciccone. Current trends in cardiovascular pharmacology. Phys Ther 1996;76:481.

Table 1-C.8. Vasodilators

Category	Generic Name (Brand Name; Route of Entry)	Indications	Mechanism of Action	Side Effects
Venodilators	Amyl nitrate (Aspirol, Vaporole; inhalation) Nitroglycerin (Nitro-Bid, Nitrostat; sublingual, spray, percutaneous ointment, oral [sustained release, intravenous]) (Nitro-Dur, Transdermal-NTG, Nitrodisc; transdermal patch) Isosorbide dinitrate (Isordil, Sorbitrate; sublingual, oral, chewable) Pentaerythritol tetranitrate (Peritrate; sublingual) (Pentrinitrol, Pentafin; oral) (Vasitol; sustained release) Erythrityl tetranitrate (Tetranitrol, Erythrol retranitrate; oral) (Cardilate; sublingual)	Heart failure Hypertension	Decreases preload	Headache Hypotension Compensatory sympathetic reflex causing increased heart rate Vasoconstriction Elevated plasma renin (usually avoided with combination of medications that includes a sympathetic inhibiting agent)
Arteriodilators	Hydralazine (Apresoline; oral) Minoxidil (Loniten; oral) Nifedipine (Procardia; oral) Diazoxide (Hyperstat IV; oral)	Heart failure Hypertension	Decreases afterload	See Venodilators, above

| Combined arterio- and venodilator | Sodium nitroprusside (Nipride; IV) | Heart failure | Reduces both preload and afterload for the treatment of acute severe heart failure | See Venodilators, above |

Source: Adapted from EA Hillegass, HS Sadowsky. Essentials of Cardiopulmonary Physical Therapy. Philadelphia: Saunders, 1994;512; C Peel, KA Mossberg. Effects of cardiovascular medications on exercise responses. Phys Ther 1995;75:387; and CD Ciccone. Current trends in cardiovascular pharmacology. Phys Ther 1996;76:481.

Table 1-C.9. Angiotensin-Converting Enzyme Inhibitors

Indications
  Heart failure

Generic name (brand name)
  Captopril (Capoten)
  Enalapril (Vasotec)
  Lisinopril (Prinivil, Zestril)

Mechanism of action
  Inhibits conversion of angiotensin I to angiotensin II and therefore acts to decrease excess water and sodium retention while preventing vasoconstriction

Side effects
  Edema
  Cough
  Hypotension
  Skin rash

Source: Adapted from EA Hillegass, HS Sadowsky. Essentials of Cardiopulmonary Physical Therapy. Philadelphia: Saunders, 1994;497; C Peel, KA Mossberg. Effects of cardiovascular medications on exercise responses. Phys Ther 1995;75:387; and CD Ciccone. Current trends in cardiovascular pharmacology. Phys Ther 1996;76:481.

Table 1-C.10. Antiarrhythmic Drugs

Class	Generic Name (Brand Name)	Indications	Mechanism of Action	Side Effects
Class I Sodium channel blockers	Quinidine (Biquin, Kinidin, Durules) Disopyramide (Norpace, Rhythmodan) Procainamide (Pronestyl) Lidocaine (Xylocaine) Mexiletine (Mexitil) Phenytoin (Dilantin) Tocainide (Tonocard) Moricizine (Ethmozine) Encainide (Enkaid) Flecainide (Tambocor) Propafenone (Rhythmol)	Arrhythmia	Slows the fast sodium channels	Gastrointestinal and urinary retention Toxicity may cause central nervous system abnormality
Class II Beta blockers	See Chapter Appendix Table 1-C.1			
Class III Refractory period alterations	Amiodarone (Cordarone) Bretylium tosylate (Bretylol)	Arrhythmia	Prolongs refractory period of cardiac tissue	Can transiently increase pacemaker activity
Class IV Calcium channel blockers	See Chapter Appendix Table 1-C.2			

Source: Adapted from K Grimes, M Cohen. Cardiac Medications. In EA Hillegass, HS Sadowsky (eds), Essentials in Cardiopulmonary Physical Therapy. Philadelphia: Saunders, 1994;507.

Table 1-C.11. Lipid-Lowering Drugs

Category	Generic Name (Brand Name)	Indications	Mechanism of Action	Side Effects
Anion exchange resins	Cholestyramine (Questran) Colestipol (Colestid)	Lipid disorders	Decreases low-density lipoproteins	Constipation Diarrhea Nausea Liver function abnormalities Skin rashes
Fibric acid derivatives	Clofibrate (Atromid-S) Gemfibrozil (Lopid)	Lipid disorders	Decreases triglycerides	See Anion Exchange Resins, above
HMG-CoA reductase inhibitor	Lovastatin (Mevacor) Pravastatin	Lipid disorders	Decreases low-density lipoproteins	See Anion Exchange Resins, above
Nicotinic acid	Niacin	Lipid disorders	Decreases low-density lipoproteins and triglycerides	See Anion Exchange Resins, above
Probucol	Probucol (Lorelco)	Lipid disorders	Decreases low-density lipoproteins	See Anion Exchange Resins, above
Fish oils	Omega-3 fatty acid (SuperEPA, many other over-the-counter varieties)	Lipid disorders	Decreases triglycerides	See Anion Exchange Resins, above Increased bleeding time

Source: Adapted from K Grimes, M Cohen. Cardiac Medications. In EA Hillegass, HS Sadowsky (eds), Essentials in Cardiopulmonary Physical Therapy. Philadelphia: Saunders, 1994;515.

2

Respiratory System

Michele Panik and Jaime C. Paz

Introduction

To safely and effectively provide exercise, bronchopulmonary hygiene program(s), or both to patients with respiratory dysfunction, physical therapists require an understanding of the respiratory system and of the principles of gas exchange. The objectives for this chapter are to provide the following:

1. A brief review of the structure and function of the respiratory system

2. An overview of respiratory assessment, including physical examination and diagnostic testing

3. A description of the purpose, mechanisms of action, and side effects of common pulmonary medications

4. A description of respiratory diseases and disorders, including clinical findings, medical-surgical management, and physical therapy intervention.

Note: *Ventilation* is defined as gas (oxygen [O_2] and carbon dioxide [CO_2]) transport into and out of lungs, and *respiration* is defined as gas exchange across the alveolar-capillary and capillary-tissue interfaces. The term *pulmonary* primarily refers to the lungs, their airways, and their vascular system [1].

Structure

The primary organs and muscles of the respiratory system are outlined in Tables 2-1 and 2-2, respectively. A schematic of the pulmonary system within the thorax is presented in Figure 2-1A–C.

Table 2-1. Structure and Function of Primary Organs of the Respiratory System

Structure	Description	Function
Nose	Paired mucosal-lined nasal cavities supported by bone and cartilage	Conduit that filters, warms, and humidifies air entering lungs
Pharynx	Passageway connecting nasal cavity to larynx and oral cavity to esophagus Subdivisions naso-, oro-, and laryngopharynx	Conduit for air and food Facilitates exposure of immune system to inhaled antigens
Larynx	Connects pharynx to trachea Opening (glottis) is covered by the vocal folds or by the epiglottis during swallowing Contains true vocal cords	Passageway that prevents food from entering lower respiratory tract Voice production
Trachea	Flexible tube composed of C-shaped cartilaginous rings that are connected posteriorly to the trachealis muscle Divides into the right and left main stem bronchi	Cleans, warms, and moistens incoming air
Bronchial tree	Right and left main stem bronchi subdivide within each lung into secondary bronchi, tertiary bronchi,	Warms and moistens incoming air from trachea to alveoli Smooth muscle constriction alters airflow

Structure	Description	Function
	and bronchioles, which contain smooth muscle	
Lungs	Paired organs located within pleural cavities of thorax	Contains air passageways distal to main stem bronchi, alveoli, and respiratory membranes
Alveoli	Microscopic sacs at end of bronchial tree immediately adjacent to pulmonary capillaries	Primary gas exchange site Surfactant lines the alveoli to decrease surface tension and prevent complete closure during exhalation
Pleurae	Doubled-layered, continuous serous membrane lining the inside of the thoracic cavity	
	Divided into parietal pleura (outer) and visceral pleura (inner)	Produces lubricating fluid that allows smooth gliding of lungs in thorax

Source: Adapted from E Marieb. Human Anatomy and Physiology (3rd ed). Redwood City, CA: Benjamin-Cummings, 1995;743.

Function

To accomplish ventilation and respiration, the respiratory system is regulated by many neural, chemical, and nonchemical mechanisms, which are discussed below.

Neural Control

Respiration is regulated by two separate neural mechanisms: One controls automatic respiration and the other controls voluntary respiration. Automatic respiration is controlled by the medullary respiratory system in the brain stem, which is responsible for the rhythmicity of breathing. The pneumotaxic center located in the pons controls respiratory rate and depth. Voluntary respiration is mediated by the cerebral cortex, which sends impulses directly to the motor neurons of respiratory muscles.

Table 2-2. Primary and Accessory Respiratory Muscles
and Associated Innervation

Respiratory Muscles	Innervation
Primary inspiratory muscles	
Diaphragm	Phrenic nerve (C3, 4, 5)
External intercostals	Spinal segments T1–9
Internal intercostals	Spinal segments T1–9
Accessory inspiratory muscles	
Trapezius	Cervical nerve (C1–4)
Sternocleidomastoid	Spinal accessory nerve (cranial nerve XI)
Scalenes	Cervical/brachial plexus branches
Pectorals	Medial/lateral pectoral nerve (C5, 6, 7, 8, T1)
Serratus anterior	Long thoracic nerve (C5, 6, 7, 8)
Latissimus dorsi	Thoracodorsal nerve (C5, 6, 7, 8)
Primary expiratory muscles	
Abdominals	Spinal segments T5–12
Internal intercostals	Spinal segments T1–12
Accessory expiratory muscles	
Latissimus dorsi	Thoracodorsal nerve (C5, 6, 7, 8)

Source: Data from FP Kendall, EK McCreary. Muscles: Testing and Function (3rd ed).
Baltimore: Williams & Wilkins, 1983;40, 42–46, 262.

Chemical Control

Arterial levels of CO_2 (PCO_2), of hydrogen ions (H^+), and of O_2 (PO_2)
can modify the rate and depth of respiration. To maintain homeostasis in the body, specialized cells on the carotid arteries and aortic arch
(carotid and aortic bodies, respectively) sense a rise or fall in these
chemicals and send impulses to the respiratory centers to increase or
decrease the respiratory drive. For example, an increase in PCO_2 would
increase the respiratory drive.

Nonchemical Influences

Coughing, bronchoconstriction, and mucus secretion occur in the lungs
as protective reflexes to irritants such as smoke or dust. Emotions, stres-

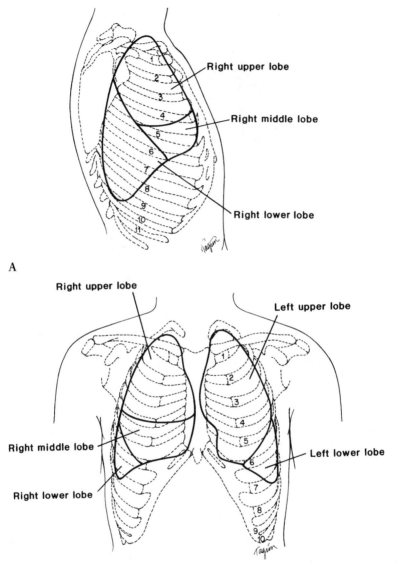

A

B

Figure 2-1. A. Right lung positioned in the thorax. Bony landmarks assist in identifying normal right lung configuration. B. Anterior view of the lungs in the thorax in conjunction with bony landmarks. Left upper lobe is divided into apical and left lingula, which matches the general position of the right upper and middle lobes.

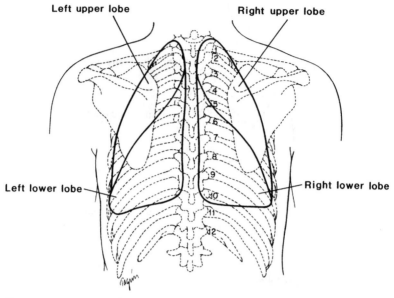

C

Figure 2-1. *Continued. C. Posterior view of the lungs in conjunction with bony landmarks. (Reprinted with permission from E Ellis, J Alison. Key Issues in Cardiorespiratory Physiotherapy. Oxford: Butterworth-Heinemann, 1992;12.)*

sors, pain, and visceral reflexes from lung tissue and other organ systems can also influence respiratory rate and depth.

Respiratory Mechanics

After the respiratory muscles receive signals from the respiratory centers, two motions (bucket and pump handle) occur simultaneously with thoracic stabilization. During inspiration, the diaphragm lowers, and the rib cage elevates and expands in anterior (pump handle) and lateral (bucket handle) directions. During expiration, the diaphragm relaxes and elevates while the rib cage lowers to its resting position. These motions are schematically outlined in Figure 2-2. The changes in shape of the thorax during inspiration and expiration result in pressure changes between the atmosphere and the alveolar spaces. Pressure

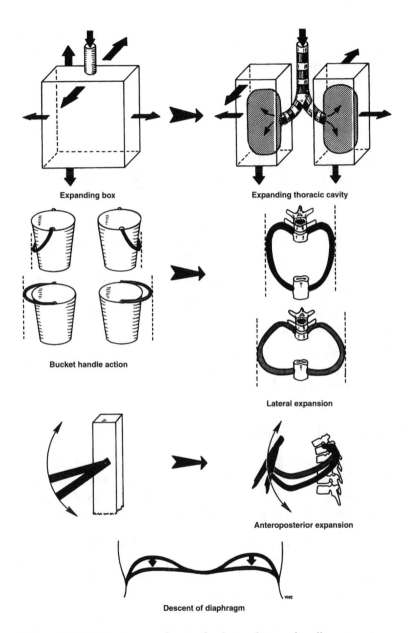

Figure 2-2. *Respiratory mechanics (bucket and pump handle motions).*
(Reprinted with permission from RS Snell. Clinical Anatomy for Medical
Students [5th ed]. Boston: Little, Brown, 1995;89.)

changes result in the bulk flow of air (ventilation) in and out of the lungs. When alveolar pressure is less than atmospheric pressure, inspiration occurs; when alveolar pressure is greater than atmospheric pressure, expiration occurs.

Gas Exchange

Once air has reached the alveolar spaces, gas exchange can occur at the alveolar-capillary membrane. Diffusion of gases through the membrane is affected by the following:

1. A concentration gradient in which gases will diffuse from areas of high concentration to areas of low concentration (e.g., alveolar O_2 = 100 mm Hg $\rightarrow$ capillary O_2 = 40 mm Hg)

2. Surface area, or the total amount of alveolar-capillary interface available for gas exchange (e.g., the breakdown of alveolar membranes that occurs in emphysema will reduce the amount of surface area available for gas exchange)

3. The thickness of the barrier (membrane) between the two areas involved (e.g., retained secretions in the alveolar spaces will impede gas exchange through the membrane)

Ventilation and Perfusion Ratio

Gas exchange is optimized when the ratio of air flow (ventilation [$\dot{V}$]) to blood flow (perfusion [$\dot{Q}$]) approaches 1 to 1. The optimal $\dot{V}/\dot{Q}$ ratio is 0.8, however, as alveolar ventilation is approximately equal to 4 liters per minute and pulmonary blood flow is approximately equal to 5 liters per minute [4].

Gravity, body position, and cardiopulmonary dysfunction can influence this ratio. Perfusion is greatest in gravity-dependent areas. For example, when a person is in a sitting position, perfusion is the greatest at the base of the lungs; when a person is in a left side-lying position, the left lung receives the most blood. Ventilation is optimized in areas of least resistance. For example, when a person is in a sitting position, the upper lobes initially receive more ventilation than the lower lobes; however, the lower lobes have the largest net change in ventilation. Two terms that are associated with $\dot{V}/\dot{Q}$ mismatch are *dead space*

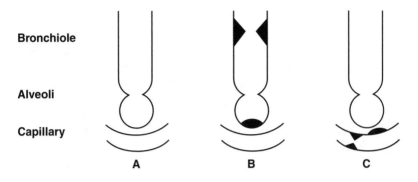

Bronchiole

Alveoli

Capillary

A   B   C

Figure 2-3. *Ventilation and perfusion mismatch. A. Normal alveolar ventilation. B. Capillary shunt. C. Alveolar dead space.*

and *shunt*. Dead space occurs when ventilation is in excess of perfusion, such as a pulmonary embolus. A shunt occurs when perfusion is in excess of ventilation, such as in alveolar collapse from secretion retention. These conditions are shown in Figure 2-3.

Gas Transport

O_2 is transported away from the lungs to the tissues in two forms: (1) dissolved in plasma or (2) chemically bound to hemoglobin on a red blood cell (oxyhemoglobin). As a by-product of cellular metabolism, CO_2 is transported away from the tissues to the lungs in three forms: (1) dissolved in plasma, (2) chemically bound to hemoglobin (carboxyhemoglobin), and (3) as bicarbonate.

The majority of O_2 and CO_2 transport occurs in the combined forms of oxyhemoglobin, carboxyhemoglobin, and bicarbonate. A smaller percentage of gases are transported in dissolved forms. Dissolved O_2 and CO_2 exert a partial pressure within the plasma and can be measured by sampling arterial, venous, or mixed venous blood [5]. See "Arterial Blood Gas Analysis" for further description of this process.

Assessment

Respiratory assessment is composed of patient history, physical examination, and diagnostic testing.

Patient History

In addition to the general chart review presented in Appendix I, relevant information to respiratory dysfunction that should be ascertained from the chart review or patient interview is listed below [5–7].

- History of smoking, including packs per day (ppd) or pack years (ppd × number of years smoked) and the amount of time that smoking has been discontinued (if applicable)

- Presence, history, and amount of O_2 therapy at rest, with activity, or both

- Exposure to environmental or occupational toxins (e.g., asbestos)

- History of thoracic procedures or surgery

- History of intubation and mechanical ventilation

- Level of activity before admittance

- Sleeping position

Physical Examination

The physical examination of the respiratory system consists of inspection, palpation, auscultation, and cough function.

Inspection
A wealth of information can be gathered by simple observation of the patient both at rest and with activity. Physical observation should proceed in a systematic fashion and include the following:

- General appearance and level of alertness

- Skin color

- Posture and chest shape

- Respiratory pattern (including assessment of rate [12–20 breaths per minute is normal], depth, ratio of inspiration to expiration [1 to 2 is normal], sequence of chest wall movement during inspiration and expiration, comfort, presence of accessory muscle use, and symmetry). Note: Respiratory patterns vary among individuals and may be influenced by (1) pain; (2) emotion; (3) body temperature; (4) sleep; (5) body position; (6) activity level; and (7) the presence of pulmonary, cardiac, metabolic, or nervous system disease. Table 2-3 provides a description of breathing patterns.

- Ease of phonation

- Presence of digital clubbing

- Presence of O_2 therapy

- Presence of lines and tubes

- Presence and location of surgical incisions

Table 2-3. Description of Breathing Patterns and Their Associated Conditions

Breathing Pattern	Description	Associated With
Apnea	Lack of airflow to the lungs for longer than 15 secs	Airway obstruction, cardiopulmonary arrest, alterations of the respiratory center, narcotic overdose
Biot's respirations	Constant increased rate and depth of respiration followed by periods of apnea of varying lengths	Elevated intracranial pressure, meningitis
Bradypnea	Respiratory rate less than 12 breaths per min	Use of sedatives, narcotics, or alcohol; neurologic or metabolic disorders; excessive fatigue
Cheyne-Stokes respirations	Increasing depth of respiration followed by a period of apnea	Elevated intracranial pressure, congestive heart failure, renal failure, narcotic overdose
Dyspnea	Subjective complaint of difficulty with respiration	Activity, pulmonary infections, congestive heart failure, anxiety
Hyperpnea	Increased depth of respiration	Activity, pulmonary infections, congestive heart failure
Hyperventilation	Increased rate and depth of respiration resulting in decreased PCO_2	Anxiety, nervousness, metabolic acidosis

Table 2-3. *Continued*

Breathing Pattern	Description	Associated With
Hypoven- tilation	Decreased rate and depth of respiration resulting in increased PCO_2	Sedation or somnolence, neurologic depression of respiratory centers, overmedication, metabolic alkalosis
Kussmaul's respir- ations	Increased regular rate and depth of respiration	Diabetic ketoacidosis, renal failure
Orthopnea	Dyspnea that occurs from being positioned in supine Relief occurs with upright sitting or standing	Chronic lung disease, congestive heart failure
Paradoxical respir- ations	Inward abdominal or chest wall movement with inspiration and outward movement with exhalation	Diaphragm paralysis, respiratory muscle fatigue, chest wall trauma
Sighing res- pirations	The presence of a sigh >2–3 times per minute	Angina, anxiety, dyspnea
Tachypnea	Respiratory rate >20 breaths per minute	Acute respiratory distress, fever, pain, emotions, anemia

PCO_2 = partial pressure of carbon dioxide.
Source: Adapted from LD Kersten. Comprehensive Respiratory Nursing: A Decision-Making Approach. Philadelphia: Saunders, 1989;119; and T Desjardins, GG Burton. Clinical Manifestations and Assessment of Respiratory Disease (3rd ed). St. Louis: Mosby, 1995;18.

Clinical tip

The optimal time, clinically, to assess a patient's breathing pattern is when he or she is unaware of the inspection. Knowledge of the physical examination can influence the patient's respiratory pattern. Therefore, compare the patient's respiratory pattern while he or she is asleep with the patient's respiratory pattern while he or she is awake, or compare the patient's respiratory pattern during conversation with his or her respiratory pattern during activity.

Palpation

The second component of the physical examination is palpation of the chest wall, which is performed in a cephalocaudal direction. Figure 2-4A–C demonstrates hand placement for chest wall palpation of the upper, middle, and lower lung fields. This is done to assess the following:

- Presence of fremitus during respirations

- Presence, location, and reproducibility of pain, tenderness, or both

- Skin temperature

- Presence of bony abnormalities, rib fractures, or both

- Chest expansion and symmetry

- Presence of subcutaneous emphysema (the presence of air in the subcutaneous tissue palpated as bubbles popping under the skin; this finding is abnormal)

Clinical tip

To decrease patient fatigue, palpation of each chest wall segment for the above assessments can be performed simultaneously.

Percussion

Mediate percussion can indirectly measure diaphragmatic excursion during respirations as well as help in assessing tissue densities within the thoracic cage. Mediate percussion can also be used to help confirm other findings in the physical examination. The procedure is shown in Figure 2-5A and B and is performed by placing the palmar surface of the index finger, middle finger, or both of one hand flatly against the surface of the chest wall in the intercostal spaces. The tips of the other index finger, middle finger, or both then strike the distal third of the fingers that are resting against the chest wall. The clinician proceeds from side to side in a cephalocaudal fashion for both anterior and posterior

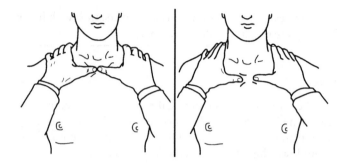

A

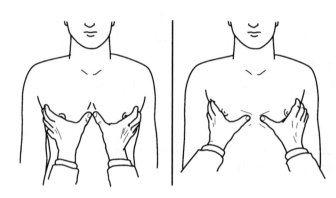

B

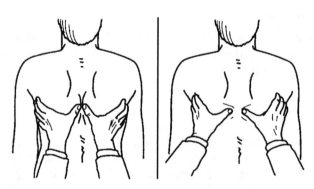

C

Figure 2-4. *A. Palpation of upper lobe motion. B. Palpation of right middle and left lingula lobe motion. C. Palpation of lower lobe motion. (Reprinted with permission from EA Hillegass, HS Sadowsky. Essentials of Cardiopulmonary Physical Therapy. Philadelphia: Saunders, 1994;577.)*

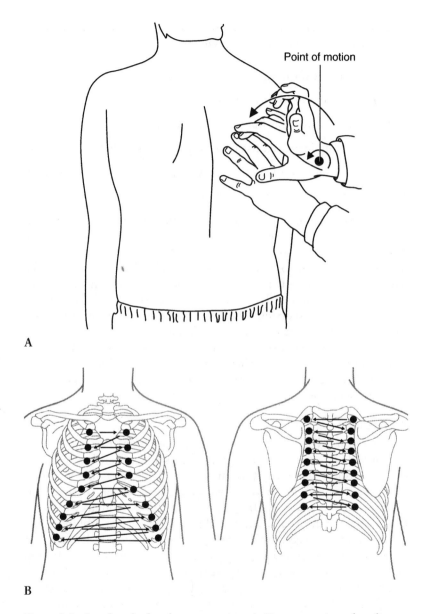

Figure 2-5. *Landmarks for chest percussion. A. Demonstration of mediate percussion technique. B. Landmarks for mediate percussion technique. (Reprinted with permission from EA Hillegass, HS Sadowsky. Essentials of Cardiopulmonary Physical Therapy. Philadelphia: Saunders, 1994;581.)*

aspects of the chest wall. Sounds produced from mediate percussion can be characterized as one of the following:

- Resonant (over normal lung tissue)
- Hyperresonant (over emphysematous lungs or pneumothorax)
- Tympanic (over gas bubbles in abdomen)
- Dull (from increased tissue density or lungs with decreased air)
- Flat (extreme dullness over very dense tissues such as the thigh muscles [6])

To assess diaphragmatic excursion with mediate percussion, the clinician first delineates the resting position of the diaphragm by percussing down the posterior aspect of one side of the chest wall until a change from resonant to dull or flat sounds occurs. The clinician then asks the patient to inspire deeply and repeats the process, noting the difference in landmarks when sound changes occur. The difference is the amount of diaphragmatic excursion. The other side is also assessed and a comparison can then be made of the hemidiaphragms.

Note: Mediate percussion is a difficult skill and is performed most proficiently by experienced therapists or physicians. Mediate percussion can also be performed over the abdominal cavity to assess tissue densities, which is described further in Chapter 8.

Auscultation

Auscultation is listening to the sounds of air passing through the tracheobronchial tree and alveolar spaces. The sounds of airflow normally dissipate from proximal to distal airways, making the sounds less audible in the periphery as compared with the central airways. Alterations in airflow and respiratory effort result in distinctive sounds within the thoracic cavity that may indicate pulmonary disease or dysfunction.

Auscultation proceeds in a systematic, cephalocaudal fashion. Breath sounds on the left and right sides are compared in the anterior, lateral, and posterior segments of the chest wall as shown in Figure 2-6. The diaphragm (flat side) of the stethoscope should be used for auscultation. The patient should be seated or lying comfortably in a position that allows access to all lung fields. Full inspirations and expirations are performed by the patient through the mouth, as the clinician listens to the entire cycle of respiration before moving the stethoscope to another lung segment. There are normal and abnormal (adventitious) breath sounds.

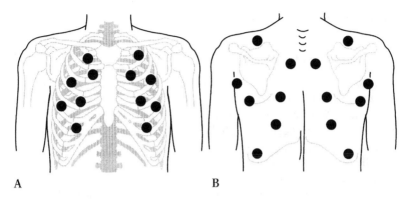

Figure 2-6. *Anterior (A) and posterior (B) auscultation locations. (Reprinted with permission from EA Hillegass, HS Sadowsky. Essentials of Cardiopulmonary Physical Therapy. Philadelphia: Saunders, 1994;571.)*

Normal Breath Sounds

Tracheal or Bronchial Sounds. Normal tracheal or bronchial breath sounds are loud, tubular sounds that are heard over the proximal airways, such as the trachea and main stem bronchi. A pause is heard between inspiration and expiration, with the expiratory phase being longer than the inspiratory phase.

Bronchovesicular or Vesicular Sounds. Normal bronchovesicular or vesicular sounds are soft, rustling sounds that are heard over the more distal airways and lung parenchyma. Inspiration is longer and more pronounced than expiration, as a decrease in airway lumen during expiration limits transmission of airflow sounds.

Note: In most reference books, a distinction between bronchovesicular and vesicular sounds is made. Bronchovesicular sounds are described as occurring in the middle airway zones, whereas vesicular sounds are heard in the peripheral airway zones, with subtle differences in sounds at inspiratory and expiratory phases. This distinction, however, is often unnecessary in the clinical setting.

Abnormal or Adventitious Breath Sounds

Alterations or turbulence in airflow result in abnormal breath sounds that can be divided into continuous or discontinuous sounds. These alterations should be documented according to the location and the phase of respiration (i.e., inspiration, expiration, or both) and in comparison with the opposite lung.

Continuous Sounds

Wheeze. Wheezes occur most commonly with airway obstruction from bronchoconstriction or retained secretions and are commonly heard on expiration. Wheezes may also be present during inspiration if the obstruction is significant enough. Wheezes can be high pitched (usually from bronchospasm or constriction, as in asthma) or low pitched (usually from secretions, as in pneumonia).

Note: Low-pitched or coarse wheezes can also be referred to as *rhonchi*, but a trend toward consistency by the American Thoracic Society and American College of Chest Physicians (ATS-ACCP) Ad Hoc Subcommittee on Pulmonary Nomenclature has moved away from this terminology [8].

Stridor. Stridor is an extremely high-pitched wheeze that occurs with upper airway obstruction and is present during both inspiration and expiration. The presence of stridor indicates a medical emergency. Stridor is also audible without a stethoscope.

Discontinuous Sounds: Crackles
Crackles are bubbling or popping sounds that represent the presence of fluid or secretions or the sudden opening of closed airways. Crackles that result from fluid (pulmonary edema) or secretions (pneumonia) are described as wet, whereas crackles that occur from the sudden opening or closed airways (atelectasis) are referred to as dry.

Note: Wet crackles can also be referred to as *rales*, but again, the ATS-ACCP has moved to eliminate this terminology.

Other Adventitious Sounds
Other adventitious breath sounds with possible sources are outlined in the following table:

Sound	Possible Etiology
Bronchial (abnormal if heard in areas where vesicular sounds should be present)	Fluid or secretion consolidation (airlessness)
Friction rub	Pleuritis (inflamed pleurae rubbing on one another)
Decreased or diminished (less audible)	Hypoventilation, severe congestion, or emphysema

Sound	*Possible Etiology*
Absent	Pneumothorax or lung collapse

Voice Sounds

Normal phonation is audible during auscultation, with the intensity and clarity of speech also dissipating from proximal to distal airways. Voice sounds that are more or less pronounced in distal lung regions, where vesicular breath sounds should occur, may indicate areas of consolidation or hyperinflation, respectively. The same areas of auscultation should be used when assessing voice sounds. The following three types of voice sound tests can be used to help confirm breath sound findings:

Whispered pectoriloquy	The patient whispers "one, two, three." The test is positive for consolidation if phrases are clearly audible in distal lung fields. This test is positive for hyperinflation if the phrases are less audible in distal lung fields.
Egophony	The patient repeats the letter "e." If the auscultation in the distal lung fields sound like "a," then fluid in the air spaces or lung parenchyma is suspected.
Bronchophony	The patient repeats the phrase "ninety-nine." The results are similar to whispered pectoriloquy.

Clinical tip

To ensure accurate auscultation, do the following:

• Make sure earpieces are pointing up and inward before placing in the ears.

• Always check proper function of the stethoscope before auscultating by listening to finger tapping on the diaphragm while the earpieces are in place.

• Apply the stethoscope diaphragm firmly against the skin.

• Observe chest wall expansion and breathing pattern while auscultating to help confirm palpatory findings of breathing pattern (e.g., sequence and symmetry).

To minimize false positive adventitious breath sound findings, do the following:

• Ensure full deep inspirations (decreased effort can be misinterpreted as decreased breath sounds).

• Be aware of the stethoscope tubing touching other objects (especially ventilator tubing) or chest hair.

• Periodically lift the stethoscope off the chest wall to help differentiate extraneous sounds (e.g., chest or nasogastric tubes, patient snoring) that may appear to originate from the thorax. To maximize patient comfort, allow periodic rest periods between deep respirations to prevent hyperventilation and dizziness.

Cough Assessment

An essential component of bronchopulmonary hygiene is cough effectiveness. The cough mechanism can be divided into four phases: (1) full inspiration, (2) closure of the glottis with an increase of intrathoracic pressure, (3) abdominal contraction, and (4) rapid expulsion of air. The inability to perform one or more portions of the cough mechanism can lead to decreased pulmonary secretion clearance.

Cough assessment includes evaluating the following components [6]:

• Effectiveness (ability to clear secretions)

• Control (ability to start and stop coughs)

• Quality (wet, dry, bronchospastic)

• Frequency (how often during the day and night cough occurs)

• Sputum production (color, quantity, odor, and consistency)

Clinical tip

Hemoptysis, the expectoration of blood during coughing, may occur for many reasons. Hemoptysis is usually benign postoperatively if it is not sustained with successive coughs. The therapist should note whether the blood is dark red or brownish in color (old blood) or bright red (new or frank blood). The presence of frank blood in sputum should be documented and the nurse or physician notified.

Cough effectiveness and secretion clearance can be enhanced with pain premedication, bronchodilator therapy, splinting, positioning, and proper hydration.

Diagnostic Testing

Pulmonary Function Tests

Pulmonary function tests (PFTs) consist of measuring a patient's lung volumes and capacities, as well as inspiratory and expiratory flow rates. Quantification of these parameters helps in distinguishing obstructive from restrictive respiratory patterns, as well as determining how the respiratory system contributes to physical activity limitations. Volume, flow, and gas dilution spirometers and body plethysmography are the measurement tools used for PFTs. A comprehensive assessment of PFT results includes comparisons with normal values and prior test results. PFT results may be skewed according to a patient's effort.

Table 2-4 outlines the measurements performed during PFTs. The respiratory system's volumes and capacities are shown in Figure 2-7. The normal range of values for PFTs is based on a person's age, sex, and height and can be extrapolated from a nomogram. Indications for PFTs are the following [9, 10]:

- Detection and quantification of respiratory disease

- Assessment of disease progression, response to bronchodilator therapy or surgery, or both

- Preoperative evaluation (high-risk patient identification)

Clinical tip

FEV, FVC, and the FEV/FVC ratio are the most commonly interpreted PFT values. These measures represent the degree of airway patency during expiration, which affects airflow in and out of the lung.

Table 2-4. Description and Clinical Significance of Pulmonary Function Tests

Test	Description	Significance
Lung volume tests		
Vital capacity (VC)	The maximum amount of air that can be expired slowly and completely following a maximal inspiration	A decrease in VC can result from a decrease in lung tissue distensibility or depression of the respiratory centers in the brain.
Functional residual capacity (FRC)	The volume of air remaining in the lungs at the end of a normal expiration Calculated from body plethysmography	FRC values help differentiate between obstructive and restrictive respiratory patterns. An increased FRC indicates an obstructive respiratory pattern, and a decreased FRC indicates a restrictive respiratory pattern.
Expiratory reserve volume (ERV)	The maximum amount of air that can be exhaled following a resting expiratory level	ERV alone has no diagnostic value, but it is necessary to calculate residual volume and FRC.
Inspiratory reserve volume (IRV)	The maximum amount of air that can be inspired following a normal inspiration	IRV alone has no diagnostic value, but it helps estimate ventilatory reserve.
Residual volume (RV)	The volume of air remaining in the lungs at the end of maximal expiration	RV helps to differentiate between obstructive and restrictive disorders. An increased RV indicates an obstructive disorder, and a decreased RV indicates a restrictive disorder.
Inspiratory capacity (IC)	The largest volume of air that can be inspired in one breath from the resting expiratory level	Changes in IC usually parallel changes in VC. It is used primarily in postoperative assessments.

Term	Description	Clinical significance
Total lung capacity (TLC)	The volume of air contained in the lung at the end of maximal inspiration	TLC helps to differentiate between obstructive and restrictive disorders. A decreased TLC indicates a restrictive disorder; an increased TLC indicates an obstructive disorder.
Residual volume to total lung capacity ratio (RV:TLC × 100)	The percentage of air that cannot be expired in relation to the total amount of air that can be brought into the lungs	Values of >35% are indicative of obstructive disorders.
Ventilation tests		
Tidal volume (VT)	The volume of air inspired or expired during each respiratory cycle. Usually measured over a 1-min time frame and divided by the respiratory rate	VT is used in combination with arterial blood gas measurements, respiratory rate, and minute volume to diagnose pulmonary disorders.
Minute volume (VE)	The total volume of air inspired or expired in 1 min	VE is most commonly used in exercise or stress testing. VE can increase with hypoxia, hypercapnia, acidosis, and exercise.
Respiratory dead space (VD)	The volume of air in the lungs that is ventilated but not perfused in conducting airways and nonfunctioning alveoli	VD provides information about available surface area for gas exchange.
Alveolar ventilation (VA)	The volume of air that participates in gas exchange	VA measures the amount of oxygen available to tissues, but it should be confirmed by arterial blood gas measurements.

Table 2-4. *Continued*

Test	Description	Significance
Pulmonary spirometry tests		
Forced vital capacity (FVC)	The volume of air that can be expired forcefully and rapidly after a maximal inspiration	FVC is normally equal to VC, but FVC can be decreased in obstructive disorders.
Forced expiratory volume timed (FEV_t)	The volume of air expired over a given interval during the performance of an FVC. The interval is usually 1 sec (FEV_1). After 3 secs, FEV should equal FVC.	FEV_t is the most common screening test for obstructive airway disease. A decrease in FEV_t indicates obstructive airway disease.
FEV% (usually $FEV_1/FVC \times 100$)	The percent of FVC that can be expired over a given time interval, usually 1 sec	FEV% is a better discriminator of obstructive and restrictive disorders than FEV_t. An increase in FEV_1/FVC indicates a restrictive disorder, and a decrease in FEV_1/FVC indicates an obstructive disorder.
Forced expiratory flow 25–75% (FEF_{25-75}) or maximum midexpiratory flow rate (MMEF)	The average flow of air during the middle 50% of an FEV maneuver. Used in comparison with VC. Represents peripheral airway resistance	FEF_{25-75} is an index of the status of medium-sized airways.
Peak expiratory flow rate (PEFR)	The maximum flow rate attainable at any time during an FEV	PEFR can assist with diagnosing obstructive disorders such as asthma.
Maximum voluntary ventilation (MVV)	The largest volume of air that can be breathed per minute by voluntary effort	MVV measures status of respiratory muscles, the resistance offered by airways and tissues, and the

Flow-volume loop (F-V loop)	A graphic analysis of the maximum forced expiratory flow volume (MEFV) followed by a maximum inspiratory flow volume (MIFV). Test lasts 10–15 secs	compliance of the lung and thorax. The distinctive curves of the F-V loop are created according to the presence or absence of disease. Restrictive disease demonstrates an equal reduction in flow and volume, resulting in a vertical oval-shaped loop. Obstructive disease demonstrates a greater reduction in flow compared with volume, resulting in a horizontal tear-shaped loop.
Gas exchange		
Diffusing capacity of carbon monoxide (DL_{CO})	A known mixture of carbon monoxide and helium gas is inhaled and then exhaled after 10 secs and the amount of gases are remeasured	DL_{CO} assesses the amount of functioning pulmonary capillary bed in contact with functioning alveoli (gas exchange area).
Airway resistance (Raw) Airway conductance (Gaw)	Raw is the pressure difference required for a unit flow change. Gaw is the flow generated per unit of pressure drop in the airway. Measured with a body plethysmograph and taken in conjunction with the FRC	Raw increases with acute asthma attacks, emphysema, or other obstructive diseases. Raw and Gaw are useful in determining response to bronchodilator therapy.

Source: Reprinted with permission from JM Thompson, GK McFarland, JE Hirsch, et al. Clinical Nursing Practice. Mosby, 1993;1410.

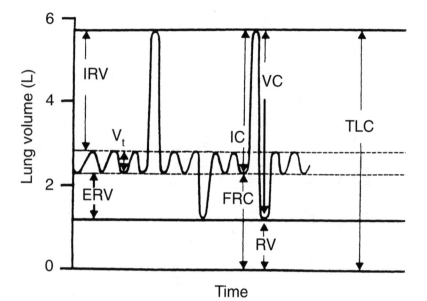

Figure 2-7. *Lung volumes. (TLC = total lung capacity; RV = residual volume; FRC = functional residual capacity; VC = vital capacity; IC = inspiratory capacity; IRV = inspiratory reserve volume; ERV = expiratory reserve volume; V_t = tidal volume.) (Reprinted with permission from E Ellis, J Alison. Key Issues in Cardiorespiratory Physiotherapy. Oxford: Butterworth–Heinemann, 1992;40.)*

Chest X-Rays

Radiographic information of the thoracic cavity in combination with a clinical history provides critical assistance in the differential diagnosis of pulmonary conditions. Indications for chest x-rays (CXRs) are the following [11, 12]:

- To assist in the clinical diagnosis of the following:
    Airspace consolidation (pulmonary edema, pneumonia, adult respiratory distress syndrome [ARDS], pulmonary hemorrhage and infarctions)
    Large intrapulmonary air spaces
    Lobar atelectasis

Mediastinal or subcutaneous air
Other pulmonary lesions such as lung nodules and abscesses
Pneumothorax
Rib fractures

- To monitor the progression or regression of pulmonary disease or dysfunction

- To determine proper placement of endotracheal tubes, central lines, chest tubes, or nasogastric tubes

- To evaluate structural features, such as the following:
  Cardiac or mediastinal size
  Diaphragmatic shape and position

Film markers for CXRs are listed below and are shown in Figure 2-8:

- Bronchopulmonary tree

- Clavicle position

- Diaphragmatic borders

- Distribution of blood flow

- Heart borders

- Pleural fluid (if collected in areas)

- Pulmonary vasculature

- Rib cage

CXRs are classified according to the direction of radiographic beam projection. The first word describes where the beam enters the body, and the second word describes the exit.
Common types of CXRs include the following:

Posterior-anterior (P-A)	Taken while the patient is upright sitting or standing
Anterior-posterior (A-P)	Taken while the patient is upright sitting or standing, semireclined, or supine
Lateral	Taken while the patient is upright sitting or standing or decubitus (lying on the side)

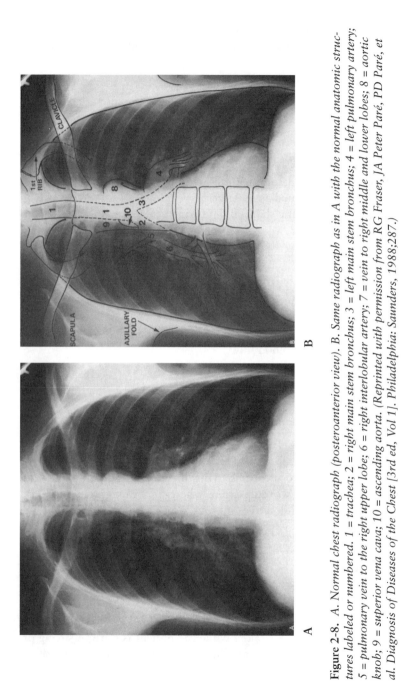

Figure 2-8. A. *Normal chest radiograph (posteroanterior view). B. Same radiograph as in A with the normal anatomic structures labeled or numbered. 1 = trachea; 2 = right main stem bronchus; 3 = left main stem bronchus; 4 = left pulmonary artery; 5 = pulmonary vein to the right upper lobe; 6 = right interlobular artery; 7 = vein to right middle and lower lobes; 8 = aortic knob; 9 = superior vena cava; 10 = ascending aorta. (Reprinted with permission from RG Fraser, JA Peter Paré, PD Paré, et al. Diagnosis of Diseases of the Chest [3rd ed, Vol 1]. Philadelphia: Saunders, 1988;287.)*

Upright positions are preferred to allow full expansion of lungs without visceral hindrance and to visualize gravity-dependent fluid collections. Lateral films aid in three-dimensional, segmental localization of lesions and fluid collections not visible in P-A or A-P views.

Clinical tip

Diagnosis cannot be made by CXR alone. Use CXRs as a guide for decision making and not as an absolute parameter for bronchopulmonary hygiene assessment and treatment. CXRs sometimes lag behind significant clinical presentation (e.g., symptoms of pulmonary infection may resolve clinically while CXR findings remain positive).

Flexible Bronchoscopy

A flexible, fiberoptic tube is used as a diagnostic and interventional tool to directly visualize and aspirate (suction) the bronchopulmonary tree. If a patient is mechanically ventilated, the bronchoscope is inserted through the endotracheal or tracheal tube. If the patient is spontaneously breathing, a local anesthetic is applied, and then the bronchoscope is inserted through one of the patient's nares. Table 2-5 summarizes the diagnostic and therapeutic indications of bronchoscopy. Note: Bronchoscopy can also be performed with a rigid bronchoscope. This is primarily an operative procedure [12, 13].

Table 2-5. Diagnostic and Therapeutic Indications for Flexible Bronchoscopy

Diagnostic indications
    Malignancy
    Evaluation of the patient before and after lung transplantation
    Mediastinal mass
    Endotracheal intubation
    Infection
    Tracheobronchial stricture and stenosis
    Hemoptysis

Table 2-5. *Continued*

Hoarseness or vocal cord paralysis
Unexplained chronic cough
Fistula
Localized wheezing
Persistent pneumothorax
Stridor
Foreign body aspiration
Chest trauma
Unexplained pleural effusion
Postoperative assessment of tracheal, tracheobronchial, bronchial, or
    stump anastomosis
Therapeutic indications
  Pulmonary hygiene
  Removal of foreign bodies
  Removal of obstructive endotracheal tissue
  Stent placement
  Bronchoalveolar lavage
  Aspiration of cysts
  Drainage of abscesses
  Pneumothorax
  Lobar collapse
  Intralesional injection
  Thoracic trauma
  Intubation
  Airway maintenance (tamponade for bleeding)

Source: Adapted from MR Hetzed. Minimally Invasive Techniques in Thoracic Medicine and Surgery. London: Chapman & Hall, 1995;4; and JM Rippe, RS Irwin, MP Fink, et al. Procedures and Techniques in Intensive Care Medicine. Boston: Little, Brown, 1994.

Sputum Analysis

Analysis of sputum includes culture and Gram's stain to isolate and identify organisms that may be present in the lower respiratory tract. After the organisms are identified, appropriate antibiotic therapy can be instituted. Sputum specimens are collected when a temperature spike or a change in the color or consistency of sputum occurs. They can also be used to evaluate the efficacy of antibiotic therapy. Sputum analysis can be inaccurate if a sterile technique is not maintained during sputum collection or if the specimen is contaminated with too much saliva, as noted microscopically by the presence of many squamous epithelial cells.

Clinical tip

To ensure sputum collection, have sterile sputum collection containers and equipment on hand before performing bronchopulmonary hygiene.

Arterial Blood Gas Analysis

Arterial blood gas (ABG) analysis is performed to assess acid-base balance (pH), ventilation (CO_2 levels), and oxygenation (O_2 levels), as well as to help modify respiratory interventions, such as mechanical ventilator settings [5]. For proper cellular metabolism to occur, acid-base balance must be maintained. Disturbances in acid-base balance can be caused by respiratory or metabolic dysfunction. Normally, the respiratory and metabolic systems work in synergy to help maintain acid-base balance.

The ability to interpret ABGs provides the physical therapist with valuable information regarding the current medical status of the patient, the appropriateness for bronchopulmonary hygiene or exercise treatments, and the outcomes of medical and physical therapy intervention.

ABGs are usually performed on a routine basis, which is specified according to need in the critical care setting. For the critically ill patient, ABG sampling may occur every 1–3 hours. In contrast, ABGs may be sampled one or two times a day in a patient whose pulmonary or metabolic status has stabilized. Unless specified, arterial blood is sampled from an indwelling arterial line. Other sites of sampling include venous blood from a peripheral venous puncture or catheter and mixed venous blood from a pulmonary artery catheter. Appendix IV-A describes vascular monitoring lines in more detail.

Terminology
The following terms are frequently used in ABG analysis:

PaO_2 (PO_2)	The partial pressure of dissolved O_2 in plasma
$PaCO_2$ (PCO_2)	The partial pressure of dissolved CO_2 in plasma
pH	The degree of acidity or alkalinity in blood

HCO_3 level	The level of bicarbonate in the blood
Percentage of SaO_2 (O_2 saturation)	A percentage of the amount of hemoglobin sites filled (saturated) with O_2 molecules (PaO_2 and SaO_2 are intimately related but are not synonymous)

Normal Values

The normal values for ABGs are as follows [8]:

PaO_2	greater than 80 mm Hg
$PaCO_2$	35–45 mm Hg
pH	7.35–7.45
HCO_3	22–28 mEq/liter

ABGs are generally reported in the following format: PaO_2/$PaCO_2$/pH/HCO_3 (e.g., 96/42/7.38/26).

Arterial Blood Gas Interpretation

Interpretation of ABGs includes the ability to determine deviation from normal values and hypothesize a cause (or causes) for the acid-base disturbance in relation to the patient's clinical history.

The following terms are associated with ABG interpretation:

- *Acidemia* occurs when the pH is less than 7.4
- *Acidosis* is the process that causes acidemia
- *Alkalemia* occurs when the pH is greater than 7.4
- *Alkalosis* is the process that causes alkalemia
- *Hypoxia* occurs when PO_2 is less than 80 mm Hg
- *Hypercarbia* occurs when PCO_2 is greater than 50 mm Hg

The following are concepts of ABG interpretation:

1. Respiratory or metabolic disorders can cause states of acidemia or alkalemia.

2. If respiratory or metabolic disorders cause acid-base imbalances, they are called the *primary process*.

3. Acid-base imbalances can be *compensated* for by the non-primary system. For example, a primary respiratory acidosis can be compensated for by the metabolic system.

4. If the nonprimary system fails to compensate for the primary system, the disorder is referred to as *uncompensated*.

5. Acid-base imbalances can be also be *corrected* by addressing the primary process involved. For example, a primary metabolic alkalosis can be corrected by administering medical therapy to the renal system.

Knowledge of uncompensated, compensated, or corrected acid-base disturbances provides insight into the patient's current medical status. The following outline provides basic guidelines for ABG interpretation:

1. Look at the patient's pH level to determine acid-base balance.

    a. If the patient's pH = 7.4, acid-base balance is normal.

    b. If the patient's pH <7.4, the patient is acidotic.

    c. If the patient's pH >7.4, the patient is alkalotic.

2. To determine if the patient's pH change is due to a primary respiratory process, look at PCO_2. For every 10-point change in PCO_2, there is a 0.08 change in pH in the opposite direction.

    a. A low pH and a high PCO_2 indicate uncompensated respiratory acidosis.

    b. A high pH and a low PCO_2 indicate uncompensated respiratory alkalosis.

3. To determine if the patient's pH change is due to a primary metabolic process, look at HCO_3. For every 10-point change in HCO_3, there is a 0.15 change in pH in the same direction.

    a. A low pH and a low HCO_3 indicate uncompensated metabolic acidosis.

    b. A high pH and a high HCO_3 indicate uncompensated metabolic alkalosis.

4. To determine if the patient's primary respiratory process has been compensated for by the renal system, look at HCO_3.

a. A high HCO_3 in respiratory acidosis indicates compensated respiratory acidosis.

b. A low HCO_3 in respiratory alkalosis indicates compensated respiratory alkalosis.

5. To determine if the patient's primary metabolic process has been compensated for by the respiratory system, look at PCO_2.

a. A low PCO_2 in metabolic acidosis indicates compensated metabolic acidosis.

b. A high PCO_2 in metabolic alkalosis indicates compensated metabolic alkalosis.

The possible causes for these disorders are summarized in Table 2-6. Decreased levels of alertness may result from retained CO_2. A list of signs and symptoms of CO_2 retention is shown in Table 2-7.

Clinical tip

• Mixed or complex acid-base disorders may not appear as straightforward as the above examples demonstrate.

• Acid-base balance or pH is the most important ABG value to be within normal limits. It is important to relate ABG values with medical history and clinical course. ABG values and vital signs are generally documented on a daily flow sheet, an invaluable source of information. Changes in ABG values over time are more informative than a single ABG reading. Single ABG readings should be correlated with previous ABG readings, medical status, supplemental O_2 or ventilator changes, and medical procedures.

• Bicarbonate (HCO_3) levels are not routinely reported unless requested.

• Be sure to note if an ABG sample is drawn from mixed venous blood, as the normal O_2 value is lower. $P\bar{v}O_2$ of mixed venous blood is 35–40 mm Hg.

Table 2-6. Causes of Acid-Base Imbalances

Causes of respiratory acidosis
    Obstructive lung disease
    Airway obstruction
    Neuromuscular disorders
    Central nervous system depression
    Hypoventilation from pain, oversedation, chest wall deformities, secretion retention
    Cardiopulmonary arrest

Causes of respiratory alkalosis
    Hyperventilation from nervousness and anxiety, fever, pain, or mechanical ventilation
    Hypoxia
    Pulmonary embolus
    Pulmonary fibrosis
    Pregnancy
    Brain injury
    Salicylates
    Gram-negative septicemia
    Hepatic insufficiency
    Congestive heart failure
    Asthma
    Severe anemia

Causes of metabolic alkalosis
    Fluid losses from upper gastrointestinal tract (e.g., vomiting or nasogastric tube aspiration of acid)
    Rapid correction of chronic hypercapnia
    Diuretic therapy
    Cushing's disease
    Corticosteroid therapy
    Hyperaldosteronism
    Severe potassium depletion
    Excessive ingestion of licorice
    Bartter's syndrome
    Alkali administration
    Nonparathyroid hypercalemia

Causes of metabolic acidosis
    Ketoacidosis from diabetes, starvation, or alcohol
    Poisonings from salicylates, ethylene glycol, methyl glycol, paraldehyde
    Lactic acidosis
    Renal failure

Table 2-6. *Continued*

Diarrhea
Drainage of pancreatic fluid
Ureterosigmoidostomy
Obstructed ileal loop
Therapy with acetazolamide (Diamox) or with ammonium chloride
  (NH_4Cl)
Renal tubular acidosis
Intravenous hyperalimentation
Dilutional acidosis

Source: Adapted from CM Hudak, BM Gallo. Critical Care Nursing, A Holistic
Approach (6th ed). Philadelphia: Lippincott, 1994.

Table 2-7. Clinical Presentation of Carbon Dioxide Retention and Narcosis

Altered mental status
  Lethargy
  Drowsiness
  Coma
Headache
Tachycardia
Hypertension
Diaphoresis
Tremors
Redness of skin, sclera, conjunctiva

Source: Adapted from LD Kersten. Comprehensive Respiratory Nursing: A Decision-
Making Approach. Philadelphia: Saunders, 1989;351.

Oximetry

Oximetry is a noninvasive method of determining oxyhemoglobin saturation (SaO_2). It also indirectly assesses partial pressure of O_2. Finger or ear sensors are generally applied to a patient on a continuous or intermittent basis. Oxyhemoglobin saturation is an indication of pulmonary reserve and is driven by the PO_2 level in the blood. Figure

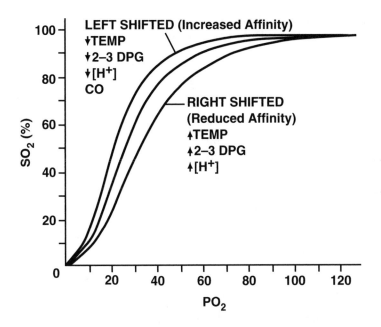

Figure 2-9. *The oxyhemoglobin dissociation curve and variables that affect oxygen-hemoglobin affinity. 2-3 DGP = 2,3-diphosphoglycerate; CO = carbon monoxide; [H⁺] = hydrogen concentration; TEMP = temperature. (Reprinted with permission from MH Kryger. Pathophysiology of Respiration. New York: Wiley, 1981.)*

2-9 demonstrates the direct relationship of oxyhemoglobin saturation and partial pressures of O_2. As shown on the curve, PO_2 levels of approximately 55 mm Hg result in an oxygen saturation below 87%, which is considered moderately hypoxic. The relationship between oxygen saturation and PO_2 levels are further summarized in Table 2-8. The affinity or binding of O_2 to hemoglobin is affected by changes in pH, PCO_2, temperature, and 2,3-diphosphoglycerate (a by-product of red blood cell metabolism) levels.

Physical therapists can use oximetry to help assess physical activity tolerance and the need for supplemental O_2 during exercise or bronchopulmonary hygiene sessions. O_2 saturation should be monitored before, during, and after a therapy session [3, 6, 15].

Table 2-8. Relationship Between Oxygen Saturation and Oxygen Partial Pressure on the Oxygen Dissociation Curve

Oxyhemoglobin Saturation (SaO_2 [percentage])	Oxygen Partial Pressure (PaO_2 [mm Hg])
97–99	90–100
95	80
90	60
85	50
80	45
75	40

Clinical tip

To ensure accurate O_2 saturation readings, do the following: (1) check for proper waveform or pulsations, which indicate proper signal reception, and (2) compare pulse readings on O_2 saturation monitor with the patient's peripheral pulses or electrocardiograph readings (if available). O_2 saturation readings can be affected by nail polish, sunlight, poor circulation (cool digits), movement of sensor cord, and the cleanliness of the sensors.

Ventilation-Perfusion Scan

The ventilation-perfusion ($\dot{V}/\dot{Q}$) scan is used to rule out the presence of pulmonary embolism and other acute abnormalities of oxygenation and gas exchange and as pre- and postoperative evaluation of lung transplantation.

In the perfusion lung scan, a radioisotope is injected intravenously into a peripheral vessel, and six projections are taken (i.e., anterior, posterior, both laterals, and both posterior obliques). The scan is very sensitive to diminished or absent blood flow, and lesions of 2 cm or greater are detected.

Perfusion defects can occur with pulmonary embolus, asthma, emphysema and virtually all alveolar filling, destructive or space-occupying lesions in lung, and hypoventilation. A CXR a few hours after the perfusion scan helps the differential diagnosis.

In a ventilation scan, inert radioactive gases or aerosols are inhaled, and three subsequent projections (i.e., after first breath, at equilibrium, and during washout) of airflow are recorded.

Ventilation scans are performed first, followed by perfusion scan. The two scans are then compared to determine extent of V/Q matching [13, 19].

Pathophysiology

Respiratory disorders can be classified as obstructive or restrictive. A patient may also present with multiple obstructive or restrictive processes or with a combination of both as a result of environmental, drug-induced, traumatic, neuromuscular, nutritional, or orthopedic factors.

These disorders may be vascular, neoplastic, or infectious in nature or involve the connective tissue of the thorax [4–6, 17, 18, 20, 21].

Obstructive Pulmonary Conditions

Obstructive lung diseases or conditions may be described by onset (acute versus chronic), severity (mild, moderate, or severe) and location (upper or lower airway). Obstructive pulmonary patterns are characterized by decreased air flow as a result of narrowing of the airway lumen. Table 2-9 outlines obstructive disorders, their physical and diagnostic findings, and their general clinical management.

Asthma

Asthma is an immunologic response that can result from allergens (e.g., dust, pollen, smoke, pollutants), food additives, bacterial infection, gastroesophageal reflux, stress, cold air, and exercise. The asthmatic response may be immediate or delayed, resulting in air entrapment and alveolar hyperinflation during the episode with symptoms disappearing between attacks. The primary characteristics of an asthma attack are the following:

- Bronchial smooth muscle constriction

- Mucus production

- Bronchial mucosa inflammation

Table 2-9. Characteristics and General Management of Obstructive Disorders

Disorder	Observation	Palpation	Auscultation	Cough	Chest X-Ray	Medical Management
Asthma	Increased respiratory rate Accessory muscle use Pursed lip breathing Fatigue Anxiety Cyanosis if severe	Increased HR Increased BP with pulsus paradoxus Decreased tactile and vocal fremitus Increased A-P chest diameter	Wheeze (high-pitch) Diminished breath sounds	Tight, nonproductive, then slightly productive	During attack: Translucent lung fields, flattened diaphragms, increased A-P diameter of chest, horizontal ribs Not during an attack: Chest x-ray is WNL	Removal of causative agent Bronchodilators Supplemental O_2 Corticosteroids IV fluid administration
Bronchiectasis	Increased respiratory rate Accessory muscle use Pursed lip breathing Fatigue Anxiety Cachexia Clubbing	Increased HR Increased BP Decreased tactile and vocal fremitus Hyperresonant percussion	Rhonchi Crackles Diminished breath sounds	Purulent, odorous sputum Hemoptysis is variable	± Atelectasis Patchy infiltrates ± Cystic changes ±Air fluid level	Antibiotics IV fluid administration Supplemental O_2 Nutritional support Bronchopulmonary hygiene

Chronic bronchitis	"Blue bloater" Increased respiratory rate with prolonged expiratory phase Accessory muscle use often with fixed upper extremities Pursed lip breathing Elevated shoulders Fatigue Anxiety JVD	See Bronchiectasis, above Increased A-P chest diameter	Rhonchi Crackles Diminished breath sounds	Sputum ranges from clear to purulent Most productive in the morning Audible wheeze	Translucent lung fields Translucent lung fields Flattened diaphragms Increased heart size	Smoking cessation Antibiotics Supplemental O_2 Bronchopulmonary hygiene
Cystic fibrosis	Increased respiratory rate Accessory muscle use Barrel chest Cachexia Clubbing Fatigue	See Bronchiectasis, above Increased A-P chest diameter	Rhonchi Crackles Diminished breath sounds	Usually very viscous, green sputum that may be tannish or blood-streaked	Translucent lung fields Flattened diaphragms Fibrosis Atelectasis Enlarged right ventricle	Antibiotics Supplemental O_2 Bronchopulmonary hygiene Nutritional support Lung transplantation

Table 2-9. *Continued*

Disorder	Observation	Palpation	Auscultation	Cough	Chest X-Ray	Medical Management
Emphysema	"Pink puffer" Increased respiratory rate Pursed lip breathing Elevated ribs Barrel chest	See Bronchiectasis, above Increased A-P chest diameter	Diminished breath sounds Wheeze Crackles	Usually nonproductive	Translucent lung fields Flattened diaphragms Bullae Increased heart size	Supplemental O$_2$ Nutritional support

A-P = anteroposterior; CXR = chest x-ray; WNL = within normal limits; IV = intravenous; ± = with or without; HR = heart rate; BP = blood pressure; JVD = jugular venous distention.

Bronchiectasis

Bronchiectasis is an obstructive, restrictive disorder characterized by the following:

- Destruction of the elastic and muscular bronchiole walls

- Destruction of the mucociliary escalator (in which normal epithelium is replaced by nonciliated mucus-producing cells)

- Bronchial dilation

- Bronchial artery enlargement

Bronchiectasis results in fibrosis and ulceration of bronchioles, chronically retained pulmonary secretions, atelectasis, and infection. The etiology of bronchiectasis includes previous bacterial respiratory infection, postoperative infections, cystic fibrosis, tuberculosis, and immobile cilia syndromes. Bronchiectatic changes occur most frequently in the lower lobes (left more often than right) either unilaterally or bilaterally.

Chronic Bronchitis

Chronic bronchitis is the presence of cough and pulmonary secretion expectoration for at least 3 months, 2 years in a row. Chronic bronchitis is usually linked to cigarette smoking or, less likely, to air pollution or infection. It begins with the following:

- Narrowing of large then small airways due to inflammation of bronchial mucosa

- Bronchial mucous gland hyperplasia and bronchial smooth muscle cell hypertrophy

- Decreased mucociliary function

These changes result in air trapping, hyperinflated alveoli, bronchospasm, and excess secretion retention.

Cystic Fibrosis

Cystic fibrosis is a lethal, autosomal recessive trait (chromosome 7) affecting the exocrine glands of the entire body, particularly of the respiratory, gastrointestinal, and reproductive systems. Soon after birth an initial pulmonary infection occurs that leads to the following changes throughout life:

- Bronchial and bronchiolar walls become inflamed

- Bronchial gland and goblet cells hypertrophy to create tenacious pulmonary secretions

- Mucociliary clearance is decreased

These changes result in bronchospasm, atelectasis, $\dot{V}/\dot{Q}$ mismatch, increased airway resistance, hypoxemia, and recurrent pulmonary infections.

Emphysema

Emphysema may be genetic (α_1–antitrypsin protein deficiency) in origin, in which the lack of proteolytic inhibitors allows the alveolar interstitium to be destroyed, or it may be caused by cigarette smoking, air pollutants, or infection. Two types of emphysema occur: panlobular and centrilobular. Panlobular emphysema affects the respiratory bronchioles, alveolar ducts and sacs, and the alveoli. Centriacinar emphysema affects the respiratory bronchioles and the proximal acinus. Both types of emphysema have progressive destruction of alveolar walls and adjacent capillaries secondary to the following:

- Decreased pulmonary tissue elasticity

- Premature airway collapse

- Bullae formation

These changes result in decreased lung elasticity, air trapping, and lung hyperinflation.

Restrictive Pulmonary Conditions

Restrictive lung diseases or conditions may be described by onset (acute versus chronic) or by location (i.e., pulmonary or extrapulmonary). Restrictive patterns are characterized by low lung volumes that result from decreased lung compliance and distensibility and increased lung recoil. The end result is increased work of breathing. Table 2-10 outlines restrictive disorders, their physical and diagnostic findings, and their general clinical management.

Adult Respiratory Distress Syndrome

ARDS is an acute inflammation of the lung that is generally associated with aspiration, drug toxicity, inhalation injury, pulmonary trauma, shock, systemic infections, and multisystem organ failure. Characteristics of ARDS include the following:

1. An exudative phase (hours to days) characterized by increased capillary permeability, interstitial and alveolar edema, hemorrhage, and alveolar consolidation with leukocytes and macrophages

2. Proliferative stage (days to weeks) characterized by hyaline formation on alveolar walls and intra-alveolar fibrosis resulting in atelectasis, $\dot{V}/\dot{Q}$ mismatch, severe hypoxemia, and pulmonary hypertension

Atelectasis

Atelectasis involves the partial or total collapse of alveoli, lung segment(s), or lobe(s). It most commonly results from hypoventilation or infective pulmonary secretion clearance. The following conditions may contribute to atelectasis:

• Compression of lung parenchyma

• Diaphragmatic restriction from weakness or paralysis

• Inactivity

• Postobstructive pneumonia

• Presence of foreign body

• Upper abdominal or thoracic incisional pain

The result is hypoxemia from $\dot{V}/\dot{Q}$ mismatch, transpulmonary shunting, and pulmonary vasoconstriction.

General risk factors for the development of atelectasis include smoking or pulmonary disease, obesity, and increased age. Peri- or postoperative risk factors include altered surfactant function from anesthesia, hypotension, sepsis, altered consciousness or prolonged narcotic use, and emergent or extended operative time.

Table 2-10. Characteristics and General Management of Restrictive Disorders

Disorder	Observation	Palpation	Auscultation	Cough Assessment	Chest X-Ray	Medical Management
Adult respiratory distress syndrome	Labored breathing Increased HR and BP Increased pulmonary artery pressure	Decreased chest wall expansion Dull percussion	Diminished breath sounds Crackles, wheezes, or rhonchi	Generally without pulmonary secretions, although may be with other pulmonary dysfunction	Pulmonary edema with diffuse bilateral patchy opacities	Mechanical ventilation Hemodynamic monitoring IV fluid administration Nitrous oxide therapy Antibiotics
Atelectasis	Increased RR ± Fever ± Shallow respirations	Increased HR and BP Decreased tactile fremitus and vocal resonance	Crackles at involved area Diminished breath sounds If lobar collapse exists, absent or bronchial breath sounds	Dry or wet Generally clear or white sputum	Linear opacity of involved area If lobar collapse exists, white triangular-shaped density fissure and diaphragmatic displace-	Supplemental O_2 if needed Incentive spirometry

						ment
Pneumonia	See Atelectasis, above Increased white blood cell count Fatigue	See Atelectasis, above Decreased chest expansion at involved area Dull percussion	Crackles Rhonchi Bronchial breath sounds over area of consolidation	Initially dry to more productive Sputum may be yellow, tan, green, or rusty	Well-defined density at the affected area ± Air bronchogram ± Pleural effusion	Antibiotics Supplemental O_2 IV fluid administration or hydration Bronchopulmonary hygiene
Pulmonary edema	Orthopnea Increased RR Anxiety	Increased tactile and vocal fremitus	Symmetric wet crackles (especially at bases) ± Wheezes	Thin; pink, clear, or white, frothy sputum	Increased hilar vascular markings Kerley B lines (short, horizontal lines at lung field periphery) ± Pleural effusion Left ventricular hypertrophy Cardiac silhouette Fluffy opacities	Dependent on etiology Monitor cardiac output Maximize gas exchange Minimize anxiety

Table 2-10. *Continued*

Disorder	Observation	Palpation	Auscultation	Cough Assessment	Chest X-Ray	Medical Management
Pulmonary embolism	Rapid onset of increased RR ± Chest pain Increased pulmonary artery pressure Anxiety Dysrhythmia Lightheadedness	Hypotension Decreased chest expansion on involved side	Decreased or absent breath sounds distal to pulmonary embolism Wheeze Crackles	Nonproductive cough	Density at infarct area with lucency distal to the infarct Dilated pulmonary artery with increased vascular markings Decreased lung volume ± Linear atelectasis or pleural effusion Hemidiaphragm	Anticoagulation Supplemental O$_2$ Inferior vena cava filter Thrombolysis

RR = respiratory rate; ± = with or without; HR = heart rate; BP = blood pressure; IV = intravenous.

Interstitial Pulmonary Fibrosis

Interstitial pulmonary fibrosis (IPF) is the destruction of the respiratory membranes in one or more lung regions that occurs after an inflammatory phase in which the alveoli become infiltrated with macrophages and mononuclear cells and a fibrosis phase in which the alveoli become scarred with collagen. There are more than 100 suspected predisposing factors for IPF, such as infectious agents, environmental and occupational inhalants, and drugs; however, no definite etiology is known. $\dot{V}/\dot{Q}$ mismatch and increased pulmonary artery pressures are the clinical sequelae of IPF.

Lung Contusion

Lung contusion is the result of a sudden compression and decompression of lung tissue against the chest wall from a direct blunt or blast chest trauma. There is a diffuse accumulation of blood and fluid in the alveoli and interstitium that causes arteriovenous shunting. The resultant degree of hypoxemia is dependent on the size of contused tissue. Lung contusion is usually located below rib fracture(s).

Pneumonia

Pneumonia is the multistaged inflammatory reaction of the distal airways from the inhalation of a variety of irritants (e.g., bacteria, viruses, microorganisms, foreign substances, gastric contents, dusts and chemicals) or as a complication of radiation therapy. Pneumonia is often described as community or hospital (nosocomial) acquired. The consequences of pneumonia are $\dot{V}/\dot{Q}$ mismatch and hypoxemia. The phases of pneumonia are the following:

1. Alveolar edema with exudate formation

2. Alveolar infiltration with white blood cells, red blood cells, macrophages, and fibrin

3. Resolution with expectoration or enzymatic digestion of infiltrative cells

Pulmonary Edema

The etiology of pulmonary edema can be categorized as either cardiogenic or noncardiogenic. Cardiogenic pulmonary edema is an imbalance of hydrostatic and oncotic pressures within the pulmonary vasculature that results from backflow of blood from the heart. This backflow increases the movement of fluid from the pulmonary capillaries to the alveolar spaces. Initially, the fluid fills the interstitium and then progresses to the alveolar spaces, bronchioles, and ultimately the bronchi. A simultaneous decrease in the lymphatic drainage of the lung may occur, exacerbating the problem. Cardiogenic pulmonary edema can be very acute (flash pulmonary edema) or occur insidiously in association with left ventricular hypertrophy, mitral regurgitation, or aortic stenosis. Cardiogenic pulmonary edema results in atelectasis, $\dot{V}/\dot{Q}$ mismatch, and hypoxemia.

Noncardiogenic pulmonary edema can result from alterations in capillary permeability (as in ARDS or pneumonia), intrapleural pressure from airway obstruction(s), or lymph vessel obstruction. The results are similar to those of cardiogenic pulmonary edema.

Clinical tip

Be aware of a flat position in bed or other positions that exacerbate dyspnea during physical therapy intervention in patients with pulmonary edema.

Pulmonary Embolism

Pulmonary embolism (PE) is the partial or full occlusion of the pulmonary vasculature by one large or multiple small emboli from one or more of the following possible sources: thromboembolism originating from the lower extremity, air entering the venous system through catheterization or needle placement, fat droplets from traumatic origin, tumor fragments.

A PE results in the following:

- Decreased blood flow to the lungs distal to the occlusion

- Possible pulmonary infarction

- Atelectasis

- Parenchymal necrosis

- Bronchospasm

The onset of a PE is usually extremely acute and may be a life-threatening emergency. Emboli size and location determine the extent of hypoxemia and hemodynamic instability. Refer to the discussion of arterial pathophysiology in Chapter 6 for further discussion of PE.

Clinical tip

Physical therapy intervention should be discontinued if the signs and symptoms of PE arise during treatment (see Table 2-10).

Restrictive Extrapulmonary Conditions

Disorders peripheral to the visceral pleura may affect pulmonary function. Table 2-11 outlines restrictive extrapulmonary disorders, their physical findings, and their general management.

Chylothorax

Chylothorax is the presence of thoracic duct lymph (chyle) in the pleural space that results from congenital malformation, trauma to the thoracic duct from thoracic surgery or hyperextension injury of the spine, or thoracic duct obstruction or compression by neoplasm.

Empyema

Empyema is the presence of anaerobic bacterial pus in the pleural space resulting from underlying infection (such as pneumonia or lung abscess) that crosses the visceral pleura, or chest wall and parietal pleura penetration from trauma, surgery, or chest tube placement. Empyema formation involves pleural swelling and exudate formation, continued bacterial accumulation, fibrin deposition on pleura, or chronic fibroblast formation.

Hemothorax

Hemothorax is characterized by the presence of blood in the pleural space from damage to the pleura and great or smaller vessels (such as interstitial arteries). Causes of hemothorax are penetrating or blunt chest wall injury, draining aortic aneurysms, pulmonary arteriovenous malformations, and extreme coagulation therapy for PE.

Table 2-11. Characteristics of Extrapleural Disorders

Disorder	Observation	Palpation	Auscultation	Cough	Chest X-Ray	Medical Management
Chylothorax	Dyspnea	Increased heart rate and BP Tracheal shift to the opposite side	Diminished breath sounds at the site	Nonproductive cough	Homogenous density at area involved	See Pleural Effusion, below Nutritional support Pleuroperitoneal shunt Thoracic duct ligation
Empyema	See Pleural Effusion, below	See Pleural Effusion, below	See Pleural Effusion, below	Nonproductive cough	Homogenous density at area involved	See Pleural effusion, below Antibiotics
Flail chest	Increased RR Cyanosis Bony thorax discontinuity Ecchymosis at site	Increased HR and BP Dull percussion Point tenderness at site Crepitus at fracture sites	Diminished breath sounds Crackles	Blood-streaked sputum See Hemothorax, below	Opacity at site of associated lung contusion in nonsegmental or nonlobar pattern Appears immediately and resolves in 24–72 hrs	Stabilization of thorax with mechanical ventilation Pain control Fluid balance Observe for dysrhythmia or decreased cardiac output

Hemothorax	See Pneumothorax, below	See Pneumothorax, below	See Pneumothorax, below	Nonproductive cough unless associated with significant lung contusion in which hemoptysis may occur	Rib fractures at site See Pleural effusion, below	See Pleural effusion, below Monitor and treat for shock Blood transfusion as needed
Pleural effusion	Dyspnea Discomfort from pleuritis Decreased chest expansion on involved side	Decreased tactile fremitus Dull percussion	Normal to decreased breath sounds or bronchial sounds at the level of the effusion	Nonproductive cough	Homogenous density in dependent lung Fluid shifts with the patient's position Fluid obscures diaphragm and fills costophrenic angle Mediastinal shift to opposite side	Supplemental oxygen (O_2) Thoracentesis Chest tube placement Pleurodesis Workup to determine cause if unknown

Table 2-11. *Continued*

Disorder	Observation	Palpation	Auscultation	Cough	Chest X-Ray	Medical Management
Pneumothorax	Dyspnea	Increased HR and BP Tracheal shift to the opposite side	Diminished breath sounds at the pneumothorax site Absent sounds if tension pneumothorax	Nonproductive cough	Translucent area usually at apex of lung ± Associated depressed diaphragm, lung collapse, atelectasis, mediastinal shift	If pneumothorax is small and respiratory status is stable, monitor only If pneumothorax is moderate-size or large, chest tube placement Supplemental O_2

HR = heart rate; BP = blood pressure; RR = respiratory rate; ± = with or without.

Pleural Effusion

A pleural infusion is the presence of transudative or exudative fluid in the pleural space. Transudative fluid results from a change in the hydrostatic/oncotic pressure gradient of the pleural capillaries, which is associated with congestive heart failure, cirrhosis, PE, or pericardial disease. Exudative fluid (containing cellular debris), occurs with pleural or parenchymal inflammation or altered lymphatic drainage, which is associated with neoplasm, tuberculosis, pneumonia, pancreatitis, rheumatoid arthritis, or systemic lupus erythematosus. Pleural effusions may result in compressive atelectasis.

Pneumothorax

Pneumothorax (PTX) is the presence of air in the pleural space that can occur from (1) visceral pleura perforation with movement of air from within the lung (referred to as a *spontaneous pneumothorax*), (2) chest wall and parietal pleura perforation with movement of air from the atmosphere (referred to as a *traumatic* or *iatrogenic pneumothorax*), or (3) formation of gas by microorganisms associated with empyema.

Pneumothoraces may be also be described as follows:

Closed   Without air movement into the pleural space during respiration

Open   With air moving in and out of the pleural space during respiration

Tension   With air moving into the pleural space only with inspiration

Complications of PTX include atelectasis or lung collapse, V̇/Q̇ mismatch, mediastinal shift (displacement of the mediastinum), and cardiac tamponade (altered cardiac function secondary to decreased venous return to the heart) in cases in which the mediastinal shift is significant.

Flail Chest

Flail chest is caused by the double fracture of three or more adjacent ribs resulting from a crushing chest injury or vigorous cardiopulmonary resuscitation. The sequelae of this injury are

- A paradoxical breathing pattern, with the discontinuous ribs moving inward on inspiration and outward on expiration as a result of alterations in atmospheric and intrapleural pressure gradients

- Contused lung parenchyma under the flail portion

- In severe cases, mediastinal shift to the contralateral side occur as air from the involved side is shifted and rebreathed (pendelluft)

Chest Wall Restrictions

A restrictive respiratory pattern may be caused by abnormal chest wall movement.

Ankylosing Spondylitis

Ankylosing spondylitis is the fusion of the posterior intervertebral, costovertebral, and sacroiliac joints and ossification of spinal ligaments. It results in the following:

- Decreased thoracic cage mobility with the ribs fixed in an inspiratory position eliminating intercostal muscle function

- Increased diaphragmatic muscle work

- In severe cases, upper lobe atelectasis from hypoventilation, fibrotic changes of lung parenchyma from unknown etiology, or both

Kyphoscoliosis

Kyphoscoliosis, abnormal spinal curvature in varying degrees, can result in the following:

- Atelectasis from decreased thoracic cage mobility

- Respiratory muscle insufficiency

- Parenchymal compression

Other consequences of kyphoscoliosis are progressive alveolar hypoventilation, increased dead space, $\dot{V}/\dot{Q}$ mismatch, hypoxemia with eventual pulmonary artery hypertension, cor pulmonale, or mediastinal shift (in severe cases) toward the direction of the lateral curve of the spine.

Obesity

Obesity, defined as body weight 20–30% above age-predicted weight and sex, can cause the following:

- Abnormally elevated diaphragm position secondary to the upward displacement of abdominal contents
- Inefficient respiratory muscle use
- Noncompliant chest wall

These factors result in early airway closure (especially in dependent lung areas), altered respiratory rate and pattern, $\dot{V}/\dot{Q}$ mismatch, and secretion retention.

Management

Pulmonary Medications

Pulmonary medications are outlined in the Chapter Appendix 2-A, which includes a description of their mechanisms of action, purpose, and common side effects.

Clinical tip

- Generally, nebulized medications are optimally active 15–20 minutes after administration.

- If a patient has an inhaler, it may be beneficial for the therapist or the patient to bring it to physical therapy sessions in case of activity-induced bronchospasm.

Thoracic Procedures

The most common thoracic operative and nonoperative procedures for respiratory disorders are described below.

Bronchoplasty	Also called *sleeve resection*. Resection and reanastomosis (reconnection) of a bronchus;

most commonly performed for bronchial carcinoma (a concurrent pulmonary resection may or may not be performed as well)

Laryngectomy   The partial or total removal of one or more vocal cords; most commonly performed for laryngeal cancer

Laryngoscopy   Direct visual examination of the larynx with a fiberoptic scope; most commonly performed to assist with differential diagnosis of thoracic disorders or to assess the vocal cords

Mediastinoscopy   Endoscopic examination of the mediastinum; most commonly performed for precise localization and biopsy of a mediastinal mass or for the removal of lymph nodes

Pleurodesis   The obliteration of the pleural space, most commonly performed for persistent pleural effusions or pneumothoraces (A chemical agent is introduced into the pleural space via thoracostomy tube or with a thorascope.)

Pneumonectomy   Removal of an entire lung, most commonly performed as a result of bronchial carcinoma, emphysema, multiple lung abscesses, bronchiectasis, or tuberculosis

Reduction   The unilateral or bilateral removal of one or pneumoplasty   more portions of emphysematous lung parenchyma, resulting in increased alveolar surface-area

Rib resection   Removal of a portion of one or more ribs for accessing underlying pulmonary structures, as a treatment for thoracic outlet syndrome or for bone grafting

Segmentectomy   Removal of a segment of a lung; most commonly performed for a peripheral bronchial or parenchymal lesion

Thoracentesis   Therapeutic or diagnostic removal of pleural fluid via percutaneous needle aspiration

Thorascopy (video-assisted thorascopic surgery [VATS])	Examination, through the chest wall with a thorascope, of the pleura or lung parenchyma for pleural fluid biopsy or pulmonary resection
Tracheal resection and reconstruction	Resection and reanastomosis (reconnection) of the trachea, main stem bronchi, or both; most commonly performed for tracheal carcinoma, trauma, stricture, or tracheomalacia
Tracheostomy	Incision of the second and third tracheal rings or the creation of a stoma or opening for a tracheostomy tube; preferred for airway protection and prolonged ventilatory support or after laryngectomy, tracheal resection, or other head and neck surgery
Wedge resection	Removal of lung parenchyma without regard to segment divisions (a portion of more than one segment but not a full lobe); most commonly for peripheral parenchymal carcinoma

Physical Therapy Intervention

Goals

The primary physical therapy goals in treating patients with primary lung pathology include promoting independence in functional mobility and maximizing gas exchange (by improving ventilation and airway clearance), endurance, and patient knowledge of his or her condition. General treatment techniques to accomplish these goals are breathing retraining exercises, secretion clearance techniques, positioning, functional activity and exercise with vital sign monitoring, and patient education.

Basic Concepts for the Treatment of Patients with Respiratory Dysfunction

Bronchopulmonary Hygiene
The following are basic concepts for implementing a bronchopulmonary hygiene program for patients with respiratory dysfunction:

- The bronchopulmonary hygiene treatment plan will vary in direct correlation to the patient's respiratory or medical status. The physical therapist must be cognizant of the potential for rapid decline in patient status and modify treatment accordingly.

• A basic understanding of respiratory pathophysiology is necessary, as bronchopulmonary hygiene is not indicated for certain respiratory (e.g., pleural effusion) or medical conditions (e.g., pulmonary edema).

• Bronchopulmonary hygiene requires constant reassessment before, during, and after physical therapy intervention as well as on a daily basis.

• Bronchopulmonary hygiene consists of a few basic techniques. The appropriate combination and timing of these techniques based on constant reassessment are key to effective treatment.

• Bronchopulmonary hygiene may be enhanced by the use of supplemental O_2 and medications.

Activity Progression
The following are basic concepts of activity progression for patients with respiratory dysfunction:

• Rating perceived exertion (see Chapter 1 for Borg's Scale) is a better indicator of exercise intensity than heart rate because a patient's pulmonary limitations generally supersede cardiac limitations. Monitoring O_2 saturation can also assist in monitoring activity intensity.

• Shorter, more frequent sessions of activity are often better tolerated than longer treatment sessions. Patient education regarding energy conservation and paced breathing contribute to increased activity tolerance.

• Bronchopulmonary hygiene before an exercise session may optimize activity tolerance.

• Although O_2 may not be needed at rest, supplemental O_2 with exercise may decrease dyspnea and prolong exercise tolerance.

Table 2-12 provides some suggested treatment interventions based on common respiratory assessment findings.

Table 2-12. Respiratory Assessment Findings and Physical Therapy Treatment Intervention

Assessment	Finding	Physical Therapy Intervention
Inspection	Dyspnea or increased respiratory rate Asymmetric respiratory pattern	Reposition for comfort Use relaxation techniques Use diaphragmatic or lateral costal expansion exercise Administer or request supplemental O_2
Palpation	Asymmetric respiratory pattern Palpable fremitus as a result of retained pulmonary secretions	Use bronchial drainage positions (see Appendix VIII) Use manual techniques to mobilize pulmonary secretions Use diaphragmatic or lateral costal expansion exercise
Percussion	Increased dullness as a result of retained pulmonary secretions	See Palpation, above
Auscultation	Diminished or adventitious breath sounds as a result of retained pulmonary secretions	See Palpation, above
Cough effectiveness	Ineffective cough	Position for comfort or to maximize expiratory force Use incisional splinting if applicable Instruct in huffing technique Use functional activity or exercise Use external tracheal stimulation Use naso/endotracheal suctioning Request bronchodilator or mucolytic treatment

References

1. Thomas CL. Taber's Cyclopedic Medical Dictionary (17th ed). Philadelphia: FA Davis, 1989;701, 1635, 2121.
2. Ganong WF. Review of Medical Physiology (16th ed). Norwalk, CT: Appleton & Lange, 1993;587.
3. Vander AJ, Sherman JH, Luciano DS. Human Physiology, The Mechanisms of Body Function (4th ed). New York: McGraw-Hill, 1985;379.
4. Desjardins T. Clinical Manifestations of Respiratory Disease (3rd ed). St. Louis: Mosby, 1995.
5. Hillegass EA, Sadowsky HS. Essentials of Cardiopulmonary Physical Therapy. Philadelphia: Saunders, 1994.
6. Frownfelter DL. Chest Physical Therapy and Pulmonary Rehabilitation, An Interdisciplinary Approach (2nd ed). Chicago: Year Book, 1987.
7. Humberstone N. Respiratory Assessment. In S Irwin, JS Tecklin (eds), Cardiopulmonary Physical Therapy. St Louis: Mosby, 1985;208.
8. American College of CP & ATS Joint Committee on Pulmonary Nomenclature. Pulmonary terms and symbols. Chest 1975;67:583.
9. Thompson JM, Hirsch JE, MacFarland GK, et al. Clinical Nursing Practice. St. Louis: Mosby, 1986;136.
10. Wilson AF. Pulmonary Function Testing, Indications and Interpretations. Orlando, FL: Orvine & Stratton, 1985.
11. Forrest JV, Feigin DS. Essentials of Chest Radiology. Philadelphia: Saunders, 1982.
12. George RB, Matthay MA, Light RW, Matthay RA. Chest Medicine: Essentials of Pulmonary and Critical Care Medicine (3rd ed). Baltimore: Williams & Wilkins, 1995;110.
13. Hetzed MR. Minimally Invasive Techniques in Thoracic Medicine and Surgery. London: Chapman & Hall Medical, 1995;4.
14. Rippe JM, Irwin RS, Fink MP, et al. Procedures and Techniques in Intensive Care Medicine. Boston: Little, Brown, 1994.
15. Hudak CM, Gallo BM. Critical Care Nursing, A Holistic Approach (6th ed). Philadelphia: Lippincott, 1994;413.
16. Smeltzer SC, Bare BG. Brunnar and Suddarth's Textbook of Medical-Surgical Nursing (8th ed). Philadelphia: Lippincott, 1996;454.
17. Thelan LA, Davie JK, Urden LD, Lough ME. Critical Care Nursing, Diagnosis and Management (2nd ed). St. Louis: Mosby, 1994;404, 436.
18. Kersten LD. Comprehensive Respiratory Nursing: A Decision Making Approach. Philadelphia: Saunders, 1989.
19. Lilington GA. A Diagnostic Approach to Chest Diseases (3rd ed). Baltimore: Williams & Wilkins, 1987;23.
20. Farzan S. A Concise Handbook of Respiratory Diseases (3rd ed). Norwalk, CT: Appleton & Lange, 1992.
21. Brannon FJ, Foley MW, Starr JA, Geyer Black MJ. Cardiopulmonary Rehabilitation: Basic Theory and Application (2nd ed). Philadelphia: FA Davis, 1993.

22. Baue AE, Geha AS. Glenn's Thoracic and Cardiovascular Surgery (6th ed, Vol. 1). Stamford, CT: Appleton & Lange, 1996.
23. Sabiston DC, Spencer FC. Surgery of the Chest (6th ed, Vol. 1 and 2). Philadelphia: Saunders, 1995.
24. Waldhausen JA, Pierce WS. Johnson's Surgery of the Chest (5th ed). Chicago: Year Book, 1985.

Appendix 2-A:
Pulmonary Medications

Table 2-A.1. Bronchodilators

Mechanism of action
  Reduce smooth muscle bronchoconstriction by altering receptor sensitivity
Purpose
  To enhance secretion clearance, improve alveolar ventilation, and optimize
  gas exchange
General side effects
  Blood pressure changes, anxiety, tachycardia, tremor, headache, dysrhythmia,
  nervousness, dizziness, chest pain, nausea, vomiting, increased respira-
  tory rate, irritability, insomnia, restlessness, nasal congestion, joint
  swelling, wheezing, and muscle cramps
Sympathomimetic bronchodilators
  Beta-1 and beta-2 nonselective
    Ephedrine (Ectasule, Efedron, Ephedsol, Vatronol)
    Epinephrine (Adrenalin Chloride, AsthmaHaler, Asthma Nefrin, Bronkaid
      Mistometer, Bronkaid Mist, Bronkaid Mist Suspension, Brontin Mist
      Suspension, Dey-Dose Epinephrine, Dysne-Inhal, Epifrin, EpiPen Auto-
      Injector, Epitrate, Glaucon, Medihaler-Epi, microNefrin, Primatene Mist
      Suspension, S-2 Inhalant)
    Isoproterenol (Medihaler-Iso, Isuprel)
  Beta-2 selective
    Albuterol (Ventolin, Proventil)
    Isoetharine (Arm-a-Med Isoetharine, Beta-2, Bronkometer, Bronkosol,
      Dey-Lute)

Table 2-A.1. *Continued*

Terbutaline (Brethaire, Brethine, Bricanyl)
Metaproterenol (Alupent, Metaprel)
Bitolterol (Tornalate)
Pirbuterol (Maxair)
Salmeterol xinafoate (Serevent)
Parasympatholytics
Ipratropium (Atrovent)
Theophylline (Theo-Dur, Slo-Bid, Elixophyllin, Slo-Phyillin, Theo-24, Aerolate, Bronkodyl)
Aminophylline (Phyllocontin, Somophyllin)
Dyphylline (Dilor, Dyflex, Lufyllin, Neothylline, Thylline)
Oxtriphylline (Choledyl)
Cromolyn (Intal, Gastrocrom, Nasalcrom, Opticrom)

Source: Data from ME Shannon, BA Wilson, CL Strang. Goroni and Hayes Drugs and Nursing Implications (8th ed). Norwalk, CT: Appleton & Lange, 1995.

Table 2-A.2. Corticosteroids

Mechanism of action
Stabilize and limit inflammatory responses in airways
Purpose
To decrease inflammation and bronchoconstriction
General side effects
Decreased healing, hypotension, hypertension, tachycardia, osteoporosis, fractures, muscle weakness, immunosuppression
Generic name (brand name)
Prednisone (Deltasone, Orasone, Meticorten)
Dexamethasone (Decadron)
Hydrocortisone (Solu-Cortef)
Beclomethasone dipropionate (Beclovent, Vanceril)
Methylprednisolone (Solu-Medrol)

Source: Data from ME Shannon, BA Wilson, CL Strang. Goroni and Hayes Drugs and Nursing Implications (8th ed). Norwalk, CT: Appleton & Lange, 1995.

Table 2-A.3. Inhaled Corticosteroids

Mechanism of action
  Stabilize and limit inflammatory responses in airways
  Direct action via inhalation
Purpose
  To decrease inflammation and bronchoconstriction
General side effects
  Mucosal irritation, hoarseness, sore throat, bronchospasm, headache, nausea, vomiting, upper respiratory tract infections
Generic name (brand name)
  Triamcinolone (Azmacort)
  Beclomethasone (Beclovent, Vanceril, Vancenase, Beconase)
  Flunisolide (AeroBid, Nasalide)

Source: Data from ME Shannon, BA Wilson, CL Strang. Goroni and Hayes Drugs and Nursing Implications (8th ed). Norwalk, CT: Appleton & Lange, 1995.

Table 2-A.4. Antitussives

Mechanism of action
  Symptomatically relieve dry, irritating, and ineffective coughs by blocking the cough receptors, increasing the cough threshold in the brain, or both
Purpose
  To prevent throat irritation and soreness (short-term use only)
  Contraindicated for coughs due to retained secretions
General side effects
  Lightheadedness, dizziness, sedation, sweating, orthostatic hypotension, nausea, vomiting, constipation, palpitations, decreased respiratory function, seizures, tachycardia, drowsiness, headache, chills
Generic name (brand name)
  Codeine (numerous brand names)
  Hyaluronidase (Hydocan tablets and syrup)
  Dextromethorphan (Benylin DM, Robitussin DM, Romilar)
  Diphenhydramine (Benadryl)
  Benzonatate (Tessalon)

Source: Data from ME Shannon, BA Wilson, CL Strang. Goroni and Hayes Drugs and Nursing Implications (8th ed). Norwalk, CT: Appleton & Lange, 1995.

Table 2-A.5. Expectorants and Mucolytics

Mechanism of action
 Expectorants facilitate secretion removal by increasing the production of
 respiratory secretions to induce the cough reflexes
 Mucolytics decrease the viscosity of secretions by disrupting the chemical
 bonds within mucoid and purulent sputum
Purpose
 To enhance secretion clearance
General side effects
 Drowsiness, nausea, anorexia, burning mouth and throat, central nervous
 system depression, hyperreflexia, tremors, apnea, hyperventilation,
 bradycardia
Generic name (brand name)
 Guaifenesin (Triaminic, Robitussin, Breonesin, Anatyss)
 Potassium iodide (SSKI, Pima)
 Ammonium chloride
 Iodinated glycerol (Organidin, Isophen)
 Terpin hydrate
 Acetylcysteine (Mucomyst, Mucosil)

Source: Data from ME Shannon, BA Wilson, CL Strang. Goroni and Hayes Drugs and
Nursing Implications (8th ed). Norwalk, CT: Appleton & Lange, 1995.

Table 2-A.6. Antihistamines

Mechanism of action
 Decrease the inflammatory response of histamine reactions that occur from
 respiratory tract irritation such as in allergies or asthma
Purpose
 To decrease inflammation and bronchoconstriction
General side effects
 Dizziness, decreased coordination, hypotension, palpitations, increased
 thickness of secretions, nausea, vomiting
Generic name (brand name)
 Diphenhydramine (Benadryl)
 Promethazine (Phenergan)
 Terfenadine (Seldane)
 Chlorpheniramine (Aller-Chlor, Chlo-Amine, Chlor-Pro, Chlor-Trimeton,
 Telachlor, Teldrin)

Source: Data from ME Shannon, BA Wilson, CL Strang. Goroni and Hayes Drugs and
Nursing Implications (8th ed). Norwalk, CT: Appleton & Lange, 1995.

3

Orthopedics

Cheryl L. Maurer and Marie R. Reardon

Introduction

An understanding of musculoskeletal pathology and medical-surgical intervention is often the basis of physical therapy evaluation and treatment planning for patients with acute orthopedic impairments. The primary goal of the physical therapist working with a patient in the acute care setting is to initiate rehabilitative techniques that foster early restoration of maximum functional mobility and reduce the risk of secondary complications.

This chapter provides the information specific to acute orthopedic pathology needed to facilitate and direct the thought process of the clinician new to the acute care setting. The objectives for this chapter are to provide the following:

1. A brief description of the structure and function of the musculoskeletal system

2. An overview of musculoskeletal assessment, including physical examination and diagnostic tests

3. A description of orthopedic fractures, including medical-surgical management, clinical findings, and physical therapy intervention

4. A description of joint replacement surgery, including etiology, surgical management, and physical therapy intervention

5. An overview of common soft tissue injuries, including surgical management and physical therapy intervention

6. A brief overview of equipment commonly used in the acute care setting, including casts, braces, and fixation and traction devices

Structure and Function of the Musculoskeletal System

The musculoskeletal system is made up of the bony skeleton and contractile and noncontractile soft tissues, including muscles, tendons, ligaments, joint capsules, articular cartilage, and nonarticular cartilage. This matrix of soft tissue and bone provides the dynamic ability of human movement, giving individuals the agility to move through space, absorb shock, convert reactive forces, generate kinetic energy, and perform fine motor tasks. The musculoskeletal system also provides housing and protection for vital organs and the central nervous system. As a result of its location and function, the musculoskeletal system commonly sustains traumatic injuries and degenerative changes. The impairments that develop from injury or disease can significantly affect an individual's ability to remain functional without further pathologic compromise.

Physical Therapy Examination

The initial evaluation of a patient with orthopedic dysfunction is invaluable to clinical management in the acute care setting. The true challenge for the physical therapist lies in his or her ability to complete a thorough yet efficient examination. The following evaluation schema [1, 2] is structured for patients with primary orthopedic impairments. This schema is sequenced to yield the information needed to develop a functionally based treatment program.

Patient History

In addition to a standard medical review (see Appendix I) and patient interview, questions pertaining to the patient's musculoskeletal history should include the following:

- What was the cause of injury?

- Is there a history of other musculoskeletal or neurologic injury or surgery in the past? (Preexisting impairments may limit the use of assistive devices or transfer techniques.)

- Does the patient have any additional medical problems (concurrent arm, leg, or back pathology) that may limit the use of assistive devices?

- Has the patient used crutches, a walker, or a cane before? (An awareness of the patient's functional capabilities can be helpful and can direct the functional assessment to establish the appropriate short-term goals.)

- What are the physician-dictated precautions or contraindications to treatment (e.g., weight-bearing status)?

- What are the most recent hematologic test values (e.g., hematocrit level)?

Questions related to the patient's social history and discharge planning should include the following:

- Will the patient have help when discharged from the hospital?

- Where will the patient be going when discharged from the hospital?

- Will there be stairs to enter the house, stairs in the house, or both that the patient must negotiate? If so, how many? Which side is the railing on if there is any railing?

- Where is the bathroom and how is it set up? Is the bathroom already equipped with assistive devices such as grab bars, raised toilet seat, tub bench, or shower chair? Is there room to extend the leg when sitting on the toilet?

- Was the patient able to get into and out of the shower or tub independently before the injury?

Evaluation

The objective examination includes an evaluation of the patient's posture, limb position, skin integrity, subjective report of pain, upper- and lower-quarter screens, and ability to observe safety precautions.

1. Posture. The therapist should observe the patient's resting posture and look for anomalies that may result in additional impairments (e.g., forward shoulder could result in abnormal scapulothoracic rhythm).

2. Limb position. In patients with an injury involving an extremity, the therapist should observe the resting limb position. The therapist should be aware that limbs positioned in a dependent posture will increase swelling. It is important to maintain joints in a neutral resting position to preserve motion and maintain soft tissue length.

3. Skin integrity. The patient's skin integrity should be inspected at the level of and distal to the injury. The therapist should note the presence of bruising, edema, discoloration, muscle atrophy, scars, the vascularity of nail beds, the skin temperature to touch, and the presence of peripheral pulses.

4. Pain. The therapist should determine the location of the patient's pain as well as the pain rating using subjective patient report.

5. Upper- and lower-quarter screen. Upper- and lower-quarter screening is the brief evaluation of range of motion (ROM), muscle strength, sensation, and deep tendon reflexes. The therapist should perform an upper- or lower-quarter screen, depending on the extremity involved. In a patient with lower-extremity involvement who will require the use of an assistive device for functional mobility, both functional range and strength of the upper extremities must also be assessed. Tables 3-1 and 3-2 describe a modified version of an upper- and a lower-quarter screen. Table 3-3 outlines normal ROMs. Peripheral nerve innervations for the upper and lower extremities are shown in Tables 4-8 and 4-9, respectively. Dermatomal innervation is shown in Figure 4-6.

The sequencing of the upper- and lower-quarter screen is as follows:

a. The therapist should observe active ROM, progressing from proximal to distal and beginning at the spinal level and moving distally to the extremities.

b. The therapist should screen the patient's sensation to light touch over both extremities.

Table 3-1. Upper-Quarter Screen

Nerve Root	Myotome	Dermatome	Deep Tendon Reflex
C1	Cervical rotation	No innervation	No identifiable reflex
C2	Shoulder shrug	Posterior head	No identifiable reflex
C3	Shoulder shrug	Posterior neck	No identifiable reflex
C4	Shoulder shrug	Acromioclavicular joint	No identifiable reflex
C5	Shoulder abduction	Lateral arm	Biceps
C5 and C6	Elbow flexion		No identifiable reflex
C6	Wrist extension	Lateral forearm and palmar tip of thumb	Brachioradialis
C7	Elbow extension and wrist flexion	Palmar distal phalanx of middle finger	Triceps
C8	Thumb extension and grasp	Palmar distal phalanx of little finger	No identifiable reflex
T1	Abduction little finger	Medial forearm	No identifiable reflex
T2	Finger intrinsics	Medial arm	No identifiable reflex

Source: Data from S Hoppenfield. Physical Examination of the Spine and Extremities. East Norwalk, CT: Appleton-Century-Crofts, 1976; and DJ Magee. Orthopedic Physical Assessment. Philadelphia: Saunders, 1987.

c. The therapist should assess myotomes, peripheral nerve innervation, or both. He or she should remember that it is imperative to assess the peripheral nerve innervation, myotomes, and dermatomes below the level of injury, as neurologic impairments may exist.

d. The therapist should assess the patient's strength using manual muscle testing. Break testing may also be performed as a modified way to assess isometric capacity of motor performance.

Table 3-2. Lower-Quarter Screen

Nerve Root	Myotome	Dermatome	Deep Tendon Reflex
L1	Hip flexion		No identifiable reflex
L2	Hip flexion	2.5 in. below anterior superior iliac spine	No identifiable reflex
L3	Knee extension with L4	Middle one-third ventral thigh	No identifiable reflex
L4	Knee extension with L3 and L5	Patella and medial malleolus	Patellar tendon
L4 and L5	Ankle dorsiflexion		No identifiable reflex
L5	Great toe extension	Fibula head and dorsum of foot	Posterior tibialis
S1	Ankle plantar flexion	Lateral side and plantar surface of foot	Achilles tendon

Source: Adapted from S Hoppenfield. Physical Examination of the Spine and Extremities. East Norwalk, CT: Appleton-Century-Crofts, 1976; and DJ Magee. Orthopedic Physical Assessment. Philadelphia: Saunders, 1987.

    e. The therapist should complete a functional assessment to determine the patient's skill level with functional mobility, including bed mobility, transfers, and ambulation on level surfaces and stairs as appropriate.

  6. Safety. The therapist should evaluate the patient's willingness to observe safety precautions during transfers and ambulation. He or she should look for loss of balance, early fatigue, poor coordination, failure to maintain weight-bearing status, and compliance with other precautions.

Clinical tip

• Often, fear may cause the patient to rush or move unsafely. The clinician should use strategies to ease the patient's fears and pace his or her activity.

Table 3-3. Normal Ranges of Motion Most Applicable in the Acute Care Setting

Joint	Normal Range of Motion (Degrees)
Shoulder	
Flexion	0–180
Extension	0–60
Abduction	0–180
Medial Rotation	0–70
Lateral Rotation	0–90
Elbow	
Flexion	0–150
Forearm	
Pronation	0–80
Supination	0–80
Wrist	
Extension	0–70
Flexion	0–80
Hip	
Flexion	0–120
Extension	0–30
Abduction	0–45
Lateral Rotation	0–45
Medial Rotation	0–45
Knee	
Flexion	0–135
Ankle	
Dorsiflexion	0–20

Source: Adapted from CA Norton, DJ White. Measurement of Joint Motion: A Guide to Goniometry. Philadelphia: FA Davis, 1985;138.

- The patient may demonstrate but not realize poor body awareness and judgment. The physical therapist may observe that the patient turns quickly or walks briskly and loses balance. The therapist may notice that the patient leans on a rolling bed table, unaware that it may move; sways when standing; or leans into the wall when walking. These actions may strongly suggest the need for external stability.

Because fractures can often be the final insult of other medical problems (e.g., balance disorders, visual or sensory impairments, decreased cardiac capacities), it is important that the clinician take a thorough history and musculoskeletal screen and critically observe the patient's functional mobility. Such medical problems may be subtle in presentation but may dramatically influence the patient's capabilities and require skilled management. In the acute care setting, it may be the physical therapist who will first appreciate a neurologic deficit, additional fractures, or a pertinent piece of medical or social history. Any and all abnormal evaluation findings should be reported to the physician.

Diagnostic Tests

Listed below are the most commonly used diagnostic tests in orthopedics [3]. The results of these tests assist in the differential diagnosis of musculoskeletal dysfunction and help determine the medical or surgical intervention indicated. Test results should be incorporated into the physical therapy evaluation and used in decision making for treatment.

Arthrogram	An arthrogram is a radiograph with dye contrast to provide visualization of joint structures. The joint suspected of pathology is injected with dye that outlines the joint surfaces and demonstrates leakage from the joint cavity and capsule if soft tissue disruption is present.
Bone scan	A bone scan is a radiographic visualization of musculoskeletal absorption of injected chemical isotopes. Bone scans are used to detect subtle fractures not visible on standard x-rays, stress fractures, infection, tumors, and lytic lesions.
Computed tomography scans	See Chapter 4
Magnetic resonance imaging	See Chapter 4
Myelogram	See Chapter 4
Venogram or arteriogram	Venograms and arteriograms are radiographs that visualize the distribution of radiopaque dye

X-rays that has been injected into blood vessels. They are used to detect arteriosclerosis, tumors, blockages, and disruption secondary to trauma.

X-rays X-rays are radiographic photographs used in orthopedics to detect fractures, dislocations, foreign bodies, and bone loss. Serial x-rays in multiple planes can be taken to visualize a lesion's location and size. Three-dimensional views are used to visualize metal implants, bone, soft tissue, water, fat, and air.

Fracture Management

Types of Fractures

Fractures can be described according to the following:

1. The maintenance of skin integrity

   a. An *open fracture* is a bony fracture with open laceration of the skin or protrusion of the bone through the skin.

   b. A *closed fracture* is a bony fracture without disruption of the skin.

2. The direction or line of the fracture (Figure 3-1)

   a. A *transverse fracture* is perpendicular to the long axis of the bone.

   b. An *oblique fracture* is a diagonal or slanted fracture in the shaft of long bones.

   c. A *spiral fracture* is circular and follows the long axis of the bone.

   d. A *linear fracture* resembles a straight line following the long axis of the bone.

3. The energy impact of the fracture

   a. A *burst fracture* is an impacted fracture with fragment displacement (Figure 3-2).

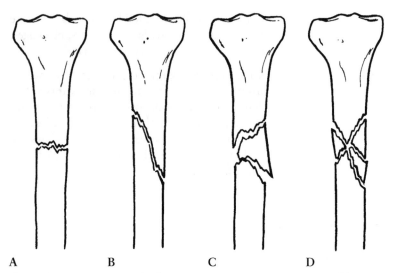

A   B   C   D

Figure 3-1. *Orientation of a fracture pattern. A. Transverse. B. Oblique. C. Segmental. D. Comminuted. (Reprinted with permission from A Unwin, K Jones. Emergency Orthopaedics and Trauma. Oxford: Butterworth–Heinemann, 1995;22.)*

    b. A *compression fracture* is an impacted fracture without fragment displacement.

  4. The number of fracture segments

    a. A *two-part fracture* has two fracture fragments.

    b. A *comminuted fracture* has multiple fracture fragments (see Figure 3-1).

  5. The relative position of the fragments:

    a. A *nondisplaced fracture* is characterized by anatomic alignment of fracture fragments.

    b. A *displaced fracture* is characterized by abnormal anatomic alignment of fracture fragments (Figure 3-3).

    c. An *angulated fracture* is characterized by abnormal anatomic alignment of fracture fragments with relative twisting (see Figure 3-3).

  6. The fracture site relative to adjacent joints

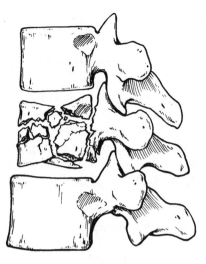

Figure 3-2. *Burst fracture. (Reprinted with permission from A Unwin, K Jones. Emergency Orthopaedics and Trauma. Oxford: Butterworth–Heinemann, 1995;88.)*

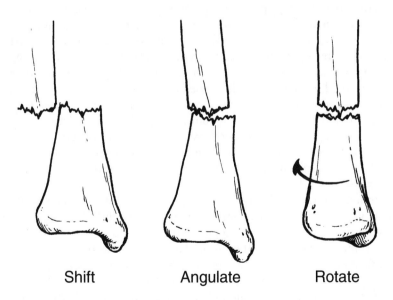

Shift   Angulate   Rotate

Figure 3-3. *A bone may displace in three ways: displace (shift), angulate, or rotate. (Reprinted with permission from A Unwin, K Jones. Emergency Orthopaedics and Trauma. Oxford: Butterworth–Heinemann, 1995;23.)*

a. An *intra-articular fracture* involves the articulating surface or surfaces of a joint.

b. An *extra-articular fracture* occurs outside of the articulating joint surfaces.

Fractures are often complicated by a wide variety of soft tissue injuries, including trauma to skin, muscles, nerves, blood vessels, and internal organs. These associated injuries often complicate or even delay orthopedic medical management and surgical repair. They may also require separate medical or surgical intervention, modification of physical therapy intervention, or both [4–6].

The Clinical Goal of Fracture Management

The goal of fracture management is early restoration of maximal function [4]. Early restoration of function minimizes cardiopulmonary compromise, muscle atrophy, and the loss of functional ROM. It also minimizes impairments associated with limited skeletal weight bearing (e.g., osteoporosis).

For proper fracture healing, the fracture site must develop a callus. This scab-like formation requires approximation of the bone fragments. If the fracture fragments are displaced by any means, the fracture must be reduced by a physician. Fracture reduction is the process of aligning and approximating fracture fragments. Reduction may be achieved by either closed or open methods. *Closed reduction* is noninvasive and is accomplished by manual manipulation or traction. *Open reduction internal fixation (ORIF)* techniques require surgery and fixation devices (e.g., screws, rods, plates) commonly referred to as hardware and are the treatment of choice when closed reduction cannot be achieved or when closed methods cannot maintain adequate fracture fixation throughout the healing phase.

Immobilization of the fracture is required to maintain reduction and viability of the fracture site. Immobilization is accomplished through both noninvasive and invasive techniques. Noninvasive devices include casts and splints. A cast is a rigid dressing that provides the greatest stability for joint immobilization. Casts are custom fit to each patient and provide the optimal circumferential conformity of a body region. A splint can be fabricated from either semirigid or flexible materials and can provide either complete immobilization or a combination of immobilization and joint motion. Splints offer donning and doffing capabilities and may be chosen in situations that require monitoring of skin integrity. Splints can be prefabricated or custom made and weigh less than casts, therefore reducing energy expenditure during functional mobility.

Invasive devices include external fixators, rods, pins, screws, and plates. Invasive devices are the specific support structures used to approximate fractures and maintain bony alignment during fracture healing [7].

Fracture Management According to Body Region

Pelvis and Lower Extremity

Pelvic Fractures

Fractures of the pelvis are the result of high-velocity trauma such as a motor vehicle accident (MVA) and often present with significant secondary or potentially life-threatening internal injuries such as the following:

- Abdominal injuries, including the hemorrhage, contusion, rupture, or tear of one or more abdominal organs, most commonly the bladder, liver, spleen, or lower intestine

- Lumbosacral plexus injury, which may involve the traction or laceration of peripheral nerves

Fracture classification, medical management, and physical therapy intervention for pelvic fractures are described in Chapter Appendix Table 3-A.1. Medical management is directed by the degree of posterior ring disruption; whereas physical therapy intervention is directed by the level of fracture stability [8, 9]. The medical management includes reduction of the fracture to anatomic alignment, along with serial radiographs being performed to monitor fracture healing.

External fixation is used for stable fractures only and can decrease post-traumatic hemorrhage. It is a good choice if other injuries (e.g., abdominal) are present, and the patient must be mobilized early. External fixation will not stabilize vertical displacement [10].

ORIF techniques are the optimal choice of treatment for anterior and posterior pelvic displacement. Risks are high and should be taken only when benefits of anatomic reduction and rigid fixation outweigh problems of hemorrhage and postoperative infection [10].

Hip Dislocation

Hip dislocations are caused by high-energy forces loading the long axis of the lower extremity and are often associated with fractures of the femoral

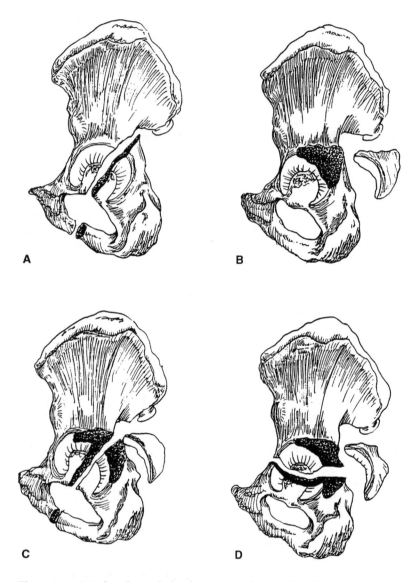

Figure 3-4. *Displaced acetabular fractures with or without hip dislocation. A. Posterior column fracture. B. Posterior wall fracture. C. Posterior wall and column fractures. D. Posterior wall and transverse fractures. (Reprinted with permission from SH Kozin, AC Berlet. Handbook of Common Orthopaedic Fractures [2nd ed]. Westchester, PA: Medical Surveillance, 1992;97.)*

neck, pelvis, and acetabulum (Figure 3-4) [11]. Posterior pelvic fracture and hip dislocations, anterior hip dislocations, and central acetabular fractures are types of pelvic fractures and combined hip dislocations. Posterior acetabular fracture with hip dislocation is the result of a direct blow to the lower extremity while the hip is flexed and adducted [10] (Chapter Appendix Table 3-A.2).

Anterior dislocations result from forced lower extremity abduction and lateral rotation of the lower extremity; injuries associated with anterior dislocations include rupture and tear of femoral artery and nerve. Medical treatment for an anterior dislocation involves closed reduction with maintenance of anterior hip precautions (i.e., 0-degree hip extension and external rotation) during functional mobilization.

Central acetabular fractures result from compressive forces transmitted through the femoral head to the acetabulum. They are located in the concavity of the arch formed by the anterior column (iliopubic articulation) and the posterior column (ilioischial articulation) (Chapter Appendix Table 3-A.3). Diagnosis of central acetabular fractures is based on the integrity of the acetabular dome and the relationship of the femoral head to the weight-bearing surface of the dome.

Clinical tip

• A continuous passive motion (CPM) machine placed at the knee joint can be used to assist with ROM of the hip. By moving the knee, the CPM machine will indirectly provide mobility into flexion at the hip.

• The therapist should elevate the height of the head of the bed to assist with sit-to-stand transferring of tall patients or to ensure maintenance of posterior hip precautions.

• The patient should use a shoe lift or foot insert on the uninvolved limb to help facilitate maintenance of non-weight-bearing status.

Complications of hip dislocation can be characterized as either acute or chronic [11]. Acute complications involve sciatic nerve injury, which occurs in 10% of posterior hip fracture and dislocations. Chronic complications are avascular necrosis and post-traumatic arthritis. Avascular necrosis of the femoral head can occur approximately 18–24 months after the injury. Fifteen percent of patients with posterior dislocation develop avascular necrosis; 4% of people with anterior dislocation develop avascular necrosis [11].

Femur Fractures

Femoral Neck Fractures. Femoral neck fractures (Figure 3-5) are often referred to as *hip fractures*. They can be classified as either intracapsular or extracapsular. Femoral neck fractures often occur with surprisingly little force applied to the hip while the hip is positioned in external rotation with or without concomitant hip abduction [12].

Intracapsular femoral neck fractures are located within the hip capsule and are also called subcapital fractures (Chapter Appendix Table 3-A.4). The four-stage Garden Scale is used to classify femoral neck fractures and is based on the amount of displacement and the degree of angulation. Garden III and IV hip fractures can be complicated by a disruption of the blood supply to the femoral head as a result of extensive capsular trauma. Poor blood supply can lead to avascular necrosis of the femoral head, which can often cause collapse of the femoral head, fracture nonunion, or both [13].

Extracapsular fractures occur outside of the hip capsule and are most prevalent in people older than 60 years of age [14]. They can be further classified as intertrochanteric or subtrochanteric. Intertrochanteric fractures occur between the greater and lesser trochanters and are summarized in Chapter Appendix Table 3-A.5. Subtrochanteric fractures occur in the proximal one-third of the femoral diaphysis and can occur with intertrochanteric or shaft fractures [15]. Subtrochanteric fractures are summarized in Chapter Appendix Table 3-A.6.

Femoral Shaft Fractures. Femoral shaft fractures result from high-energy trauma and are often associated with major abdominal or pelvic injuries. Femoral shaft fractures can be accompanied by life-threatening systemic complications such as hypovolemia, shock, or fat emboli. These fractures are most commonly repaired by ORIF techniques, unless the fracture is open or severe comminution is present [16] (Chapter Appendix Table 3-A.7).

Clinical tip

• Avoid rotation of the lower extremities of patients who have intramedullary (IM) rods, as microrotation of the IM rod can occur and place stress on the interlocking screws.

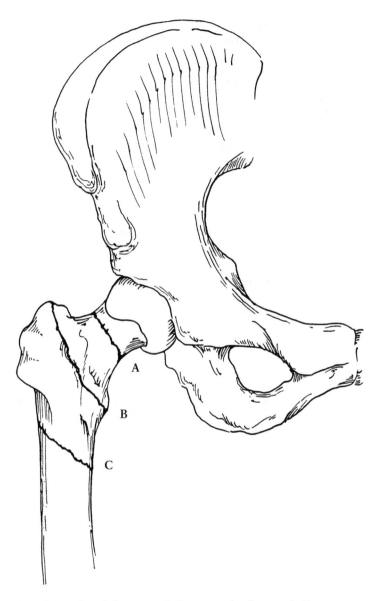

Figure 3-5. *Femoral neck fractures. A. Intracapsular fracture B. Extracapsular (intertrochanteric) fractures. C. Extracapsular (subtrochanteric) fractures. (Reprinted with permission from SH Kozin, AC Berlet. Handbook of Common Orthopaedic Fractures [2nd ed]. Westchester, PA: Medical Surveillance, 1992;107.)*

- Instruct patients to take small steps when they turn during ambulation. The physical therapist should also instruct them not to pivot on the involved lower extremity.

- Knee ROM can be difficult to regain in the involved extremity secondary to quadriceps splinting. Adherence of quadriceps tissues over the healing fracture site can also be difficult. The use of a CPM at the knee can be helpful to regain and maintain range. Soft tissue massage will also assist in decreasing muscle splinting, adhesion formation, and pain.

- Instruct the patient to use the uninvolved limb to assist the involved limb in and out of bed. Patients can also use a single crutch as a tool to assist the limb.

Distal Femoral Fractures. Distal femoral fractures result from direct trauma to the distal femur or a direct force that drives the tibia cranially into the intercondylar fossa. In the elderly, the fracture is often a result of minor trauma to osteoporotic bone [17] (Chapter Appendix Table 3-A.8).

The following are complications associated with distal femoral fractures:

- Limited knee ROM

- Myositis ossificans in the quadriceps (Myositis ossificans is the development of heterotopic bone within a muscle as a result of severe muscle contusion or hemorrhage [18].)

- Abnormal patellofemoral mechanics

Patellar Fractures
Patellar fractures result from direct trauma to the patella (e.g., dashboard injury) or, more rarely, as the result of muscle force with the knee partially flexed (Chapter Appendix Table 3-A.9) [19].

Clinical tip

The therapist should instruct the patient to use the uninvolved lower extremity or single crutch to assist the involved limb when getting in and out of bed by hooking the uninvolved leg under the ankle of the involved limb.

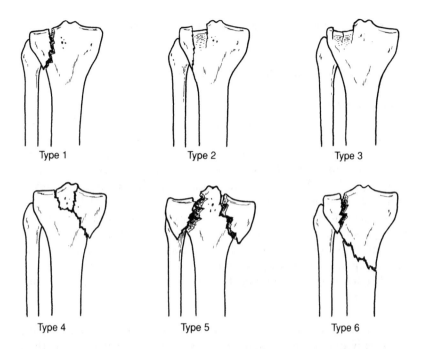

Type 1   Type 2   Type 3

Type 4   Type 5   Type 6

Figure 3-6. *Classification of tibial plateau fractures. Type 1 is a wedge fracture of the lateral tibial plateau. Type 2 is a wedge fracture of the lateral plateau with depression of the adjacent plateau. Type 3 is a central depression of the articular surface of the lateral plateau without a wedge fragment. Type 4 is a fracture of the medial tibial plateau. Type 5 is a bicondylar fracture. Type 6 is a tibial plateau fracture with separation of metaphysis from diaphysis [44]. (Reprinted with permission from A Unwin, K Jones. Emergency Orthopaedics and Trauma. Oxford: Butterworth–Heinemann, 1995;226.)*

Tibial Plateau Fractures
Tibial plateau fractures result from direct force on the proximal tibia (e.g., when a pedestrian is hit by an automobile), as shown in Figure 3-6. This high-force injury often presents with soft tissue injuries and ligamentous disruption. Ligamentous injuries are most common in nondisplaced and split compression fractures and are less common in central compression fractures [20] (Chapter Appendix Table 3-A.10).

The following are complications associated with tibial plateau fractures:

• Limited knee ROM

- Post-traumatic arthritis throughout the tibial articular surface
- Knee instability
- Abnormal patellofemoral mechanics

Tibial Shaft and Fibula Fractures
Because of their location and exposure, the tibia and fibula are very susceptible to injury and thus two of the most frequently fractured long bones [21]. Tibial shaft and fibula fractures result from high-energy trauma (e.g., MVAs, gunshot wounds, skiing accidents) (Chapter Appendix Table 3-A.11 and Figure 3-7). The higher the energy of impact, the more soft tissue and bone damage occur. Tibia fracture management is very complicated because the associated injuries (i.e., compression syndrome, nerve trauma, degloving injury) require additional surgical management, decompression fasciotomies, neurovascular repairs, skin graft procedures, or any combination of these.

The following are complications associated with tibial and fibular fractures:

- Infection (Infection in tibial and fibular fractures is most commonly due to open fractures and significant tissue injury with or without resultant tissue loss [21].)

- Delayed union, nonunion, or malunion [21]

- Peroneal nerve injury (Peroneal nerve injury is usually a result of stretch injury occurring during initial trauma or compartment syndrome.)

- Amputation

Fibula Fractures. Fibula fractures result from direct trauma to the fibula. They often occur with tibial fractures (e.g., crush injuries). The distal lower extremity must be thoroughly evaluated to rule out concomitant ankle trauma (e.g., trimalleolar fractures, syndesmotic disruption, or talar dome fractures). The fibula absorbs 10% of the weight-bearing force. These fractures tend to be very painful and often involve complications with the peroneal nerve [21] (Chapter Appendix Table 3-A.12).

Distal Tibial Fractures. Distal tibial fractures are often referred to as tibial pylon fractures and extend into the talocrural mortise. These fractures are the result of high vertical loading forces, such as

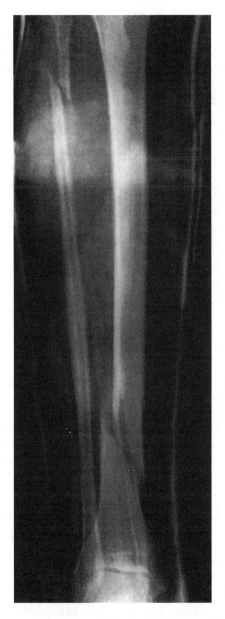

Figure 3-7. *Fracture of the tibia and fibula. (Reprinted with permission from A Unwin, K Jones. Emergency Orthopaedics and Trauma. Oxford: Butterworth–Heinemann, 1995;228.)*

with parachuting accidents, falls, sporting injuries, and MVAs [22]. As discussed in "Pelvic Fractures" and "Femoral Shaft Fractures," high-energy fractures are often accompanied by extensive trauma to surrounding soft tissue and damage to the articular cartilage. Often, the patient will demonstrate long-axis compression throughout the proximal lower extremity and present with tibial plateau fractures, hip dislocations, or acetabular fractures (Chapter Appendix Table 3-A.13).

Clinical tip

- The physical therapist can use a foot plate attached to the external fixator to help maintain 0 degrees of ankle dorsiflexion with a distal tibial fracture.

- Distal tibial fractures are often associated with post-traumatic arthritis, resulting in joint arthrodesis secondary to chronic pain.

Ankle Fractures
Ankle fractures result commonly from torque caused by abnormal loading of the talocrural joint with body weight. Fractures may be simple, involving avulsion of a portion of the distal fibula, or complicated, involving the entire mortise (trimalleolar fracture) with disruption of the syndesmosis. Stability of the ankle depends on joint congruity and ligamentous integrity [23] (Chapter Appendix Table 3-A.14).

The following are complications associated with ankle fractures:

- Nonunion or malunion
- Hypomobility throughout the talocrural, subtalar, and forefoot
- Post-traumatic arthritis with potential talocrural fusion
- Peroneal nerve injury

Calcaneal Fractures
Calcaneal fractures result from high falls and may be associated with spiral fractures throughout the lower extremity (Chapter Appendix Table 3-A.15) [24].

Forefoot Fractures
Forefoot fractures and dislocations are the result of crush injuries (Chapter Appendix Table 3-A.16) [25].

Spinal Fractures
Cervical Fracture
Cervical fractures result from abnormal loading to the head and neck as seen with low-load/high-velocity accidents (e.g., whiplash) or with the high-loading forces of direct impact to the head and neck (e.g., diving accidents, sports-related accidents). The central and peripheral nervous systems may not incur direct trauma; however, patients must be monitored closely, as swelling may result in transient neurologic involvement known as neurapraxia. Without medical intervention, permanent damage can occur [26] (Chapter Appendix Table 3-A.17).

Thoracolumbar Fractures
Thoracolumbar fractures are hyperflexion-forced fractures of the vertebral bodies that result from excessive spinal loading into flexion [27, 28] (Chapter Appendix Table 3-A.18).

The following are complications associated with thoracolumbar fractures:

- Loss of neurologic homeostasis

- Pseudoarthrosis, also known as a *false joint* (A pseudoarthrosis is caused by fracture nonunion, which allows abnormal motion to occur.)

- Chronic back pain

Upper-Extremity Fractures
Shoulder Girdle Fractures
Shoulder girdle fractures result from high-energy trauma, which is commonly sustained in automobile and motorcycle accidents. Little treatment is needed to manage scapula body and spine fractures because the surrounding musculature serves to protect and immobilize these fractures. Fractures involving the articulation of the glenohumeral joint or coracoid process are more complicated and may result in post-traumatic arthritis. These fractures are commonly associated with spine and rib fractures, pulmonary injuries, trauma to the brachial plexus, and shoulder dislocations [29] (Chapter Appendix Table 3-A.19).

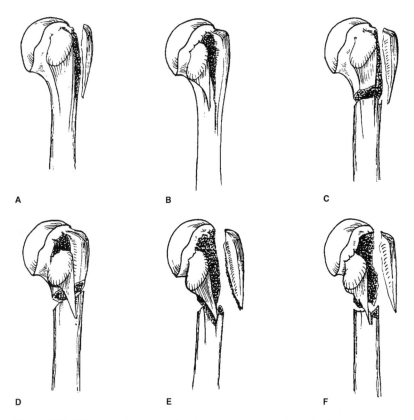

Figure 3-8. *Humerus fractures. A. Two-part greater tuberosity fracture. B. Two-part lesser tuberosity fracture. C. Three-part greater tuberosity and shaft fracture. D. Three-part lesser tuberosity and shaft fracture. E. Four-part fracture. F. Four-part fracture. (Reprinted with permission from SH Kozin, AC Berlet. Handbook of Common Orthopaedic Fractures [2nd ed]. Westchester, PA: Medical Surveillance, 1992;45.)*

Humeral Fractures
Proximal humeral fractures and humeral shaft fractures (Figure 3-8) occur when the humerus is subjected to direct and indirect trauma and can be associated with glenohumeral dislocation, rotator cuff injuries, and brachial plexus or peripheral nerve damage (Chapter Appendix Tables 3-A.20 and 3-A.21).

The following are complications associated with proximal humeral fractures:

- Nonunion
- Avascular necrosis of humeral head
- Hypomobility of the glenohumeral joint
- Abnormal posture (usually anteriorly tilted and downwardly rotated scapula)
- Abnormal scapulothoracic rhythm

The following are complications associated with humeral shaft fractures:

- Radial nerve injury
- Nonunion or malunion
- Glenohumeral hypomobility

Clinical tip

- A Rowe sling (which maintains the shoulder in slight flexion, 0 degrees of abduction, and internal rotation across the abdomen by use of an adduction strap across the trunk and a flexion strap placed around the neck) offers better stability than standard slings. This type of sling is used for rotator cuff and anterior ligamentous injuries and repairs.

- When the patient is lying supine, placing a pillow under the humeral shaft will help maintain neutral alignment with the trunk and reduce pain.

Olecranon Fractures
Olecranon fractures result from direct trauma, commonly a fall onto a flexed upper extremity. These are typically associated with humeral fractures and elbow dislocations [30]. Medical management and physical therapy interventions for olecranon fractures are presented in Chapter Appendix Table 3-A.22.
 The following are complications associated with olecranon fractures:

- Nonunion
- Hypomobility

- Ulnar nerve injury

- Myositis ossificans

Forearm Fractures
Forearm fractures occur with a wide variety of injuries, often high-velocity falls and sports injuries. Most adult forearm fractures are displaced and affect both the ulna and radius [31]. Dorsally displaced radial fractures are referred to as *Colles' fractures* (Figure 3-9); volarly displaced radial fractures are referred to as *Smith's fractures* [32]. Medical management and physical therapy interventions for forearm fractures are presented in Chapter Appendix Table 3-A.23.
The following are complications of forearm fractures:

- Nonunion or malunion

- Redisplacement of proximal and distal radioulnar units

- Malalignment and length discrepancy between radius and ulna

- Hypomobility of the elbow, forearm, and wrist

Carpal Fractures
Carpal fractures result from forced wrist extension with radial deviation and result in disruption of both the proximal and distal carpal rows, affecting wrist biomechanics. Medical management and physical therapy interventions are presented in Chapter Appendix Table 3-A.24.
The following are complications of carpal fractures:

- Nonunion or malunion

- Post-traumatic arthritis of radioscaphoid and scaphocapitate joints

- Avascular necrosis, which leads to intracarpal collapse and can lead to wrist fusion

- Wrist hypomobility

- Median nerve injury

Clinical tip

For patients who have concurrent lower- and upper-extremity involvement (e.g., fracture or hematoma) and need to use

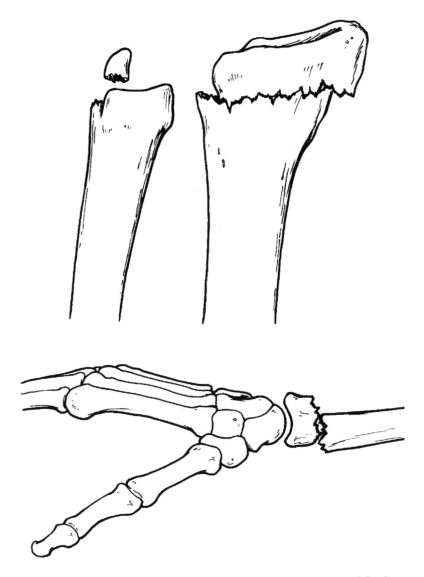

Figure 3-9. *Colles' fracture. Note the dorsal and radial deviation of the distal fragment and the ulna styloid avulsion. (Reprinted with permission from A Unwin, K Jones. Emergency Orthopaedics and Trauma. Oxford: Butterworth–Heinemann, 1995;138.)*

a walker or crutches, a platform attachment placed on the ambulatory assistive device will allow weight bearing to occur through the upper extremity proximal to the wrist.

Metacarpal Fractures
Metacarpal fractures result from direct trauma, such as a crush injury, or by long-axis loading, as is seen with punching injuries. The fracture may be accompanied by severe soft tissue injuries that can result in a treatment delay of 3–5 days to allow edema to resolve [32]. Definitive treatment depends on the exact location of the metacarpal involved (Chapter Appendix Table 3-A.25).

The following are complications of metacarpal injuries:

- Limited metacarpal motion
- Malunion
- Extensor tendon adhesions, which may require extensor tenolysis
- Reflex sympathetic dystrophy
- Cosmetic deformities

Phalangeal Fractures
Phalangeal fractures result from crush forces and consequently are usually compounded by soft tissue damage of the skin, tendons, and ligaments (Chapter Appendix Table 3-A.26) [32].

The following are complications of phalangeal fractures:

- Hypomobility
- Malunion with rotatory malalignment
- Tendon adhesions
- Cosmetic deformity

Clinical tip

Sterile whirlpool treatments can facilitate wound healing. This treatment must be approved by the physician.

Joint Replacement Surgeries

Joint replacement surgeries provide caregivers with some of the most predictable postoperative course information and expected outcomes in the orthopedic acute care setting. As a result, there is a high level of expectation for all patients to accomplish specific short- and long-term goals. The following sections provide basic surgical information as well as clinical techniques and tips.

Hip Replacement Surgery

Hip replacement surgery involves the replacement of either the femoral head, the acetabulum, or both with prosthetic components. A total hip replacement (THR) consists of replacing both the femoral head and the acetabulum, as shown in Figure 3-10. The components may or may not be cemented into the bone. The benefit of cement is immediate stability, which often allows full weight bearing. The disadvantage of cement is that it often loosens over time and with activity; therefore, cement may not be used in young or very active patients. Surgical approaches and precautions for hip replacement surgery are presented in Table 3-4.

A good understanding of the surgical approach taken to expose the hip joint for repair is necessary because the approach will determine the precautions and help prevent the complication of postoperative hip dislocation. In the acute care setting, the risk of hip dislocation is significant. The joint is positioned deep within the pelvic girdle; therefore, both muscle masses and joint capsular structures are incised and reflected to expose the area for surgery. Consequently, the hip remains at high risk for dislocation until the supporting muscle and joint structures are healed. The priority of physical therapy intervention becomes early functional mobilization accompanied by good precaution awareness. When in doubt about the surgical approach, the physical therapist should consult with the surgeon.

Physical Therapy Intervention for Hip Replacement Surgery

- The priority of treatment is to achieve safe functional mobility (i.e., bed mobility, sit-to-stand transfers, and ambulation with assistive devices) and maximize independence. The therapist accomplishes this by calming the patient's fears about the use of the limb

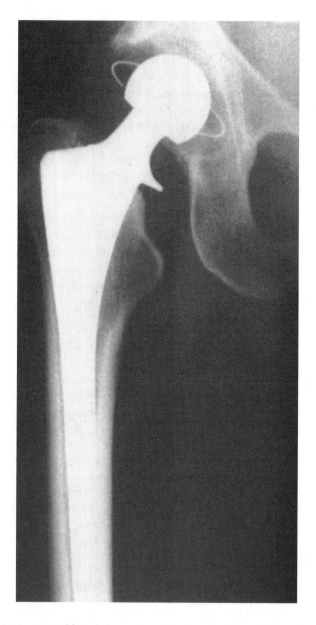

Figure 3-10. *A total hip replacement. (Reprinted with permission from A Unwin, K Jones. Emergency Orthopaedics and Trauma. Oxford: Butterworth–Heinemann, 1995;196.)*

Table 3-4. Surgical Approaches and Precautions for Hip Replacement Surgeries*

Type of Surgical Approach	Precautions
Posterior (most common approach)	No hip flexion beyond 90 degrees No hip IR past neutral No hip adduction past neutral
Lateral (more complicated surgical technique, allows more hip stability immediately after the operation)	No combined hip flexion beyond 90 degrees with adduction, IR, or both
Anterior (rare secondary to the high risks associated with the neurovascular structures passing through the femoral triangle)	Hip extension and external rotation are to be avoided

IR = internal rotation.

*Hip replacement surgery done in conjunction with a trochanteric osteotomy will warrant additional limitation with no active hip abduction and may often result in more limited weight-bearing parameters. Trochanteric osteotomies are commonly done in complex hip replacement surgery and in hip revision surgery.

Source: Data from GJ Benke. Joint Replacement. In PA Downie (ed), Cash's Textbook of Orthopaedics and Rheumatology for the Physiotherapist. Philadelphia: Lippincott, 1984;427.

that has undergone surgery. The therapist should also assure the patient that movement will help decrease pain.

• ROM at the patient's hip should be maintained within the parameters of hip precautions.

• Isometric gluteal and quadriceps contractions should be initiated on the first postoperative day. Clinicians must remember to always assess distal peripheral motor innervation on initial evaluation, because nerve injury may have occurred. Before establishing an advanced strengthening exercise program, it is necessary to consult with the physician because excessive strain could hinder healing of surgically involved structures.

• Patient education is a key factor in achieving a successful outcome. Precautions must be reiterated throughout all treatment sessions. Verbal and tactile cueing can be useful in assisting patients in precaution maintenance, because failure to adhere to all precautions can lead to THR dislocation.

Clinical tip

• Knee immobilizers reduce hip flexion by maintaining knee extension. This can be helpful in preventing THR dislocation in patients who are unable to maintain posterior hip precautions without assistance.

• Instruct the patient to avoid pivoting when turning. Turns should be initiated by moving the feet and taking many small steps.

• Elevation of the height of the bed reduces the degree of hip flexion and work of the hip abductors and extensors, facilitating sit-to-stand transfers.

Knee Replacement Surgery

Knee replacement surgery can be classified as total or partial. *Total knee replacement* (TKR) is the replacement of the femoral condyles and the tibial articulating surface. The dorsal surface of the patella may or may not be replaced depending on the extent of the degenerative changes. *Partial knee replacement* (also known as a *unicondylar* or *unicompartmental knee replacement*) is the replacement of the worn femoral and tibial articulating surfaces in either the medial or lateral knee compartment.

The goal of a unicompartmental knee replacement is to maximize the preservation of unaffected articular cartilage in the healthier compartment. Patients undergoing this surgery may demonstrate associated impairments, such as a valgus deformity or soft tissue contractures. These impairments can be corrected by surgical release of the soft tissues or with tibial osteotomy at the time of surgery [33]. The therapist must take into account any additional procedures performed (e.g., lateral release or tibial osteotomy) because additional procedures can reduce patient tolerance and capabilities immediately after the operation, prolong length of stay, and result in decreased functional mobility on discharge [34].

Physical Therapy Intervention for Knee Replacement Surgery

Physical therapy intervention techniques for knee replacement surgeries include ROM exercises, soft tissue mobilization, and positioning techniques.

Range-of-Motion Exercises
Inadequate knee ROM is one of the most common postoperative complications of TKR. Consequently, regaining joint mobility becomes the priority. ROM at the knee is most effectively achieved by both active and passive techniques. Passive ROM (PROM) includes manual assistance as well as the use of a CPM. The CPM should be initiated within 24–48 hours postoperatively (per physician). With active-assistive ROM (AAROM), the major limitation to knee range is post-traumatic muscle guarding and associated swelling.

Note: At least 90 degrees of flexion is achieved in the operating room. Swelling, muscle guarding, pain, and apprehension are the only factors limiting knee motion. Physical therapy can affect all of these in positive ways.

Clinical tip

With AAROM, the use of hold relax techniques to the hamstrings works well to decrease muscle guarding and increase knee flexion by reciprocal inhibition of the quadriceps muscle. This technique also provides a dorsal glide of the tibia, which prepares the posterior capsule for flexion. Gentle massaging of the quadriceps mechanism over the muscle belly or throughout the peripatellar region will improve range and reduce muscle guarding.

With lateral release procedures (surgical release of the lateral patella soft tissue), there is an increased risk of lateral patellar subluxation with flexion; therefore, flexion parameters should be clarified with the surgeon. There is also an increase in edema and pain that will inhibit quadriceps performance.

Patients who have undergone a lateral release are slightly more compromised in their mobility after surgery and often benefit from the use of a knee immobilizer to improve stability and tolerance with functional mobility. They may also tend to require bracing longer than after a standard knee replacement procedure. Sit-to-stand transfers are also often more difficult for patients who have lateral-release procedures. By simply elevating the height of the bed both the degree of knee flexion and work load are reduced, allowing the patient an advantage and improving his or her level of functional mobility. As the patient progresses, the height of the bed should be lowered to simulate his or her home environment.

Soft Tissue

The therapist should assess the level of the inflammatory response of the knee and the condition of the surgical incision during treatment. Inflamed knees will respond better to less aggressive treatment techniques.

Clinical tip

• For inflamed and reactive knees, the therapist should alter the treatment plan to include more frequent, shorter sessions (e.g., one to two times a day for 20–30 minutes as opposed to one 40- to 60-minute session).

• The use of ice in conjunction with the CPM at submaximal ROM settings for a prolonged duration will maintain knee motion and assist in edema reduction.

Positioning Techniques

It is important to implement positioning techniques early in physical therapy intervention after TKR in order to facilitate full knee extension. Pillows should not be placed under the patient's knee but rather under the distal calf.

Clinical tip

• Faulty knee braces or immobilizers can keep the knee positioned in as much as 10 degrees of knee flexion. (The therapist should inspect the knee immobilizer; often, the brace will have a moderate bend into flexion. The brace must be straightened to 0 degrees by adjusting the hinge, reverse bending the metal insert, or by obtaining a new brace.)

• The therapist should place a blanket roll along the lateral femur-trochanter to maintain neutral positioning of the lower extremity because patients often externally rotate their hips in bed, which results in slight knee flexion.

Strengthening Exercises
Quadriceps retraining is best initiated with isometric exercise. The use of contralateral limb or distal limb overflow techniques can improve quadriceps recruitment. When the knee presents with significant effusion or edema, 0 degrees of extension may not be available secondary to capsular distention. As a result, pain and swelling may inhibit quadriceps recruitment.

Clinical tip

The therapist should place a pillow or folded blanket under the knee in the degree of available range toward extension while performing isometric exercises. This will allow the quadriceps to succeed by reducing passive stretch on joint receptors and pain receptors as well as provide posterior support to the knee for feedback.

Functional Mobility
Functional mobility includes bed mobility; transfer training sit-to-stand from a chair, commode, or low seat; and gait training. Gait training on level surfaces is done with assistive devices (e.g., walker or crutches), knee immobilizer (for 2–3 days), and weight-bearing parameters (per physician). Gait training involving stair ambulation is also done with assistive devices.

Total Shoulder Replacement

Total shoulder replacement (TSR) surgery involves the replacement of the glenoid fossa and proximal humeral head with prosthetic components. Indications for shoulder replacement are osteoarthritis, rheumatoid arthritis, or the destruction of glenoid fossa secondary to trauma, which results in significant degenerative changes to both joint surfaces. Table 3-5 describes the types of surgical approaches performed and the physical therapy intervention techniques.

Rehabilitation depends on the extent of soft tissue destruction surrounding the joint before TSR, as well as the surgical approach and muscle dissection performed.

Table 3-5. Surgical Approaches, Assistive Devices, and Physical Therapy Intervention for Total Shoulder Replacement Surgery

Surgical Approach	Assistive Device	Physical Therapy Intervention
Deltopectoral (most common) Lateral retraction of deltoid, allowing for removal of distal clavicle or anterior deltoid	Rowe sling	Pendulum exercises
Anterior-medial Offers increased exposure by taking the deltoid down from the anterior clavicle and acromion, which delays physical therapy	Rowe sling	Postural training with focus on scapula positioning Scapulothoracic and distal (elbow, wrist, and hand) isometric exercises
Posterior (rarely performed) Removal of the deltoid muscle from the posterior spine with risk of supraspinous nerve injury	Abduction brace	Distal range-of-motion exercises only (elbow and below)

Source: Data from The Shoulder, Arm, and Elbow. In CM Evarts, Surgery of the Musculoskeletal System. New York: Churchill Livingstone, 1983.

Proximal Humeral Hemiarthroplasty

Proximal humeral hemiarthroplasty is performed secondary to degenerative changes affecting the humeral head or as the result of traumatic displaced fractures of the humeral head. In surgery, the proximal head is replaced with a prosthetic component. The rehabilitation following a proximal humeral hemiarthroplasty is similar to that of a TSR (see Table 3-5).

Experimental Total Joint Replacement

There are two types of experimental total joint replacement surgeries currently in the developmental and research stages: total ankle replacement and total elbow replacement (Table 3-6). The indication for these surgeries is to maintain functional mobility, which may be compromised as the result of severe degenerative changes and pain associated with rheumatoid arthritis and osteoarthritis of the elbow and ankle joints.

Table 3-6. Medical Management and Physical Therapy Interventions for Experimental Joint Replacement

Type	Medical Management	Physical Therapy Intervention
Total ankle replacement	Short-leg rigid immobilization	Edema management Functional mobility NWB status ROM exercises per physician's orders only
Total elbow replacement	Immobilization in slight flexion	Proximal and distal ROM exercises Edema management

NWB = non–weight-bearing; ROM = range of motion.

The following are complications of total ankle and total elbow replacement surgeries [35, 36]:

- Dislocation

- Infection

- Loosening or failing of prosthetic hardware

- Failure of bony ingrowth around and throughout the prosthesis

- Chronic pain of undetermined etiology

- Limb length discrepancy

- Fracture

Surgeries of the Spine

Disorders of the spine can be extremely debilitating and can limit a patient's ability to work and complete activities of daily living (ADLs). Because the axioskeleton is the core structure of the torso and is involved in all movement patterns of the upper and lower extremities, it commonly compensates for impairments of strength, muscle length, and joint mobility throughout the body. Over time, chronic compensation will abnormally load the spine and result in degenerative changes of the discs, vertebral bodies, facets, and intervertebral foramen. The chief complaint of most people with back dysfunctions is pain, which may be caused by the following [37]:

- Ligamentous sprain or muscle strain as the result of acute injury or repetitive chronic strain

- Rupture of intervertebral disc or herniated nucleus pulposus

- Spinal stenosis (narrowing of the spinal canal resulting in neural compression)

- Progressive degeneration of the vertebral disc, vertebral bodies, facet joints, or any combination of these

Medical management always looks to conservative treatment options first. These include the following:

- Bed rest with bathroom privileges up to 4 weeks

- Use of anti-inflammatory, antispasmodic, and analgesic medications

- Outpatient physical therapy, including patient education, bracing, body mechanics re-education, strengthening, stretching, manual techniques (e.g., joint mobilization), mechanical techniques (e.g., traction), and modalities (e.g., electrical stimulation, ultrasound)

- Lifestyle modification for completion of ADLs and participation in recreational and leisure activities

- Ergonomic modifications to occupational, home, and automobile environments

If dysfunction persists, surgery may be considered (Table 3-7). The role of the physical therapist in the acute care setting is to maximize the patient's functional mobility while maintaining neutral spinal alignment. Spinal alignment and reduction of biomechanical stresses caused by positioning (sitting places the greatest compressive stress on the lumbar spine) allow for optimal healing.

The following are complications associated with surgeries of the spine:

- Nerve damage commonly involving the nerve root

- Persistent back pain

- Infection

- Fusion

- Nonunion

Table 3-7. Medical Indications and Physical Therapy Interventions for Surgeries of the Spine

Surgery	Medical Indications	Physical Therapy Intervention
Laminectomy (removal of bone at the interlaminar space)	Spinal stenosis Nerve root compression	Lower-extremity strengthening Functional transfer techniques (log rolling optional*) Gait training (assistive devices as indicated) Patient education (body mechanics, postural awareness)
Discectomy (partial or complete removal of the intervertebral disc [may be done in conjunction with laminectomy])	HNP	See Laminectomy, above
Spinal fusion (fusion of the facet joints at a given vertebral level by either iliac bone graft or the use of mechanical hardware)	Segment instability Fractures Facet joint arthritis	Functional mobility with strict log rolling* Limited mobility (flexion not allowed) Limited lifting per physician Brace or corset per physician
Foraminotomy (removal of the spinous process and entire laminae to the level of the pedicle [will usually require fusion to retain spinal stabilization])	Spinal stenosis Multiple HNP Multiple nerve root compression	See Spinal fusion, above

HNP = herniated nucleus pulposus.
*Log rolling is a technique used for bed mobility that limits the patient's trunk rotation by having the patient turn as a single segment. The patient is instructed to move the shoulders and hips as one unit, or "as a log."

Clinical tip

- Patients commonly experience persistent and possibly new radicular symptoms immediately after surgery. These symptoms tend to be transient and are thought to be a result of the acute inflammatory response to the surgery. A significant increase in the patient's report of pain is abnormal and should be reported to the physician.

• Elevating the height of the bed and the use of tall chairs can facilitate sit-to-stand transfers. This also minimizes trunk flexion and fosters an upright posture.

• As a splinting mechanism for pain after spinal surgery, patients often forward bend when using assistive devices. Forward bending results in increased biomechanical strain and work of the spine. It is optimal to encourage ambulation without use of an assistive device.

• Rolling walkers are helpful during initial stages of gait training because the patient will not need to lift the walker to advance in gait.

• Corsets can be useful to minimize pain and serve as a reminder to maintain proper posture and body mechanics.

• Patients should be educated in alternative lifting and bending techniques. Demonstration is an effective way to teach body mechanics with ADLs, as most patients do not have the tolerance to perform all activities with the therapist.

• The therapist should be sure to confirm the exact amount of weight a patient can lift to accurately educate him or her before discharge. Adaptive devices are useful to avoid excessive bending and reaching.

Soft Tissue Surgeries

Soft tissue surgeries encompass a wide variety of procedures to repair or reconstruct contractile and noncontractile tissues. The primary goals of surgery are to improve joint stability or repair disruption of muscles and tendons and to improve functional muscle or tendon length. Common soft tissue surgeries include muscle repairs, tendon transfers, fasciotomies, cartilage resections, and ligament reconstructions. Patients are often discharged from the hospital within 24–48 hours after surgery. Consequently, the primary role of physical therapy is to educate and train the patient to maximize his or her own functional mobility and minimize postoperative complications. Technologic advancement of surgical techniques and early initiation of rehabilitation have resulted in a wide variety of protocols and a lack of standardized parameters. Tables 3-8 and 3-9 and Figures 3-11 and 3-12 describe the most common soft tissue surgeries performed on the knee and shoulder. Infection and joint hypomobility are complications associated with knee and shoulder soft tissue surgeries.

Orthopedic Equipment for Fracture and Soft Tissue Injury Management

Cast

A cast is a circumferential rigid dressing used to provide the immobilization necessary for musculoskeletal healing. Casts can be made of plaster or fiberglass material and can be used on almost any body part. The rigidity of the cast allows for fracture stabilization with maintenance of the deformity realignment and pain reduction [38]. Casts can also be used to provide low-load, prolonged, passive stretch to soft tissue to improve ROM. This is known as *serial casting*. Specific joint positioning is determined by the physician. Table 3-10 lists the common types of casts and immobilization positions.

The following are complications associated with casts:

• Neurovascular compromise or compartment syndrome are conditions caused by decreased venous return, the constriction of edematous tissues within a muscle compartment, or both. This may be caused by excessive swelling or the improper fit of a cast. Venous pressure of more than 30 mm Hg will compromise arterial blood flow leading to ischemia. Venous pressures must be relieved immediately by elevation, splitting or bivalving the cast, cast removal, or surgical fasciotomy (surgical release of fascia dividing muscle compartments to allow tissue expansion and increase arterial blood flow), depending on the source of pressure constriction and the physical examination [38].

• Nerve compression is compression of a peripheral nerve over bony prominence (i.e., peroneal nerve next to the fibula head) by the cast. This form of nerve entrapment can result in transient or permanent nerve damage depending on how long the nerve is compressed.

Table 3-8. Types of Repair and Reconstruction and Physical Therapy Interventions for Soft Tissue Surgeries of the Knee

Surgery	Type of Repair and Reconstruction	Physical Therapy Intervention
Ligamentous repairs and reconstruction Anterior cruciate ligament avulsion (either treated as a fracture, in which the bone segment that avulsed is reattached and fixed with a screw, or the remaining ligament is removed, in which case reconstruction is performed)	Reattachment of bony avulsion if possible	Immobilization with brace or cast per physician Edema management Proximal and distal ROM exercises Functional mobility with weight-bearing parameters per physician

Anterior cruciate ligament reconstruction [40] or posterior cruciate ligament reconstruction (Postoperative course is dependent on physician preferences.)	Autograph
	  Middle one-third patellar tendon
	  Hamstring tendon
	Allograft
	  Patellar or hamstring tendon
	Prosthetic
	  Synthetic ligament
		Edema management
		Proximal and distal joint ROM exercises
		Functional mobility with weight-bearing parameters per physician
		Bracing per physician (The patient should be independent in donning and doffing the brace as appropriate.)
		Knee ROM exercises per physician (The physician should determine whether the patient performs AROM or PROM exercises.)
		Quadriceps and hamstring strengthening per physician

Cartilage surgery Meniscal repair (reattachment of	Usually done in conjunction with	See Anterior and posterior cruciate recon-

torn meniscus)	ligamentous reconstruction	struction, above
Meniscectomy (removal of part or all of meniscus)	See Meniscal repair, above	See Anterior and posterior cruciate reconstruction, above
Extensor mechanism surgery		
Lateral retinacular release	Patellofemoral soft tissue Tibiofemoral soft tissue	See Anterior and posterior cruciate reconstruction, above
Quadricepsplasty	Separation of quadriceps mechanism, lengthening of the quadriceps mechanism, or both	See Anterior and posterior cruciate reconstruction, above

ROM = range of motion; AROM = active range of motion; PROM = passive range of motion.

Table 3-9. Soft Tissue Surgeries of the Shoulder

	Type of Repair or Reconstruction	Physical Therapy Intervention
Anterior shoulder instability		
Anterior capsulo-labral recon-struction [41]	Anterior capsular shift	Patient instruction in donning and doffing sling
	Anterior capsular shift with labral repair	Scapulothoracic isometrics Postural education Distal edema management Wrist and hand strengthening
Muscle and tendon repair		
Rotator cuff repair [42]	Including but not limited to the following:	Upper-extremity pendulum exercises per physician (The physician determines
	Biceps tendon repair Supraspinatus repair Rotator cuff avulsion	whether the exercise is done with the sling off or on.)

- Skin breakdown can occur secondary to increased pressure, moisture development in the cast (causing blister formation), open skin lesions, or any combination of these.

Clinical tip

The following tips are helpful for minimizing secondary complications of casts and in the promotion of maximal comfort:

- The therapist should elevate all distal extremities 4–5 inches above the heart to allow gravity to assist venous return. Elevation of more than 5 inches can increase venous pressure, causing increased cardiovascular work load [38].

- Casts should not get wet. The therapist should instruct the patient to wrap the cast in a waterproof bag during bathing or showering. Exposing casting materials to water

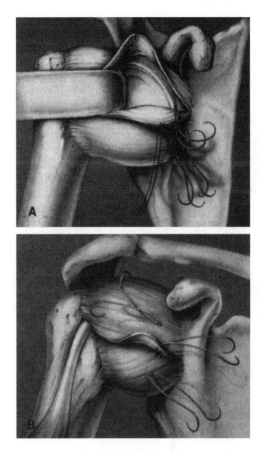

Figure 3-11. *Anterior capsulolabral reconstruction procedure with sutures in place. A. Inferior flap will be brought superiorly. B. Superior flap is brought inferiorly. (Reprinted with permission from FW Jobe, M Pink. Classification and treatment of shoulder dysfunction in the overhead athlete. J Orthop Sports Phys Ther 1993,18:427.)*

weakens the structure and traps moisture against the skin. Patients in body casts cannot shower and must be instructed to sponge bathe.

- The therapist should instruct the patient to contact the physician if the following develop: symptoms of burning,

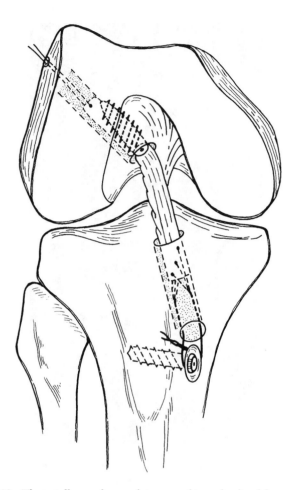

Figure 3-12. *The patellar tendon graft is secured into the distal femur with an interference screw and into the tibia with a bicortical screw. (Reprinted with permission from KE Wilk, JR Andrews. Current concepts in the treatment of anterior cruciate ligament disruption. J Orthop Sports Phys Ther 1992,15:279.)*

numbness, or tingling; movement of the limb within the cast; or a strong odor from within the cast.

• The therapist should discourage patients from sliding objects in the cast to scratch itchy skin. Such objects can

Table 3-10. Types of Casts

Type	Location	Immobilization
Short-arm	Forearm and wrist	Forearm supination and pronation Wrist flexion and extension Wrist radial and ulna deviation
Long-arm	Upper arm, forearm, and wrist	Fixed elbow flexion Forearm supination and pronation Wrist flexion and extension Wrist radial and ulnar deviation
Body	Thoracic and lumbar spine	All thoracic and lumbar motions
Minerva jacket	Head, neck, and thoracic spine	All cervical motions
Body spica	Thoracic and lumbar spine with single or bilateral hip joints	All thoracic and lumbar motions Fixed hip motion into flexion, extension, abduction, and adduction
Thumb spica	Thumb and wrist	Wrist flexion and extension Wrist radial and ulnar deviation Thumb flexion and extension Thumb abduction and adduction
Shoulder spica	Shoulder and upper thoracic spine	Fixed shoulder flexion, abduction and rotation Fixed scapula position
Long-leg	Upper leg, lower leg, and foot	Fixed knee flexion and extension Fixed ankle dorsiflexion Fixed foot position with neutral inversion and eversion
Short-leg	Lower leg and foot	Fixed ankle dorsiflexion Fixed foot position with neutral inversion and eversion

be lost in the cast, increasing the risk of pressure sore formation, or the skin may be broken, increasing the risk of infection. Because the cast provides a moist and warm environment, bacterial growth can develop at an accelerated rate and develop into a gangrenous lesion.

- Most casts are not rigid enough to withstand the forces of weight bearing. Weight-bearing parameters must be clarified by the physician.

- For patients who have casts encompassing the foot and are allowed to weight bear with transfers and ambulation, a nonslip cast boot should be provided.

- It is important to reinforce the importance that the patient move all joints proximal and distal to the cast to maintain functional ROM.

Traction

Traction involves the use of a distractive force on the bone to restore alignment of a fracture or joint [39]. Types of traction are presented in Table 3-11. The weight is applied distal to the area of involvement by either direct (skeletal traction) or indirect (skin traction) means. Skeletal traction uses pins or wires placed through the bone to provide distractive force. It is maintained continuously; therefore, the patient is on strict bed rest. Skeletal traction is more effective as a distraction tool than skin traction. Skin traction can be removed for intermittent use of the involved extremity per physician's orders.

The following are complications associated with traction:

- Decreased joint mobility after the joint is removed from immobilization

- Generalized muscle atrophy of the immobilized limbs

- Deconditioning of the cardiovascular system

- Pulmonary compromise secondary to bed rest

- Skin breakdown or decubitus ulcer formation of the immobilized limb and high pressure areas secondary to bed rest (see Chapter 7, "The Pathophysiology of Wounds")

- Infection of the traction pin sites

- Delayed union or nonunion of the fracture

- Joint hypermobility (at the joint closest to the skeletal pin site)

Table 3-11. Types of Traction

Type	Description and Use
Skin traction	Used intermittently on less severe injuries; helps relieve pain secondary to muscle spasm
Buck's traction	Provides distraction of the lower extremity
Russell traction or pillow suspension	Positioning device to maintain neutral alignment of the lower extremity
Bryant traction	Used in children younger than 3 yrs of age with congenital hip dislocation
Dunlop traction	Humeral fractures
Skeletal traction	Continuous application for prolonged period of time (days to weeks); used to treat severe injuries
Skeletal tongs	Cervical or upper thoracic fractures
Skeletal Dunlop	Humeral fractures
Halo traction	Cervical fractures
90–90 traction	Pediatric femoral fractures
Positioning devices	
Balanced suspension	A positioning system suspended from the bed frame; used in conjunction with skeletal traction
Pillow suspension	A positioning system suspended from the bed frame

---

Clinical tip

• The therapist must have good working knowledge of the traction apparatus to allow removal and reapplication during the treatment session. Physician orders must be received to remove or adjust the traction unit.

• The patient's position in bed allows for proper alignment of the traction forces; therefore, the therapist must maintain neutral alignment of the limb in traction.

- It is important to monitor the lower extremity's position when in traction because external rotation of the hip can cause compression of the peroneal nerve against the suspension device and result in nerve palsy.

External Fixation Devices

An external fixation device is a device consisting of pins that insert at an oblique or right angle to the long axis of the bone and that are connected externally to the skin by a frame. The frame provides the alignment forces to fracture ends and maintains reduction while healing occurs [39]. External fixation devices are used in severely comminuted fractures, open fractures, fractures with severe soft tissue or vascular injuries, or when infection is present. An additional use of external fixation is to lengthen a long bone when a space between fracture ends remains. This technique is performed using an Ilizarov frame. The advantage of external fixation devices is that they allow medical management of associated injuries, such as skin grafts, and areas of debridement. They also provide fracture stability with early mobilization. External fixation devices can be placed on the upper extremity, lower extremity, pelvis, and cervical spine.

The following are complications of external fixation devices:

- Infection of the pin sites
- Cutaneous nerve damage secondary to pin placement
- Muscle impingement
- Loss of fracture reduction
- Nonunion or malunion

Clinical tip

- It is important to maintain full ROM of all joints proximal and distal to the external fixator. Foot plates can be attached to the lower leg fixator to maintain neutral ankle dorsiflexion.

- Elevation of the extremity will decrease edema by assisting in venous return and reducing pain.

- The external fixator is very sturdy and can be used to assist in moving the involved limb (grasping the fixator frame to lift the involved extremity is allowed).
- Clear drainage, as well as slight bleeding at the pin sites, is normal.

Braces and Splints

Braces are used in conjunction with medical and surgical intervention techniques for management of musculoskeletal dysfunctions. Functional bracing is based on the concept that continued function during healing promotes osteogenesis (bone growth) and enhances soft tissue healing while preventing joint hypomobility and disuse atrophy [39]. Bracing can be used to maintain fracture alignment during healing, joint stabilization, and anatomic joint alignment and to minimize weight-bearing forces on the bone. Braces can be applied immediately at the time of injury or used as part of a progressive treatment course following conventional casting or traction. They may be prefabricated or custom made. Education must be provided to any patient receiving a brace orthosis regarding the functional parameters of the brace, donning and doffing, and brace maintenance. An orthotist is the best resource regarding the benefit of bracing, bracing options, and brace hygiene and should be consulted if questions or the need for modification arises. Table 3-12 lists custom-made bracing options and indications.

The following are complications associated with braces and splints:

- Improper fit
- Skin breakdown
- Improper use or poor compliance

Clinical tip

Training is vital for any patient receiving a brace or orthosis. The patient should have a good working knowledge of the function and purpose of the orthosis, as well as knowledge of donning, doffing, and hygiene.

Table 3-12. Types of Custom-Made Braces

Type of Brace	Indications and Description
Lower-extremity braces	
Long-leg cast brace (also known as a knee-ankle-foot orthosis)	Distal femur fractures Complex knee procedures Tibial plateau fractures
Patellar tendon brace or Sarmiento tibial brace	Tibial fractures Complex tibial reconstructions
Thigh braces with pelvic band or hip-knee-ankle-foot orthosis	Proximal femoral fractures Unilateral pelvic reconstruction Complex total hip replacement
Upper-extremity braces	
Sarmiento brace	Humeral shaft fractures
Spinal braces [43]	
Corset	Thoracolumbar and sacral support To limit extreme motion in the sagittal and frontal planes To remind patients of movement parameters (primary role)
Thoracolumbar orthosis	See Corset, above Encompassing the thoracic and lumbar spine and distally to the sacrum Can be extended proximally to cover the scapula and sternum with additional shoulder straps
Lumbosacral orthosis	See Corset, above Encompassing the abdomen, thoracolumbar region, and extending distally to the sacrum Rigid or flexible struts can be added for support
Sacroiliac orthosis	See Corset, above Encompassing the pelvis from iliac crests and extending distally to the greater trochanters
Rigid braces (constructed on a metal based frame that is firmly supported on the pelvis. The metal upright supports serve to provide correc-	

Type of Brace	Indications and Description
tive forces to aid in alignment corrections [i.e., posture])	
Taylor Norton Brown brace (TLSO brace)	Limits movement in the sagittal plane (flexion and extension) and frontal plane (side bending)
Fishers brace (TLSO brace)	See Taylor Norton Brown brace, above
Molded brace (TLSO brace)	See Taylor Norton Brown brace, above Consists of a body jacket extending from sternum to pubic symphysis
Anterior hyperextension brace (Jewett Brace)	See Taylor Norton Brown brace, above Provides positioning into hyperextension bases on three points of force
Correctional orthosis (rigid braces worn for years to correct spinal deformity)	
Milwaukee brace	Corrects structural scoliosis or management of ankylosing spondylitis
Boston brace	Corrects lumbar or thoracic scoliosis occurring below the eighth thoracic vertebral level
Cervical orthosis Temporary collar	Acute cervical sprains Will not control cervical movement
Thomas collar	Restricts cervical and occipital mobility Made of metal or thick plastic
Molded cervical orthosis	Restricts cervical motion Supports chin and occipital region while extending distally to the thorax
Sterno-occipital-mandibular immobilizer	Limits flexion between the first and fourth cervical vertebrae
Four-poster cervical brace	Limits flexion in the midcervical spine Supports the chin and the occipital region and extends distally to the sternum
Halo body jacket	Restricts cervical and upper thoracic motion in all planes Consists of oval halo band encircling the head and extending via body jacket to encompass the thorax

Table 3-12. *Continued*

Type of Brace	Indications and Description
Minerva jacket	Restricts cervical and upper thoracic motion in all planes Fabricated from plaster of paris, creating a body cast that encircles the chin and head and extends distally to the waist

TLSO = thoracolumbosacral orthosis.

References

1. Hoppenfeld S. Physical Examination of the Spine and Extremities. East Norwalk, CT: Appleton-Century-Crofts, 1976.
2. Principles and Concepts. In DJ Magee, Orthopedic Physical Assessment. Philadelphia: Saunders, 1987;1.
3. Magee DJ. Orthopedic Physical Assessment. Philadelphia: Saunders, 1987;25.
4. Ross ERS. Fractures. In PA Downie (ed), Cash's Text Book of Orthopedics and Rheumatology for the Physiotherapist. Philadelphia: Lippincott, 1984;451.
5. CL Thomas (ed). Taber's Cyclopedic Medical Dictionary (16th ed). Philadelphia: FA Davis, 1985.
6. Principles of Fractures. In A Apley, L Solomon, Apley's System of Orthopedics and Fractures (7th ed). Boston: Butterworth–Heinemann, 1993;515.
7. Musculoskeletal Trauma. In LA Mourad, Orthopedic Disorders: Mosby's Clinical Nursing Series. Boston: Mosby–Year Book, 1991;50.
8. Fracture of the Pelvic Ring. In RW Bucholz, MB Ezaki, FG Lipport, DR Wenger, Orthopaedic Decision Making. Philadelphia: BC Decker, 1984;28.
9. Injuries of the Pelvis. In A Apley, L Solomon, Apley's System of Orthopedics and Fractures (7th ed). Boston: Butterworth-Heinemann, 1993;639.
10. Laros GS. Dislocations of the Hip and Fractures of the Acetabulum. In CM Evarts (ed), Surgery of the Musculoskeletal System (Vol. 2, Sec. 5). New York: Churchill Livingstone, 1983;53.
11. Orthopedic Trauma. In RW Bucholz, MB Ezaki, FG Lipport, DR Wenger, Orthopaedic Decision Making. Philadelphia: BC Decker, 1984;34.
12. Pankovich AM. Intracapsular Fractures of the Femur. In CM Evarts (ed), Surgery of the Musculoskeletal System (Vol. 2, Sec. 5). New York: Churchill Livingstone, 1983;76.

13. Femoral Neck Fracture. In RW Bucholz, MB Ezaki, FG Lipport, DR Wenger, Orthopaedic Decision Making. Philadelphia: BC Decker, 1984;36
14. Laro GS. Intertrochanteric Fractures. In CM Evarts (ed), Surgery of the Musculoskeletal System (Vol. 2, Sec. 5). New York: Churchill Livingstone, 1983;123.
15. Spiegal PG, van der Schilden J. Subtrochanteric Fractures. In CM Evarts (ed), Surgery of the Musculoskeletal System (Vol. 2, Sec. 5). New York: Churchill Livingstone, 1983;149.
16. Femoral Shaft Fracture. In RW Bucholz, MB Ezaki, FG Lipport, DR Wenger, Orthopaedic Decision Making. Philadelphia: BC Decker, 1984;40.
17. Injuries of the Lower Limb. In A Apley, L Solomon, Apley's System of Orthopedics and Fractures (7th ed). Boston: Butterworth–Heinemann, 1993;670.
18. Zachazewski JE, Magee DJ, Quillen WS. Athletic Injuries and Rehabilitation. Philadelphia: Saunders, 1996;613.
19. McBreath A. The Patellofemoral Joint. In CM Evarts (ed), Surgery of the Musculoskeletal System (Vol. 3, Sec. 7). New York: Churchill Livingstone, 1983;185.
20. Tibial Plateau Fracture. In RW Bucholz, MB Ezaki, FG Lipport, DR Wenger, Orthopaedic Decision Making. Philadelphia: BC Decker, 1984;54.
21. Chapman MW. Fractures of the Tibial and Fibular Shafts. In CM Evarts (ed), Surgery of the Musculoskeletal System (Vol. 3, Sec. 8). New York: Churchill Livingstone, 1983;5.
22. Tibial Pylon Fracture. In RW Bucholz, MB Ezaki, FG Lipport, DR Wenger, Orthopaedic Decision Making. Philadelphia: BC Decker, 1984;60.
23. Yablon IG, Segal D. Ankle Fractures. In CM Evarts (ed), Surgery of the Musculoskeletal System (Vol. 3, Sec. 8). New York: Churchill Livingstone, 1983;87.
24. Fracture of the Calcaneus. In RW Bucholz, MB Ezaki, FG Lipport, DR Wenger, Orthopaedic Decision Making. Philadelphia: BC Decker, 1984;66.
25. Forefoot Fracture of Dislocation. In RW Bucholz, MB Ezaki, FG Lipport, DR Wenger, Orthopedic Decision Making. Philadelphia: BC Decker, 1984;72.
26. Stauffer ES. Management of Cervical Spine Injuries. In CM Evarts (ed), Surgery of the Musculoskeletal System (Vol. 2, Sec. 4). New York: Churchill Livingstone, 1983;259.
27. Thoracolumbar Fracture and Dislocation. In RW Bucholz, MB Ezaki, FG Lipport, DR Wenger, Orthopaedic Decision Making. Philadelphia: BC Decker, 1984;8.
28. Injuries of the Spine. In A Apley, L Solomon, Apley's System of Orthopedics and Fractures (7th ed). Boston: Butterworth–Heinemann, 1993;615.
29. Fracture of the Scapula. In RW Bucholz, MB Ezaki, FG Lipport, DR Wenger, Orthopaedic Decision Making. Philadelphia: BC Decker, 1984;16.
30. Fracture of the Humeral Shaft. In RW Bucholz, MB Ezaki, FG Lipport, DR Wenger, Orthopaedic Decision Making. Philadelphia: BC Decker, 1984;20.

31. Fracture of the Forearm. In RW Bucholz, MB Ezaki, FG Lipport, DR Wenger, Orthopaedic Decision Making. Philadelphia: BC Decker, 1984;24.
32. Hubbard LI. Fractures of the Hand and Wrist. In CM Evarts (ed), Surgery of the Musculoskeletal System (Vol. 1, Sec. 2). New York: Churchill Livingstone, 1983;81.
33. Degenerative Joint Disease of the Knee. In RW Bucholz, MB Ezaki, FG Lipport, DR Wenger, Orthopaedic Decision Making. Philadelphia: BC Decker, 1984;140.
34. Peterson LFA. Minimally Constrained Arthroplasty of the Knee. In CM Evarts (ed), Surgery of the Musculoskeletal System (Vol. 3, Sec. 7). New York: Churchill Livingstone, 1983;267.
35. Hip Pain Following Total Hip Reconstruction. In RW Bucholz, MB Ezaki, FG Lipport, DR Wenger (eds), Orthopaedic Decision Making. Philadelphia: BC Decker, 1984;114.
36. Benke G. Joint Replacement. In PA Downie (ed), Cash's Text Book of Orthopaedics and Rheumatology for Physiotherapist. Philadelphia: Lippincott, 1984;424.
37. Wiesel SW, Rothman RH. Lumbar Disc Disease and Spinal Stenosis. In CM Evarts (ed), Surgery of the Musculoskeletal System (Vol. 2). New York: Churchill Livingstone, 1983;57.
38. Casts, Traction, and External Fixation Devices. In LA Mourad, Mosby's Clinical Nursing Series: Orthopaedic Disorders. Boston: Mosby–Year Book, 1991;179.
39. Managment of Patients in Traction. In JDM Stewart, JP Hallett, Traction and Orthopaedic Appliances (2nd ed). New York: Churchill Livingstone, 1983;105.
40. Tovin BJ, Tovin TS, Tovin M. Surgical and biomechanical considerations in rehabilitation of patients with intra-articular ACL reconstructions. J Orthop Sports Phys Ther 1992;15:317.
41. Jobe FW, Pink M. Classification and treatment of shoulder dysfunction in the overhead athlete. J Orthop Sports Phys Ther 1993;18:427.
42. Meister K, Andrews JR. Classification and treatment of rotator cuff injuries in the overhand athlete. J Orthop Sports Phys Ther 1993;18:413.
43. Equipment. In MF Somers, Spinal Cord Injury: Functional Rehabilitation. Norwalk, CT: Appleton & Lange, 1992;331.
44. Unwin A, Jones K. Emergency Orthopaedics and Trauma. Oxford: Butterworth–Heinemann, 1995.

Appendix 3-A: Medical Management and Physical Therapy Interventions for Fractures

Table 3-A.1. Medical Management and Physical Therapy Interventions for Pelvic Fractures

Type	Medical Management	Physical Therapy Intervention
Stable (i.e., fractures not involving the ring or with minimal posterior ring displacement)	External fixation (see description in "The Clinical Goal of Fracture Management") ORIF techniques (see description in "The Clinical Goal of Fracture Management")	Functional mobility PWB status* Active range-of-motion exercises, including of the hip and distal joints Lower-extremity strengthening Physical therapy education
Unstable (i.e., multiple fractures involving rotatory and vertical displacement with or without posterior ring displacement)	Skeletal traction ORIF	Functional mobility NWB status (per physician) Active range-of-motion exercises, including the hip and distal joints

ORIF = open reduction internal fixation; PWB = partial weight-bearing; NWB = non–weight-bearing
*Weight-bearing status may vary per physician.

Table 3-A.2. Medical Management and Physical Therapy Interventions for Posterior Acetabular Fractures and Hip Dislocation

Type	Medical Management	Physical Therapy Intervention
Posterior hip dislocation with one minor fracture of acetabulum	Closed reduction	Functional mobility weight bearing (per physician) Gentle hip ROM exercises[a,b]
Posterior hip dislocation with one major fracture of posterior acetabulum	Closed reduction ORIF (if unstable)	Posterior hip precautions (per physician)[c]
Posterior hip dislocation with comminution of the acetabulum in addition to another major fracture	ORIF Skeletal traction	Functional mobility Posterior hip precautions (per physician)[c] Bed rest Positioning (ROM exercises for ankle) LE isometrics
Posterior hip dislocation with fracture of acetabulum rim and floor	ORIF	Functional mobility NWB status Gentle hip ROM exercises in all planes Posterior hip precautions (per physician)[c]
Posterior hip dislocation and fracture of femoral head	ORIF of the femoral head	Functional mobility NWB status Gentle hip ROM exercises in all planes Posterior hip precautions (per physician)[c]

ROM = range of motion; ORIF = open reduction internal fixation; LE = lower extremity; NWB = non–weight-bearing.

[a]*Gentle ROM* is defined as active-assistive range-of-motion techniques that are within the patient's tolerance. Tolerance is determined in part by the subjective report of pain as well as objective limitations of muscle guarding and pattern of motion. It is critical to maintain mobility of the joint surfaces to prevent joint fusion.

[b]The therapist should note that patients tend to be fearful and convey this fear as pain. Some pain is to be expected with movement; however, one should not force range of motion with progressively increasing pain.

[c]Standard posterior hip precautions limit hip flexion to 90 degrees, internal rotation to 0 degrees, and adduction to 0 degrees.

Source: Data from BL Freeman III. Acute Dislocations. In AH Grenshaw (ed), Campbells Operative Orthopaedics (Vol 3, 7th ed). St. Louis: Mosby, 1987.

Table 3-A.3. Medical Management and Physical Therapy Interventions for
Central Acetabular Fractures and Dislocations

Type	Medical Management	Physical Therapy Intervention
Central dislocation without fracture of weight-bearing dome of the acetabulum	Closed reduction	Functional mobilization Gentle hip ROM exercises in all planes[a]
Central dislocation with fracture of weight-bearing dome of the acetabulum	Skeletal Tx with delayed ORIF	Positioning while on bed rest ROM exercises to the uninvolved limbs and joints Gentle hip ROM exercises in all planes[a]
Acetabular fracture with posterior subluxation of the femoral head		
Nondisplaced fracture	Closed reduction	Functional mobilization
Displaced anterior column	Skeletal Tx, often with delayed ORIF	Gentle hip ROM exercises[a]
Displaced posterior column	ORIF	Posterior hip precautions[b]

ROM = range of motion; ORIF = open reduction internal fixation; Tx = traction.
[a]*Gentle ROM* is defined as active-assistive range-of-motion techniques that are within
the patient's tolerance. Tolerance is determined in part by the subjective report of pain
as well as objective limitations of muscle guarding and pattern of motion. It is critical
to maintain mobility of the joint surfaces to prevent joint fusion.
[b]Standard posterior hip precautions limit hip flexion to 90 degrees, internal rotation to
0 degrees, and adduction to 0 degrees.

Table 3-A.4. Medical Management and Physical Therapy Interventions for Intracapsular Hip Fractures

Fracture Classification	Medical Management	Physical Therapy Intervention
Garden I (impacted fracture with incomplete or minimal displacement)	ORIF with pins Occasional closed reduction NWB status	Functional mobility PWB status ROM exercises (limited by pain) LE strengthening
Garden II (complete fracture without displacement)	ORIF with pins	Functional mobility PWB status ROM exercises (limited by pain) LE strengthening
Garden III (complete fracture with partial displacement, capsule partially intact)	DHS or sliding nail screw	Functional mobility PWB status ROM exercises (limited by pain) LE strengthening
Garden IV (complete fracture with full displacement and capsule disruption)	Femoral prosthesis DHS	Functional mobility (PWB status advancing to WBAT status per physician) ROM exercises (usually with posterior hip precautions) Strengthening exercises

ORIF = open reduction internal fixation; NWB = non–weight-bearing; PWB = partial weight-bearing; ROM = range of motion; LE = lower extremity; DHS = dynamic hip screw; WBAT = weight bearing as tolerated.

Table 3-A.5. Medical Management and Physical Therapy Interventions for Intertrochanteric Fractures

Type	Medical Management	Physical Therapy Intervention
Stable (noncomminuted)	ORIF	Gentle ROM exercises* Functional mobility PWB status Strengthening exercises
Unstable (comminuted or multiple fragments)	ORIF Bone grafting to bony defects	Gentle ROM exercises* Functional mobility TDWB status Strengthening exercises

ORIF = open reduction internal fixation; ROM = range of motion; PWB = partial weight-bearing; TDWB = touch down weight-bearing.
*Gentle ROM is defined as active-assistive range-of-motion techniques that are within the patient's tolerance. Tolerance is determined in part by the subjective report of pain as well as objective limitations of muscle guarding and pattern of motion. It is critical to maintain mobility of the joint surfaces to prevent joint fusion.

Table 3-A.6. Medical Management and Physical Therapy Interventions for Subtrochanteric Hip Fractures

Type	Medical Management	Physical Therapy Intervention
I (two-part minimum comminution and short fractures)	ORIF-DHS plate and screws	Gentle hip ROM exercises* Strengthening exercises Functional mobility PWB status (per physician)
II (two-part minimum comminution and long fractures)	ORIF-DHS plate and screws	Gentle hip ROM exercises* Strengthening exercises Functional mobility PWB status (per physician)
III (four or more parts with comminution)	ORIF-DHS plate and screws	May require less weight bearing

ORIF-DHS = open reduction internal fixation—dynamic hip screw; ROM = range of motion; PWB = partial weight-bearing.
*Gentle ROM is defined as active-assistive range-of-motion techniques that are within the patient's tolerance. Tolerance is determined in part by the subjective report of pain as well as objective limitations of muscle guarding and pattern of motion. It is critical to maintain mobility of the joint surfaces to prevent joint fusion.

Table 3-A.7. Medical Management and Physical Therapy Interventions for Femur Shaft Fractures

Type	Medical Management	Physical Therapy Intervention
Comminuted	Skeletal Tx with or without ORIF	Bed rest and positioning UE strengthening and LE isometrics Ankle ROM exercises
Open fracture	Skeletal Tx External fixation	See Comminuted, above Functional mobilization NWB advancing to TDWB status (per physician) Knee ROM exercises (per physician)
Closed fracture	ORIF usually IM rod* or screws	LE ROM exercises LE strengthening exercises Functional mobilization TDWB (per physician)

ORIF = open reduction internal fixation; UE = upper extremity; LE = lower extremity; ROM = range of motion; NWB = non–weight-bearing; TDWB = touch down weight bearing; IM = intramedullary; Tx = traction.
*The IM rod is a stainless steel rod that is surgically placed from proximal to distal in the intramedullary canal of the shaft of a bone. IM rods often have proximal and distal perpendicular screws, known as *interlocking screws*, to prevent migration of the rod.
Source: Data from A Apley, L Solomon. Apley's System of Orthopaedics and Fractures (7th ed). Boston: Butterworth–Heinemann, 1993.

Table 3-A.8. Medical Management and Physical Therapy Interventions for Distal Femoral Fracture and Supracondylar Fractures

Type	Medical Management	Physical Therapy Intervention
Nondisplaced (minimal fracture with anatomic alignment)	Fracture reduction Long-leg cast	Functional mobility with NWB to light PWB status (per physician) Cast care
Displaced	ORIF	May be braced for functional mobility (per physician) with light PWB status Gentle PROM exercises to knee joint with CPM AAROM exercises to knee joint (per physician)* Quadriceps strengthening Maintenance of functional range throughout hip and ankle
Comminuted displaced fracture (open and closed)	Skeletal Tx Occasionally delayed ORIF at 4–6 wks after injury	Skeletal Tx and bed rest Quadriceps strengthening Ankle ROM exercises May initiate gentle knee ROM exercises in Tx at 3–4 wks (per physician)

NWB = non–weight-bearing; PWB = partial weight-bearing; ORIF = open reduction internal fixation; PROM = passive range of motion; CPM = continuous passive motion; AAROM = active-assistive range of motion; Tx = traction.

Gentle ROM is defined as active-assistive range-of-motion techniques that are within the patient's tolerance. Tolerance is determined in part by the subjective report of pain as well as objective limitations of muscle guarding and pattern of motion. It is critical to maintain mobility of the joint surfaces to prevent joint fusion.

Table 3-A.9. Medical Management and Physical Therapy Interventions for Patellar Fractures

Type	Medical Management	Physical Therapy Intervention	Long-Term Complications
Nondisplaced	Closed reduction Casted with full knee extension	Functional mobility and PWB status Avoid straight-leg raising and quadriceps contraction because it will stress the fracture site and could result in shifting fracture site	Extension contracture Decreased quadriceps strength secondary to altered quadriceps mechanics Abnormal patellofemoral mechanics Post-traumatic osteoarthritis of the patello-femoral joint, which may in time be followed by patellectomy or prosthetic patella implantation
Displaced (fracture line) Transverse Vertical	ORIF, with immobilization with knee at 0 degrees of extension	See Nondisplaced, above	See Nondisplaced, above
Comminuted	ORIF Full or partial patellectomy depending on severity Immobilization with knee at 0 degrees of extension	See Nondisplaced, above	See Nondisplaced, above

PWB = partial weight-bearing; ORIF = open reduction internal fixation.

Table 3-A.10. Medical Management and Physical Therapy Interventions for Tibial Plateau Fractures

Type	Medical Management	Physical Therapy Intervention
Nondisplaced	Closed reduction Cast-brace application or postoperative knee brace	Initiation of gentle ROM exercises and CPM to knee joint Functional mobility with TDWB
Displaced		
Single condylar split-compression fracture	ORIF Cast-brace application or postoperative knee brace	Initiation of gentle ROM exercises/CPM to knee joint Functional mobility with TDWB to PWB status (per physician)
Severe comminuted bicondylar fraction	Skeletal traction and bed rest Delayed ORIF at 4–6 wks after injury with cast	Delayed initiation of knee ROM exercises (per physician)

ROM = range of motion; CPM = continuous passive motion; TDWB = touch down weight-bearing; ORIF = open reduction internal fixation; PWB = partial weight-bearing.

Table 3-A.11. Medical Management and Physical Therapy Interventions for Tibial Shaft Fractures

Fracture Type	Medical Management	Physical Therapy Intervention
Closed fractures		
Minimal displacement	Closed reduction Long-leg cast	Functional mobility with NWB/TDWB status Quadriceps strengthening Edema management
Displaced	ORIF Short-leg cast	Functional mobility as above Knee ROM exercises Quadriceps strengthening Edema management
Severe displacement, comminution, or both	Calcaneal traction with delayed ORIF or external fixation External fixation	Quadriceps strengthening Positioning Knee ROM exercises (per physician) Edema management Knee and ankle ROM exercises
Open fractures	External fixation	Quadriceps strengthening Positioning Knee ROM exercises (per physician) Edema management Knee and ankle ROM exercises

ORIF = open reduction internal fixation; ROM = range of motion; NWB = non–weight-bearing; TDWB = touch down weight-bearing.

Table 3-A.12. Medical Management and Physical Therapy Interventions for Fibula Fractures

Medical management
    Immobilization in long-leg cast
Physical therapy intervention
    Functional mobilization weight bearing as tolerated (per physician)
    Knee range-of-motion exercises when cast is changed to short-leg cast
    Edema management

Table 3-A.13. Medical Management and Physical Therapy Interventions for Tibial Fractures

Type	Medical Management	Physical Therapy Intervention
Minimally displaced	Closed reduction Short-leg cast application (the talocrural joint is immobilized in neutral)	Edema management Functional mobility NWB status Knee ROM exercises
Displaced	ORIF Short-leg cast	Edema management Functional mobility NWB status
Severely displaced	Calcaneal skeletal traction Delayed ORIF External fixation	Positioning of ankle in neutral dorsiflexion Lower-extremity isometrics
Open	External fixation	Functional mobilization NWB status (per physician) Ankle ROM exercises

NWB = non–weight-bearing; ROM = range of motion; ORIF = open reduction internal fixation.

Table 3-A.14. Medical Management and Physical Therapy Interventions for Ankle Fractures

Type	Medical Management	Physical Therapy Intervention
Closed fractures		
Nondisplaced fractures	Closed reduction Cast application	Functional mobility NWB status Edema management
Displaced fractures, multiple fractures, or both	ORIF Cast application	See Nondisplaced fractures, above Early motion is sometimes desirable; in this instance removable casts can be applied. (Parameters must be clarified by physician regarding dorsiflexion/plantarflexion, inversion/eversion.)
Open fractures or closed fractures with significant soft tissue trauma	External fixation Delayed ORIF and casting	Position ankle in neutral dorsiflexion* Functional mobility NWB status Edema management

NWB = non–weight-bearing; ORIF = open reduction internal fixation.

*The physical therapist should use a foot plate attached to traction or external fixator to ensure neutral positioning and prevent development of a plantarflexion contracture.

Table 3-A.15. Medical Management and Physical Therapy Interventions for Calcaneal Fractures

Type	Medical Management	Physical Therapy Intervention
Minimally displaced	Closed reduction Cast	Edema management Functional mobility NWB status Proximal lower-extremity strengthening as indicated
Avulsion fracture of the Achilles tendon at the insertion	ORIF Cast	See Minimally displaced, above
Intra-articular fracture involving the subtalar joint	Skeletal Tx Delayed cast	See Minimally displaced, above
Open	Skeletal Tx External fixation	See Minimally displaced, above

NWB = non–weight-bearing; Tx = traction; ORIF = open reduction internal fixation.

Table 3-A.16. Medical Management and Physical Therapy Interventions for Forefoot Fractures

Type	Medical Management	Physical Therapy Intervention
Minimally displaced	Closed reduction Cast or rigid dressing	Edema management Functional mobility NWB status Proximal lower-extremity strengthening as indicated
Significantly displaced, fragment angulation, or both	ORIF Cast	See Minimally displaced, above
Open	External fixation	See Minimally displaced, above

NWB = non–weight-bearing; ORIF = open reduction internal fixation.

Table 3-A.17. Medical Management and Physical Therapy Interventions for Cervical Fractures

Type	Medical Management	Physical Therapy Intervention
Stable (nondisplaced compression fracture, spinous process fracture, or both without ligament involvement)	Immobilization with cervical brace	Functional mobility (log rolling,* mobilization) Postural education
Partially unstable (ligament involvement with potential vertebral displacement with load [i.e., the weight of the head])	Closed reduction with halo vest	See Stable, above
Unstable (significant ligament damage with true instability and without neurologic involvement	Closed reduction Open reduction internal fixation or fusion Cervical brace	Physical therapy involvement only in case of complication (e.g., nerve damage)
Unstable (with neurologic compromise)	Reduction in skull traction	Bed rest Range-of-motion exercises to extremities (per physician)

*Log rolling is a technique used for bed mobility that limits the patient's trunk rotation by having the patient turn the trunk as a single segment. The patient is instructed to move the shoulders and hips as one unit, or "as a log."
Source: Data from RW Bucholz, MB Ezaki, FG Lipport, DR Wenger. Orthopaedic Decision Making. Philadelphia: BC Decker, 1984;8.

Table 3-A.18. Medical Management and Physical Therapy Interventions for Thoracolumbar Fractures Secondary to Hyperflexion

Type	Medical Management	Physical Therapy Intervention
Stable (nondisplaced; e.g., compression and burst fracture, wedge fracture resulting from flexion force across anterior body, traumatic spondylolisthesis, spinal process fracture)	Immobilization in spinal brace Bed rest	Functional mobility (e.g., log rolling,* mobilization with assistive devices) Instruction in donning and doffing spinal brace Postural education

Table 3-A.18. *Continued*

Type	Medical Management	Physical Therapy Intervention
Unstable (posterior spinal displacement with actual or potential neurologic compromise; e.g., shear fracture, which is displacement of one vertebra with all ligaments disrupted, and fracture dislocation, which is a combined flexion and rotation injury with disruption of both anterior and posterior ligaments)	ORIF Immobilization in body jacket and TLSO	Lower-quarter screen (see Table 3-2) Functional mobility (e.g., log rolling, mobilization with assistive devices)
Unstable-distraction injury or chance fracture (e.g., seat belt fracture, flexion force causing facet dislocation and interspinous spread)	ORIF with immobilization in body jacket or closed reduction with immobilization	Functional mobility (e.g., log rolling, mobilization with assistive devices) Lower-quarter screen (see Table 3-2)

ORIF = open reduction internal fixation; TLSO = thoracic-lumbar-sacral orthosis; LE = lower extremity.
*Log rolling is a technique used for bed mobility that limits the patient's trunk rotation by having the patient turn the trunk as a single segment. The patient is instructed to move the shoulders and hips as one unit, or "as a log."

Table 3-A.19. Medical Management and Physical Therapy Interventions for Shoulder Girdle Fractures

Type	Medical Management	Physical Therapy Intervention
Scapula fracture	Symptomatic rest	As indicated by the physician
Coracoid fracture	Symptomatic rest Occasional UE sling	As indicated by the physician
Acromial fracture Minimal displacement	Symptomatic sling usage	As indicated by the physician

Type	Medical Management	Physical Therapy Intervention
Displaced and impingement of glenohumeral joint or rotator cuff	ORIF	Gentle pendulums Elbow and wrist AROM exercises Education (posture, sling, and donning and doffing)
Glenoid fracture Stable (void of glenohumeral subluxation)	UE sling	Gentle pendulums Elbow and wrist AROM exercises Education (posture, sling, and donning and doffing)
Unstable (glenohumeral subluxation present)	ORIF UE sling	

UE = upper extremity; ORIF = open reduction internal fixation; AROM = active range of motion.

Table 3-A.20. Medical Management and Physical Therapy Interventions for Proximal Humeral Fractures

Type (Neer Classification)	Medical Management	Physical Therapy Intervention
One-part fracture with displacement of one segment	Closed reduction* Sling	Gentle pendulums Elbow, wrist, and hand ROM exercises Distal upper-extremity edema management
Two-part fracture with displacement of one segment	ORIF Sling	See One-part fracture, above
Three-part fracture with displacement of two or more segments		See One-part fracture, above
Four-part fracture with displacement of all segments		See One-part fracture, above
Comminution of humeral head	Prosthetic hemiarthroplasty Sling	UE-NWB status Shoulder pendulums (per physician)

Table 3-A.20. *Continued*

Type (Neer Classification)	Medical Management	Physical Therapy Intervention
		Elbow, wrist, and hand ROM exercises Distal edema management

ROM = range of motion; ORIF = open reduction internal fixation; UE-NWB = upper extremity non–weight-bearing.
*Elderly patients with osteoporotic bone and comminuted fractures achieve better functional results with closed reduction and early motion [1].

Table 3-A.21. Medical Management and Physical Therapy Interventions for Humeral Shaft Fractures

Type	Medical Management	Physical Therapy Intervention
Minimal displacement with absent fragment angulation	Closed reduction Sling for comfort	UE-NWB status Scapulothoracic isometric exercises Shoulder AAROM exercises Elbow and hand AROM exercises avoiding rotation Edema management
Displaced fracture with fragment angulation	ORIF	See Minimal displacement, above
Fractures with soft tissue injury	External fixation with delayed ORIF	See Minimal displacement, above

UE-NWB = upper extremity non–weight-bearing; AAROM = active-assistive range of motion; AROM = active range of motion; ORIF = open reduction internal fixation.

Table 3-A.22. Medical Management and Physical Therapy Interventions for Olecranon Fractures

Type	Medical Management	Physical Therapy Intervention
Displaced	ORIF	UE-NWB status
		Edema management
	Soft immobilization	Distal or proximal ROM exercises
		Check with physician to initiate gentle elbow ROM exercises*
Nondisplaced	Immobilization	See Displaced, above

UE-NWB = upper extremity non–weight-bearing; ROM = range of motion; ORIF = open reduction internal fixation.

Gentle ROM is defined as active-assistive range of motion techniques that are within the patient's tolerance. Tolerance is determined in part by the subjective report of pain as well as objective limitations of muscle guarding and pattern of motion. It is critical to maintain mobility of the joint surfaces to prevent joint fusion.

Table 3-A.23. Medical Management and Physical Therapy Interventions for Forearm Fractures

Type	Medical Management	Physical Therapy Intervention
Single-bone fracture (ulna or radius)		
Closed		
Minimal displacement	Reduction	UE-NWB status
	Immobilization	Edema management
	Long-arm cast	Distal or proximal joint ROM exercises
Displaced	ORIF	See Minimal displacement, above
	Long-arm cast	
Open	External fixation	See Minimal displacement, above
Fractures with dislocation		
Monteggia's fracture (proximal one-third ulnar with minimal radial head dislocation)	ORIF ulnar with closed reduction of the radial head Long-arm cast	Edema management Proximal or distal joint ROM exercises Cast care
Severe radial dislocation and fracture to the radial head	ORIF ulnar and radial head Long-arm cast	See Monteggia's fracture, above

Table 3-A.23. *Continued*

Type	Medical Management	Physical Therapy Intervention
Galeasso fracture with dislocation		
Distal radial fracture and dislocation of the radioulnar joint	ORIF radius and closed reduction of the radioulnar joint Long-arm cast in forearm supination	UE-NWB status Edema management Proximal or distal joint ROM exercises

ORIF = open reduction internal fixation; UE-NWB = upper extremity non–weight-bearing; ROM = range of motion.

Table 3-A.24. Medical Management and Physical Therapy Interventions for Carpal Fractures

Type	Medical Management	Physical Therapy Intervention
General carpal fractures		
Minimal displacement	Closed reduction Percutaneous pin fixation	NWB status for wrist Edema management Distal and proximal joint range-of-motion exercises
Displacement	ORIF and ligament reconstruction Immobilization in thumb spica cast	See Minimal displacement, above
Specific carpal fractures		
Lunate fracture (occurs only with severe trauma and is usually nondisplaced)	Closed reduction Immobilization	See Minimal displacement, above
Hamate fracture (caused by trauma or repetitive stress [e.g., baseball catching])	Closed reduction Immobilization Short-arm cast	See Minimal displacement, above

Type	Medical Management	Physical Therapy Intervention
Triquetrum (caused by sudden forced wrist flexion)	See Hamate fracture, above	See Minimal displacement, above

NWB = non–weight-bearing; ORIF = open reduction internal fixation.

Table 3-A.25. Medical Management and Physical Therapy Interventions for Metacarpal Fractures

Location	Medical Management	Physical Therapy Intervention
Head (articular)	ORIF	Edema management
Neck	Closed reduction Percutaneous pinning Immobilization	Edema management
Shaft	ORIF or percutaneous pinning Immobilization	Edema management
Base	Percutaneous pinning Immobilization	Edema management

ORIF = open reduction internal fixation.

Table 3-A.26. Medical Management and Physical Therapy Interventions for Fractures of Phalanx

Type	Medical Management	Physical Therapy Intervention
Nondisplaced	Reduction Splinted	Edema management Check with physician for metacarpal range-of-motion exercises secondary to tendon repair
Displaced or articular fracture	Open reduction internal fixation Splinted	See Nondisplaced, above

References

1. Fracture of the Proximal Humerus. In RW Bucholz, MB Ezaki, FG Lipport, DR Wenger, Orthopaedic Decision Making. Philadelphia: BC Decker, 1984;18.

4

Nervous System

Michele Panik

Introduction

The nervous system is linked to every system of the body and is responsible for the integration and regulation of homeostasis. It is also involved in the action, communication, and higher cortical function of the body. A neurologic insult and its manifestations therefore have the potential to affect multiple body systems. To safely and effectively prevent or improve the neuromuscular and functional sequelae of altered neurologic status in the acute care setting, the physical therapist requires an understanding of the neurologic system and the principles of neuropathology. The objectives of this chapter are to provide the following:

1. A brief review of the structure and function of the nervous system

2. An overview of neurologic assessment, including the physical examination and diagnostic tests

3. A description of the purpose, mechanism of action, and side effects of common neurologic medications

4. A description of neurologic diseases and disorders, including clinical findings, medical and surgical management, and physical therapy interventions

Structure and Function of the Neurologic System

The nervous system is divided as follows:

1. The central nervous system (CNS), consisting of the brain and spinal cord

2. The peripheral (voluntary) nervous system, consisting of efferent and afferent somatic nerves outside the CNS

3. The autonomic (involuntary) nervous system consisting of the sympathetic and parasympathetic systems

Central Nervous System

Brain

The brain may be anatomically divided into the cerebral hemispheres, diencephalon, brain stem, and cerebellum. A midsagittal view of the brain is shown in Figure 4-1A. Although each portion of the brain has its own function, it is linked to other portions via tracts and rarely works in isolation. When lesions occur, disruption of these functions can be predicted. Figure 4-1B shows the basal ganglia and the internal capsule, the major white matter tract. Tables 4-1 and 4-2 describe the basic structure, function, and dysfunction of the cerebral hemispheres, the diencephalon, brain stem, and cerebellum.

Protective Mechanisms
The brain is protected by the cranium, meninges, ventricular system, and the blood-brain barrier.

Cranium. The cranium encloses the brain. It is composed of eight cranial and 14 facial bones connected by sutures and contains approximately 85 foramen for the passage of the spinal cord, cranial nerves (CNs), and blood vessels [1]. The cranium is divided into the cranial vault, or calvaria (the superolateral and posterior aspects), and the cranial floor, which is composed of fossae (the anterior fossa supports the frontal lobes; the middle fossa supports the temporal lobes; and the posterior fossa supports the cerebellum, pons, and medulla) [2].

Meninges. The meninges are three layers of connective tissue that cover the brain and spinal cord. The dura mater, the outermost layer, lines the skull (periosteum) and has four major folds (Table 4-3). The arachnoid,

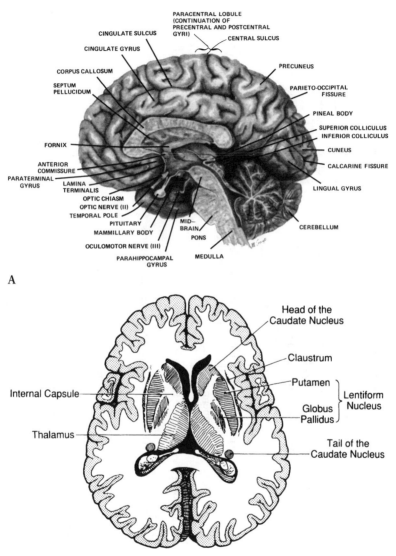

A

B

Figure 4-1. *A. Medial (midsagittal) view of a hemisected brain. (Reprinted with permission from S Gilman, SW Newman. Manter and Gatz's Essentials of Neuroanatomy and Neurophysiology [7th ed]. Philadelphia: FA Davis, 1987;9.) B. Horizontal section of the cerebrum showing the basal ganglia. (Reprinted with permission from R Love, W Webb. Neurology for the Speech-Language Pathologist [2nd ed]. Boston: Butterworth–Heinemann, 1992;22.)*

Table 4-1. Structure, Function, and Dysfunction of the Cerebral Hemispheres

Lobe of Cerebrum	Structure	Function	Dysfunction
Frontal lobe	Precentral gyrus	Voluntary motor cortex of contralateral face, arm, trunk, and leg	Contralateral mono- or hemiplegia
	Supplementary motor area	Advanced motor planning Contralateral head and eye turning (connections to CNs III, IV, VI, IX, X, and XII nuclei)	Contralateral head and eye paralysis
	Prefrontal pole	Personality center, including abstract ideas, concern for others, conscience, initiative, judgment, persistence, and planning	Loss of inhibition and demonstration of antisocial behaviors Ataxia, primitive reflexes, and hypertonicity
	Paracentral lobule	Bowel and bladder inhibition	Urinary and bowel incontinence
	Broca's area	D: motor speech expressive center ND: appreciation of intonation and gestures with vocalization	Broca's dysphagia
Parietal lobe	Postcentral gyrus	Somatosensory cortex of contralateral pain, posture, proprioception, and touch of arm, trunk, and leg	Contralateral sensation loss
	Parietal pole	D: ability to perform calculations ND: ability to construct shapes, awareness of external environment, and body image	D: acalculia, agraphia, finger agnosia ND: constructional apraxia, geographic agnosia, dressing apraxia, anosognosia

	Wernicke's area	D: sensory speech (auditory and written) comprehension center ND: appreciation of content of emotional language (e.g., tone of voice)	Wernicke's dysphagia
Temporal lobe	Visual tract	Vision	Lower homonymous quadrantanopia
	Gustatory cortex	Taste	Dysfunction is very uncommon
	Superior temporal gyrus	D: appreciation of language ND: appreciation of music, rhythm, and sound	D: decreased ability to hear ND: decreased ability to appreciate music
	Middle and inferior temporal gyri	Learning and memory centers	Learning and memory deficits
	Limbic lobe and olfactory cortex	Affective and emotion center, including mood, primitive behavior, self-preservation, short-term memory, visceral emotion processes, and interpretation of smell	Aggressive or antisocial behaviors Inability to establish new memories
	Wernicke's area	See Parietal lobe, above	Wernicke's dysphagia
	Visual tract	Vision	Upper homonymous quadrantanopia
Occipital lobe	Striate and parastriate cortices	Visual cortex	Homonymous hemianopia with or without macular damage

CN = cranial nerve; D = dominant; ND = nondominant.

Source: Data from KW Lindsay, I Bone, R Callander. Neurology and Neurosurgery Illustrated (2nd ed). Edinburgh: Churchill Livingstone, 1991; S Gilman, SW Newman. Manter and Gatz's Essentials of Clinical Neuroanatomy and Neurophysiology (7th ed). Philadelphia: FA Davis, 1989; JA Kiernan. Introduction to Human Neuroscience. Philadelphia: Lippincott, 1987; EN Marieb. Human Anatomy and Physiology. Redwood City, CA: Benjamin-Cummings, 1989; and L Thelan, J Davie, L Urden, M Lough. Critical Care Nursing: Diagnosis and Management (2nd ed). St. Louis: Mosby-Year Book, 1994.

Table 4-2. Structure, Function, and Dysfunction of the Diencephalon, Brain Stem, and Cerebellum

Brain Structure	Substructure	Function	Dysfunction
Diencephalon			
Thalamus	Specific and association nuclei	Cortical arousal	Altered consciousness
	Forms superolateral wall of third ventricle	Integrative relay station for all ascending and descending motor stimuli and all ascending sensory stimuli except smell	Signs and symptoms of increased ICP
			Contralateral hemiparesis, hemiplegia, or hemianesthesia
			Altered eye movement
		Memory	
Hypothalamus	Mamillary bodies	Autonomic center for sympathetic and parasympathetic responses	Altered autonomic function and vital signs
	Optic chiasm	Visceral center for regulation of body temperature, food intake, thirst, sleep and wake cycle, water balance	Headache
	Infundibulum (stalk) connects to the pituitary gland		Visual deficits
	Forms inferolateral wall of third ventricle	Produces ADH and oxytocin	Vomiting with signs and symptoms of increased ICP
		Regulates anterior pituitary gland	See Chapter 11 for more information on hormones and endocrine disorders
		Association with limbic system	
Epithalamus	Pineal body	Association with limbic system	Dysfunction unknown
	Posterior commissure, striae medullares, habenular nuclei and commissure		

Structure	Components	Function	Dysfunction
Subthalamus	Substantia nigra Red nuclei	Association with thalamus for motor control	Dyskinesia and decreased motor control
Pituitary	Anterior lobe Posterior lobe	Production, storage, and secretion of reproductive hormones Secretion of ADH and oxytocin	See Chapter 11 for more information on hormones and endocrine disorders
Internal capsule	Fiber tracts connecting thalamus to the cortex	Conduction pathway between the cortex and spinal cord	Deficits depend on the lesion Contralateral hemiplegia and hemianesthesia
Brain stem			
Midbrain	Superior cerebellar peduncles Superior colliculi Inferior colliculi Medial and lateral lemniscus CNs III and IV nuclei Reticular formation Cerebral aqueduct in its center	Conduction pathway between higher and lower brain centers Visual reflex Auditory reflex	Deficits depend on lesion Generally contralateral hemiplegia and hemianesthesia, altered consciousness and respiratory pattern, cranial nerve palsy

Table 4-2. *Continued*

Brain Structure	Substructure	Function	Dysfunction
Pons	Middle cerebellar peduncles Respiratory center CN V–VIII nuclei Forms anterior wall of fourth ventricle	Conduction pathway between higher and lower brain centers	See Midbrain, above
Medulla	Decussation of pyramidal tracts Inferior cerebellar peduncles Inferior olivary nuclei Nucleus cuneatus and gracilis CNs IX–XII nuclei	Homeostatic center for cardiac, respiratory, vasomotor functions	See Midbrain, above
Cerebellum			
Anterior lobe	Medial portion Lateral portion	Sensory and motor input of trunk Sensory and motor input of extremities for coordination of gait	Ipsilateral ataxia and dyscoordination or tremor of extremities

Posterior lobe	Medial and lateral portions	Sensory and motor input for coordination of motor skills and postural tone	Ipsilateral ataxia and dyscoordination of the trunk
Flocculonodular	Flocculus nodule	Sensory input from ears	Ipsilateral facial sensory loss and Horner's syndrome, nystagmus, visual overshooting
		Sensory and motor input from eyes and head for coordination of balance and eye and head movement	Loss of balance

ICP = intracranial pressure; ADH = antidiuretic hormone; CN = cranial nerve.

Source: Data from KW Lindsay, I Bone, R Callander. Neurology and Neurosurgery Illustrated (2nd ed). Edinburgh: Churchill Livingstone, 1991; S Gilman, SW Newman. Manter and Gatz's Essentials of Clinical Neuroanatomy and Neurophysiology (7th ed). Philadelphia: FA Davis, 1989; JA Kiernan. Introduction to Human Neuroscience. Philadelphia: Lippincott, 1987; EN Marieb. Human Anatomy and Physiology. Redwood City, CA: Benjamin-Cummings, 1989; and L Thelan, J Davie, L Urden, M Lough. Critical Care Nursing: Diagnosis and Management (2nd ed). St. Louis: Mosby–Year Book, 1994.

Table 4-3. Dural Folds

Falx cerebri	Vertical fold that separates the two cerebral hemispheres to prevent horizontal displacement of these structures
Falx cerebelli	Vertical fold that separates the two cerebellar hemispheres to prevent horizontal displacement of these structures
Tentorium cerebelli	Horizontal fold that separates occipital lobes from the cerebellum to prevent vertical displacement of these structures
Diaphragm sellae	Horizontal fold that separates the subarachnoid space from the sella turcica to house the pituitary gland

Source: Data from L Thelan, J Davie, L Urden, M Lough. Critical Care Nursing: Diagnosis and Management (2nd ed). St. Louis: Mosby–Year Book, 1994;477.

the middle layer, loosely encloses the brain. The pia mater, the inner layer, covers the convolutions of the brain and forms a portion of the choroid plexus in the ventricular system. The three layers create very important anatomic and potential spaces in the brain as shown in Figure 4-2 and described in Table 4-4.

Ventricular System. The ventricular system nourishes the brain and acts as a cushion by increasing the buoyancy of the brain. It consists of four ventricles and a series of foramen through which cerebrospinal fluid (CSF) passes to surround the CNS. CSF is a colorless, odorless solution produced by the choroid plexus of all ventricles. CSF circulates in a pulse-like fashion through the ventricles and around the spinal cord with the beating of ependymal cilia that line the ventricles and intracranial blood volume changes that occur with breathing and cardiac systole [3]. The flow of CSF under normal conditions, as shown in Figure 4-3, is as follows [4]:

- From the lateral ventricles via the interventricular foramen to the third ventricle

- From the third ventricle to the fourth ventricle via the cerebral aqueduct

- From the fourth ventricle to the cisterns, subarachnoid space, and spinal cord via the median and lateral apertures

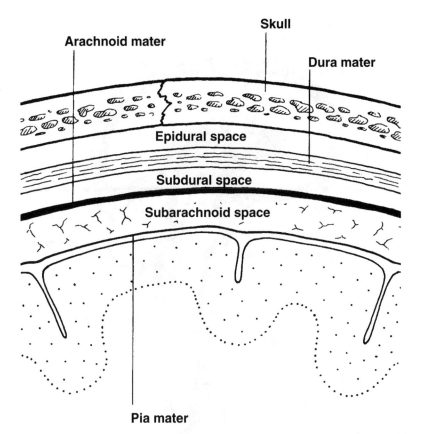

Figure 4-2. *The meninges. (Reprinted with permission from A Unwin, K Jones. Emergency Orthopaedics and Trauma. Oxford: Butterworth–Heinemann, 1995;62.)*

Table 4-4. Dural Spaces

Epidural (extradural) space	Potential space between the skull and outer dural layer
Subdural space	Anatomic space between the dura and the arachnoid mater containing the venous sinus
Subarachnoid space	Anatomic space between the arachnoid and pia mater containing cerebrospinal fluid and the vascular supply of the cortex

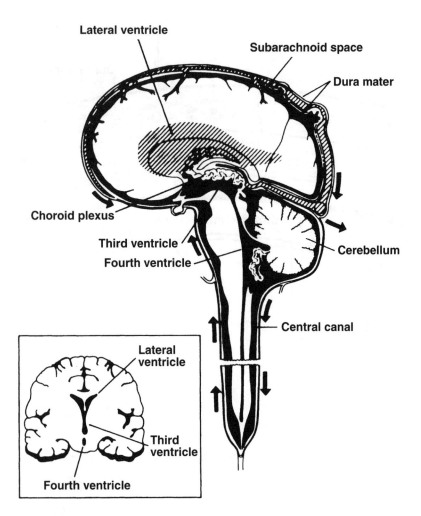

Figure 4-3. *Circulation of the cerebrospinal fluid. (Reprinted with permission from R Love, W Webb. Neurology for the Speech-Language Pathologist [2nd ed]. Boston: Butterworth–Heinemann, 1992;37.)*

When ventricular pressure is greater than venous pressure, CSF is absorbed into the venous system via the arachnoid villi, capillary walls of the pia mater, and lymphatics of the subarachnoid space near the optic nerve [2].

Blood-Brain Barrier. The blood-brain barrier is the physiologic mechanism responsible for keeping toxins, such as amino acids, hormones, ions, and urea, from altering neuronal firing of the brain. It readily allows water, oxygen, carbon dioxide, glucose, some amino acids, and substances that are highly soluble in fat (e.g., alcohol, nicotine, and anesthetic agents) to pass across the barrier [4, 5]. The barrier consists of fused endothelial cells on a basement membrane that is surrounded by astrocytic foot extensions [6]. Substances must therefore pass through rather than around these cells. The blood-brain barrier is absent near the hypothalamus, the pineal region, the anterior third ventricle, and the floor of the fourth ventricle [3].

Central Brain Systems
The central brain systems are the reticular activating system (RAS) and the limbic system. The RAS is responsible for human consciousness level and integrates the functions of the brain stem with cortical, cerebellar, thalamic, hypothalamic, and sensory receptor functions [5].

The limbic system is a complex interactive system, with primary connections between the cortex, hypothalamus, and sensory receptors [5]. The limbic system is the emotional system, mediating cortical autonomic function of internal and external stimuli.

Circulation
The brain receives blood from the internal carotid and vertebral arteries, which are linked together by the circle of Willis, as shown in Figure 4-4. Each vessel supplies blood to a certain part of the brain (Table 4-5). The circulation of the brain is discussed in terms of a single vessel or by region (usually as the anterior or posterior circulation). There are several anastomotic systems of the cerebral vasculature that provide essential blood flow to the brain. Blood is drained from the brain through a series of venous sinuses. The superior sagittal sinus with its associated lacunae and villi is the primary drainage site. The superior sagittal sinus and sinuses located in the dura and scalp then drain blood into the internal jugular vein for return to the heart.

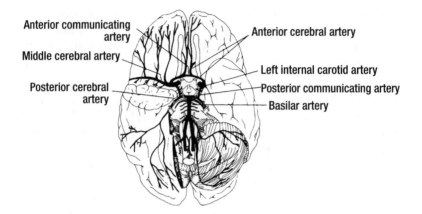

Figure 4-4. *Circle of Willis. (Reprinted with permission from R Love, W Webb. Neurology for the Speech-Language Pathologist [2nd ed]. Boston: Butterworth–Heinemann, 1992;40.)*

Spinal Cord

The spinal cord lies within the spinal column and extends from the foramen magnum to the first lumbar vertebra, where it forms the conus medullaris and the cauda equina and attaches to the coccyx via the filum terminale. Divided into the cervical, thoracic, and lumbar portions, it is protected by the mechanisms similar to those supporting the brain. The spinal cord is composed of gray and white matter and provides the pathway for the ascending and descending tracts as shown in Figure 4-5 and listed in Table 4-6.

Peripheral Nervous System

The peripheral nervous system consists of the cranial and spinal nerves and the reflex system. The primary structures include peripheral nerves, associated ganglia, and sensory receptors. There are 12 pairs of CNs, each with a unique pathway and function (sensory, motor, mixed, or autonomic). Thirty-one pairs of spinal nerves (all mixed) exit the spinal cord to form distinct plexuses (except T2–T12). The peripheral nerves of the upper and lower extremities and thorax are

Table 4-5. Blood Supply of the Brain

Artery (Abbreviation)	Area of Perfusion
Anterior circulation	
Internal carotid artery (ICA)	The dura, optic tract, basal ganglia, midbrain, uncus, lateral geniculate body, and tympanic cavity Ophthalmic branch supplies the eyes, orbits, forehead, and nose
External carotid artery (ECA)	All structures external to the skull, the larynx, and the thyroid
Anterior cerebral artery (ACA)	Medial surface of the cerebrum, including the superior surface of frontal and parietal lobes Medial lenticulostriate branch supplies the anterior portion of the internal capsule, optic chiasm and nerve, portions of the hypothalamus, and basal ganglia
Middle cerebral artery (MCA)	Lateral surface of the cerebrum, including superior and lateral surfaces of temporal lobes Lateral lenticulostriate branch supplies the internal capsule and basal ganglia
Posterior circulation	
Vertebral artery	Medulla, dura of the posterior fossa, including the falx cerebri and tentorium cerebelli
Posterior inferior cerebellar artery (PICA)	Posterior and inferior surface of cerebellum and vermis
Basilar artery	Pons and medulla
Anterior inferior cerebellar artery (AICA)	Anterior surface of the cerebellum, flocculus, and inferior vermis
Superior cerebellar artery (SCA)	Superior surface of cerebellum and vermis
Posterior cerebral artery (PCA)	Occipital lobe and medial and lateral surfaces of the temporal lobes, thalamus, lateral geniculate bodies, hippocampus, choroid plexus of the third and lateral ventricles

Source: Data from CL Rumbaugh, A Wang, FY Tsai. Cerebrovascular Disease Imaging and Interventional Treatment Options. New York: Igaku-Shoin Medical Publishers, 1995; and KL Moore. Clinically Oriented Anatomy (2nd ed). Baltimore: Williams & Wilkins, 1985.

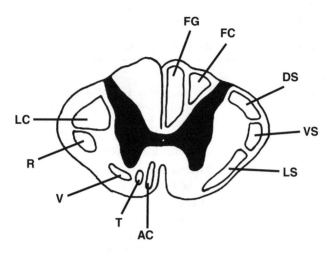

Figure 4-5. *Location of major white matter tracts in cross section. Sensory (ascending) and motor (descending) tracts are shown on the left and right sides of the spinal cord, respectively. (LC = lateral corticospinal; R = rubrospinal; T = tectospinal; V = vestibulospinal; AC = anterior corticospinal; FG = fasciculus gracilis; FC = fasciculus cuneatus; DS = dorsal spinocerebellar; VS = ventral spinocerebellar; LS = lateral spinothalamic.)*

listed in Tables 4-7 through 4-9, and the dermatomal system is shown in Figure 4-6. The reflex system includes spinal, deep tendon, stretch, and superficial reflexes and protective responses.

Autonomic Nervous System

The portion of the peripheral nervous system that innervates glands and cardiac and smooth muscle is the autonomic nervous system. The parasympathetic division is activated in time of rest, whereas the sympathetic division is activated in times of work or "fight-or-flight" situations. The two divisions work closely together, with dual innervation of most organs, to ensure homeostasis.

Neurologic Examination

The neurologic examination is initiated on hospital admission or in the field and is reassessed continuously, hourly, or daily as necessary. The

Table 4-6. Major Ascending and Descending White Matter Tracts

Tract	Function
Fasciculus gracilis	Sensory pathway for lower extremity and lower trunk joint proprioception, vibration, two-point discrimination, graphesthesia, and double simultaneous stimulation
Fasciculus cuneatus	Sensory pathway for upper extremity, upper trunk, and neck joint proprioception, vibration, two-point discrimination, graphesthesia, and double simultaneous stimulation
Lateral spinothalamic	Sensory pathway for pain, temperature, and light touch
Ventral spinocerebellar	Sensory pathway for ipsilateral subconscious proprioception
Dorsal spinocerebellar	Sensory pathway for ipsilateral and contralateral subconscious proprioception
Lateral corticospinal (pyramidal)	Motor pathway for contralateral voluntary fine muscle movement
Anterior corticospinal (pyramidal)	Motor pathway for ipsilateral voluntary movement
Rubrospinal (extrapyramidal)	Motor pathway for gross postural muscle tone
Tectospinal (extrapyramidal)	Motor pathway for contralateral gross postural muscle tone associated with auditory and visual stimuli
Vestibulospinal (extrapyramidal)	Motor pathway for ipsilateral gross postural adjustments associated with head movements

Note: Sensory tracts ascend from the spinal cord to the brain; motor tracts descend from the brain to the spinal cord.
Source: Data from S Gilman, SW Newman. Manter and Gatz's Essentials of Clinical Neuroanatomy and Neurophysiology (7th ed). Philadelphia: FA Davis, 1989; and EN Marieb. Human Anatomy and Physiology. Redwood City, CA: Benjamin-Cummings, 1989.

neurologic examination consists of patient history; mental status examination; vital sign measurement; vision, motor, sensory, and coordination testing; and diagnostic testing.

Table 4-7. Major Peripheral Nerves of the Upper Extremity

Nerve	Spinal Root	Innervation to
Dorsal scapular	C5	Levator scapulae Rhomboid major and minor
Suprascapular	C5 and C6	Supraspinatus Infraspinatus
Lower subscapular	C5 and C6	Teres major
Axillary	C5 and C6	Teres minor Deltoid
Radial	C5, C6, C7, and C8	Triceps Brachioradialis Anconeus Extensor carpi radialis longus Supinator Extensor carpi radialis brevis Extensor carpi ulnaris Extensor digitorum Extensor digiti minimi Extensor indicis Extensor pollicis longus Abductor pollicis brevis Extensor pollicis brevis
Ulnar	C8 and T1	Flexor digitorum profundus Flexor carpi ulnaris Palmaris brevis Abductor digiti minimi Flexor digiti minimi brevis Opponens digit minimi Palmar and dorsal interossei Third and fourth lumbricals
Median	C6, C7, C8, and T1	Pronator teres Flexor carpi radialis Palmaris longus Flexor digitorum superficialis Flexor digitorum profundus Flexor pollicis longus Pronator quadratus Abductor pollicis brevis Opponens pollicis Flexor pollicis brevis First and second lumbricals

Nerve	Spinal Root	Innervation to
Musculocutaneous	C5, C6, and C7	Coracobrachialis Brachialis Biceps

Source: Data from FH Netter. Atlas of Human Anatomy. Summit City, NJ: CIBA-GEIGY Corporation, 1989;446.

Table 4-8. Major Peripheral Nerves of the Lower Extremity

Nerve	Spinal Root	Innervation to
Femoral	L2, L3, and L4	Iliacus Psoas major Sartorius Pectineus Rectus femoris Vastus lateralis, intermedius, and medialis Articularis genu
Obturator	L2, L3, and L4	Obturator externus Adductor brevis Adductor longus Adductor magnus Gracilis
Sciatic	L4, L5, S1, S2, and S3	Biceps femoris Adductor magnus Semitendinosus Semimembranosus
Tibial	L4, L5, S1, S2, and S3	Gastrocnemius Soleus Flexor digitorum longus Tibialis posterior Flexor hallucis longus
Common peroneal	L4, L5, S1, and S2	Peroneus longus and brevis Tibialis anterior Extensor digitorum longus Extensor hallucis longus Extensor hallucis brevis Extensor digitorum brevis

Source: Data from FH Netter. Atlas of Human Anatomy. Summit City, NJ: CIBA-GEIGY Corporation, 1989;506.

Table 4-9. Major Peripheral Nerves of the Back, Thorax, and Abdomen

Nerve	Spinal Root	Innervation to
Spinal accessory	C3 and C4	Trapezius
Long thoracic	C5, C6, and C7	Serratus anterior
Medial pectoral	C6, C7, and C8	Pectoralis minor and major
Lateral pectoral	C7, C8, and T1	Pectoralis major
Phrenic	C3, C4, and C5	Diaphragm
Intercostal	Correspond to root level	External intercostals Internal intercostals Levatores costarum longi and brevis
Iliohypogastric and ilioinguinal	L1	Transversus abdominis Internal abdominal oblique
Inferior gluteal	L4, L5, S1, and S2	Gluteus maximus
Superior gluteal	L4, L5, and S1	Gluteus medius Gluteus minimus Tensor fascia latae

Source: Data from FH Netter. Atlas of Human Anatomy. Summit City, NJ: CIBA-GEIGY Corporation, 1989;163, 240, 241, 250.

Patient History

A detailed history, initially taken by the physician, is often the most helpful information used to delineate whether a patient presents with a true neurologic event or another process (usually cardiac or metabolic in nature). The history may be presented by the patient or, more commonly, by a family member or person witnessing the acute or progressive event(s) responsible for hospital admission. One common framework for organizing questions regarding each neurologic complaint, sign, or symptom is presented here:

- What is the patient feeling? [7]
- When did the problem initially occur and has it progressed? [7]
- What relieves or exacerbates the problem? [7]
- Are there other problems? [7]
- What is the onset, frequency, and duration of signs or symptoms? [8]

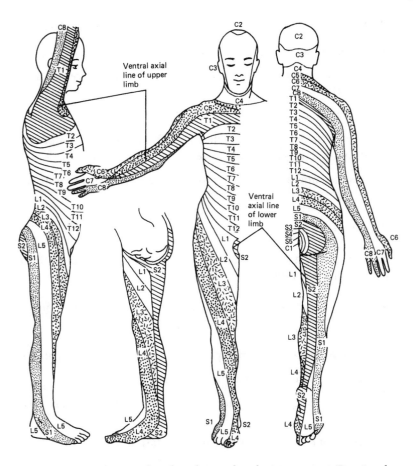

Figure 4-6. *Dermatome chart based on embryologic segments. (Reprinted with permission from GD Maitland. Vertebral Manipulation [5th ed]. Oxford: Butterworth–Heinemann, 1986;46.)*

In addition to the general medical record review (Appendix I), questions relevant to a complete neurologic history include the following:

- Does the problem involve loss of consciousness?
- Did a fall precede or follow the problem?
- Is there headache, dizziness, or visual disturbance?

- What are the functional deficits associated with the problem?
- Is there an alteration of speech?
- Does the patient demonstrate memory loss or a decreased ability to perform calculations?
- Does the patient have an altered sleep pattern?
- What is the handedness of the patient? (Handedness is a predictor of brain [language] dominance)
- Has the patient traveled to a foreign country in the recent past?

Observation

Data that can be gathered from close or distant observation of the patient include the following:

- Level of alertness, arousal, distress, or the need for restraint
- Body position
- Head, trunk, and extremity posture, including movement patterns
- Amount and quality of active movement
- Amount and quality of interaction with the environment or family members
- Degree of ease or difficulty with activities of daily living
- Presence of involuntary movements such as tremor
- Eye movement(s)
- Presence of neglect of one side of the body
- Presence of muscle atrophy
- Respiratory rate and pattern

Clinical tip

The therapist should correlate these observations with other information from the chart review and other health care team members to determine (1) if the diagnosis is consistent with the

Table 4-10. Normal and Abnormal States of Consciousness

Alert	Completely awake Aware of all stimuli Able to interact meaningfully with clinician
Lethargic or somnolent	Arousal with stimuli Falls to sleep when not stimulated Decreased awareness Loss of train of thought
Obtundent	Difficult to arouse Requires constant stimulation for all activities Confused
Stuporous	Arousal only with vigorous stimulation Unable to complete mental status examination because responses are usually incomprehensible words
Coma	Unarousable Nonverbal
Delirium	State of disorientation marked by irritability or agitation, suspicion and fear, misperception of stimuli Patient demonstrates offensive, loud, and talkative behaviors
Dementia	Alteration in mental processes secondary to organic disease that is not accompanied by a change in arousal

Source: Data from RL Strub, FW Black. Mental Status Examination in Neurology (2nd ed). Philadelphia: FA Davis, 1985; and F Plum, J Posner. The Diagnosis of Stupor and Coma (3rd ed). Philadelphia: FA Davis, 1980.

physical presentation, (2) what types of commands or tone of voice to use, (3) how much assistance is needed, and (4) how to prioritize the portions of the physical therapy evaluation.

Mental Status Examination

The mental status examination includes assessment of level of consciousness, cognition, emotional state, and speech and language ability.

Level of Consciousness

Consciousness consists of arousal and the awareness of self and environment, including the ability to interact appropriately in response to any normal stimulus [9]. Coma is often considered the opposite of consciousness. Table 4-10 describes the different states of consciousness. Evaluating a patient's level of consciousness is important because it serves as a baseline to monitor stability, improvement, or decline in the patient's condition. It also helps determine the severity and prognosis of neurologic insult or disease state, thus directing the medical plan of care.

Clinical tip

Level of consciousness is often vaguely described in medical charts; therefore, be specific when documenting a patient's mental status. Describe the intensity of stimulus needed to arouse the patient, the patient's best response, and the patient's response to the removal of the stimulus [9].

Glasgow Coma Scale

The Glasgow Coma Scale (GCS) is a widely accepted measure of level of consciousness and responsiveness and is described in Table 4-11. The GCS evaluates best eye opening (E), motor response (M), and verbal response (V). To determine a patient's overall GCS, add each score (i.e., E + M + V). Scores range from 3 to 15. A score of 8 or less signifies coma [10].

Clinical tip

Calculation of the GCS usually occurs at regular intervals. The GCS should be used to confirm the type and amount of cueing needed to communicate with a patient, determine what time of day a patient is most capable of participating in physical therapy, and delineate physical therapy goals.

Cognition

Cognitive testing includes the assessment of attention, orientation, memory, abstract thought, and the ability to perform calculations or construct figures. General intelligence and vocabulary are estimated with questions regarding history, geography, or current events. Table 4-12 lists typical methods of testing the components of cognition.

Table 4-11. The Glasgow Coma Scale

Response	Score
Eye opening (E)	
Spontaneous: eyes open without stimulation	4
To speech: eyes open to voice	3
To pain: eyes open to noxious stimulus	2
Nil: eyes do not open despite variety of stimuli	1
Motor response (M)	
Obeys: follows commands	6
Localizes: purposeful attempts to move limb to stimulus	5
Withdraws: flexor withdrawal without localizing	4
Abnormal flexion: decorticate posturing to stimulus	3
Extensor response: decerebrate posturing to stimulus	2
Nil: no motor movement	1
Verbal response (V)	
Oriented: normal conversation	5
Confused conversation: vocalizes in sentences, incorrect context	4
Inappropriate words: vocalizes with comprehensible words	3
Incomprehensible words: vocalizes with grunts, groans, and so on	2
Nil: no vocalization	1

Source: Data from B Jennett, G Teasdale. Management of Head Injuries. Philadelphia: FA Davis, 1981.

Emotional State

Emotional state assessment entails observation and direct questioning to ascertain a patient's mood, affect, perception, and thought process, as well as to evaluate for behavioral changes. Evaluation of emotion is not meant to be a full psychiatric examination; however, it provides insight to how a patient may complete the cognitive portions of the mental status examination [11].

Clinical tip

It is important to note that a patient's culture may affect particular emotional responses.

Table 4-12. Tests of Cognitive Function

Cognitive Function	Definition	Task
Attention	Ability to attend to a specific stimuli or task	Repetition of a series of numbers or letters Counting by 3s or 7s Spelling words forward and backward
Orientation	Ability to orient to person, place, and time	Identify name, age, current date, birth date, present location, state, and season
Memory	Immediate recall Short-term memory Long-term memory	Repeat three words after a few minutes Recount recent events Recount past events
Calculation	Ability to perform verbal or written mathematical problems	Add, subtract, multiply, or divide whole numbers
Constructional ability	Ability to construct two- or three-dimensional figure or shape	Draw a figure after a verbal command or reproduce a figure from a picture
Abstract ability	Ability to reason in an abstract rather than a literal or concrete fashion	Interpret proverbs Discuss how two objects are similar
Judgment	Ability to reason (according to age and lifestyle)	Demonstrate common sense and safety

Source: Data from BA Bates. A Guide to Physical Examination and History Taking (6th ed). Philadelphia: Lippincott, 1995; and HM Seidel, JW Ball, JE Dains, GW Benedict. Mosby's Guide to Physical Examination (3rd ed). St. Louis: Mosby–Year Book, 1995.

Speech and Language Ability

The physician should perform a speech and language assessment as soon as possible according to the patient's level of consciousness. The main goals of this assessment are to evaluate the patient's ability to articulate and produce voice and the presence, extent, and severity of aphasia [12]. These goals are achieved by testing comprehension and repetition of spoken speech, naming, quality and quantity of conversational speech, and reading and writing abilities [12].

A speech-language pathologist is often consulted to perform a longer, more in-depth examination of cognition, speech, and swallow using standardized tests and skilled evaluation of articulation, phonation, hearing, and orofacial muscle strength testing.

Clinical tip

• The physical therapist should be aware of and use as appropriate the speech-language pathologist's suggestions for types of commands, activity modification, and positioning as related to risk of aspiration.

• The physical therapist is often the first clinician to notice the presence or extent of speech or language dysfunction during activity, especially during tasks that cause fatigue. The physical therapist should report these findings to other members of the health care team.

Vital Signs

The brain is the homeostatic center of the body; therefore, vital signs are an indirect measure of neurologic status and the body's ability to perform basic functions such as respiration and temperature control.

Blood pressure, heart rate, respiratory rate and pattern, temperature, and other vital signs from invasive monitoring (see Appendix IV) are assessed continuously or hourly to determine hemodynamic stability and the effectiveness of medical-surgical management.

Clinical tip

The therapist should be aware of blood pressure parameters determined by the physician for the patient with neurologic dysfunction. These parameters may be set greater than normal to maintain adequate perfusion to the brain or lower than normal to prevent further injury to the brain.

Cranial Nerves

CN testing provides information about the general neurologic status of the patient and about the function of the special senses. The results assist in the differential diagnosis of neurologic dysfunction and may help in determining the location of a lesion. CNs I–XII are tested on admission, daily in the hospital, or when there is a suspected change in neurologic function (Table 4-13).

Vision

Vision testing is an important portion of the neurologic examination because alterations in vision can indicate neurologic lesions, as illustrated in Figure 4-7. In addition to the visual field, acuity, reflexive, and ophthalmoscopic testing performed by the physician during CN assessment, the pupils are further examined for the following:

- Size and equality. Pupil size is normally 2–4 mm or 4–8 mm in diameter in the light and dark, respectively [13]. The pupils should be of equal size, although up to a 1-mm difference in diameter can normally occur between the left and right pupils [14].

- Shape. Pupils are normally round but may become oval or irregularly shaped with neurologic dysfunction [14].

- Reactivity. Pupils normally constrict in response to light, as a consensual response to light shown in the opposite eye, or when fixed on a near object. Conversely, pupils normally dilate in the dark. Constriction and dilation occur briskly under normal circumstances. A variety of deviations of pupil characteristics can occur. The physician can test pupil reactivity by shining a light directly into the patient's eye. Dilated, nonreactive (fixed), malpositioned, or disconjugate pupils can signify very serious neurologic conditions (especially oculomotor compression, increased intracranial pressure [ICP], or brain herniation) [14].

Clinical tip

- If the patient's pupil size or shape changes during physical therapy intervention, discontinue the treatment and notify the nurse or physician immediately.

Table 4-13. Origin, Purpose, and Testing of the Cranial Nerves

Nerve	Origin	Purpose	How to Test
Olfactory (CN I)	Cerebral cortex	Sense of smell	Have the patient close one nostril, and ask the patient to sniff a mild-smelling material and identify it.
Optic (CN II)	Thalamus	Central and peripheral vision	Acuity: Have the patient cover one eye, and ask patient to read a visual chart. Fields: Have the patient cover one eye, and hold an object (e.g., pen) at arm's length from the patient in his or her peripheral field. Hold the patient's head steady. Slowly move the object centrally, and ask the patient to state when he or she first sees the object. Repeat the process in all quadrants.
Oculomotor (CN III)	Midbrain	Upward, inward, and inferomedial eye movement Upper eyelid elevation Pupil constriction Visual focusing	Nerves III, IV, and VI are tested together. Pupil reaction to light: Shine a light into one eye. Gaze: Hold object (e.g., pen) at arm's length from the patient, and hold the patient's head steady. Ask the patient to follow the object with a full horizontal, vertical, and diagonal gaze.

Table 4-13. *Continued*

Nerve	Origin	Purpose	How to Test
Trochlear (CN IV)	Midbrain	Inferolateral eye movement and proprioception	See Oculomotor (CN III), above.
Trigeminal (CN V)	Pons	Sensation of face Mastication Corneal reflex Jaw jerk	Conduct touch, pain, and temperature sensory testing over the patient's face. Observe for deviation of jaw. Palpate masseter as the patient clamps his or her jaw. Wisp cotton on the patient's cornea. Tap reflex hammer on the patient's chin.
Abducens (CN VI)	Pons	Lateral eye movement and proprioception	See Oculomotor (CN III), above
Facial (CN VII)	Pons	Taste (anterior two-thirds of tongue) Facial expression Autonomic innervation of lacrimal and salivary glands	Ask the patient to smile, wrinkle brow, purse lips, and close eyes.
Vestibulocochlear (CN VIII)	Pons	Vestibular branch: sense of equilibrium Cochlear branch: sense of hearing	Oculocephalic reflex (Doll's eyes): Rotate the patient's head in one direction and watch eye movement. Cochlear: Vibrate a tuning fork, place it on the midforehead, and ask patient if sound is heard louder in one ear.

Nerve	Location	Function	Test
Glossopharyngeal (CN IX)	Medulla	Gag reflex; Motor and proprioception of superior pharyngeal muscle; Autonomic innervation of salivary gland; Taste (posterior one-third of tongue); Blood pressure regulation	Test CNs IX and X together. Induce gag with tongue depressor (one side at a time) and note pitch of voice and swallowing difficulty.
Vagus (CN X)	Medulla	Swallowing; Proprioception of pharynx and larynx; Parasympathetic innervation of heart, lungs, and abdominal viscera	See Glossopharyngeal (CN IX), above.
Spinal accessory (CN XI)	Medulla	Motor control and proprioception of head rotation, shoulder elevation; Motor control of pharynx and larynx	Ask patient to rotate his or her head. Ask patient to shrug his or her shoulders.
Hypoglossal (CN XII)	Medulla	Movement and proprioception of tongue for chewing and speech	Ask patient to stick out his or her tongue. Observe patient for speech problems.

CN = cranial nerve.
Source: Data from S Goldberg. The Four-Minute Neurological Exam. Miami: Medmaster, 1992; KW Lindsay, I Bone, R Callander. Neurology and Neurosurgery Illustrated (2nd ed). Edinburgh: Churchill Livingstone, 1991; and EN Marieb. Human Anatomy and Physiology. Redwood City, CA: Benjamin-Cummings, 1989.

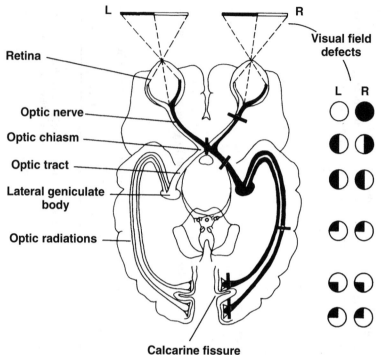

Figure 4-7. *Visual pathways with lesion sites and resulting visual-field defects. (Reprinted with permission from R Love, W Webb. Neurology for the Speech-Language Pathologist [2nd ed]. Boston: Butterworth–Heinemann, 1992;74.)*

- PERRLA is an acronym that describes pupil function: *p*upils *e*qual, *r*ound, and *r*eactive to *l*ight and *a*ccommodation.

Motor Function

The evaluation of motor function consists of strength, tone, and reflex testing.

Strength Testing

Strength is the production of tension and a static or dynamic force in a maximal effort by a muscle or muscle group [15]. Strength can be graded in the following ways:

- Graded 0–5/0–normal with manual muscle testing
- Graded as strong or weak with resisted isometrics
- Graded by the portion of a range of motion in which movement occurs (e.g., hip flexion through one-fourth of available range)
- Graded functionally

Clinical tip

The manner in which muscle strength is tested depends on the patient's ability to follow commands, arousal, cooperation, and activity tolerance, as well as constraints on the patient such as positioning, sedation, equipment, and time.

Muscle Tone

Muscle tone has been described in a multitude of ways; however, neither a precise definition nor a quantitative measure has been determined [16, 17]. It is beyond the scope of this chapter to discuss the various definitions of tone. For simplicity, muscle tone is discussed in terms of hyper- or hypotonicity. Hypertonicity, an increase in muscle contractility, includes spasticity and rigidity secondary to a neurologic lesion of the CNS or upper motor neuron system. Hypotonicity, a decrease in muscle contractility, includes flaccidity from a neurologic lesion of the lower motor neuron system (or as in the early stage of spinal cord injury [SCI]). Regardless of the specific definition of muscle tone, clinicians agree that muscle tone may change according to a variety of stimuli, including stress, febrile state, pain, body position, and medical status [18].

Muscle tone can be evaluated in the following ways:

- Passively as mild (i.e., mild resistance to movement with quick stretch), moderate (i.e., moderate resistance to movement even without quick stretch), or severe (i.e., resistance great enough to prevent movement of a joint) [19].

- Passively or actively as the ability or inability to achieve full joint range of motion

- Actively as the ability to complete functional mobility and volitional movement

- As abnormal decorticate (flexion) or decerebrate (extension) posturing. (Decortication is the result of a hemispheric or an internal capsule lesion that results in a disruption of the corticospinal tract [20]. Decerebration is the result of a brain stem lesion and is thus considered a sign of deteriorating neurologic status [20]. A patient may demonstrate one or both of these postures.)

Reflexes

A reflex is a motor response to a sensory stimulus and is used to assess the integrity of the motor system in the conscious or unconscious patient. The reflexes most commonly tested are deep tendon and superficial reflexes.

A deep tendon reflex (DTR) should elicit a muscle contraction of the tendon stimulated. Table 4-14 describes DTRs according to spinal level and expected response. DTR testing should proceed in the following manner:

1. The patient should be sitting or supine and as relaxed as possible.

2. The joint to be tested should be in midposition to stretch the tendon.

3. The tendon is then directly tapped with a reflex hammer. Both sides should be compared. Reflexes are typically graded as present (normal, exaggerated, or depressed) or absent. Reflexes can also be graded on a scale of 0–4 as described in Table 4-15. Depressed reflexes signify lower motor neuron disease or neuropathy. Exaggerated reflexes signify upper motor neuron disease.

Clinical tip

The numeric results of DTR testing may appear in a stick figure drawing in the medical record. The DTR grades are placed next to each of the main DTR sites. An arrow may

Table 4-14. Deep Tendon Reflexes of the Upper and Lower Extremities

Reflex	Spinal Level	Normal Response
Biceps	C5	Elbow flexion
Brachioradialis	C6	Elbow flexion
Triceps	C7	Elbow extension
Patellar	L4	Knee extension
Posterior tibialis	L5	Plantar flexion and inversion
Achilles	S1	Plantar flexion

Table 4-15. Deep Tendon Reflex Grades

Grade	Response
0	No response: abnormal
1+	Diminished or sluggish response: low normal
2+	Active response: normal
3+	Brisk response: high normal
4+	Very brisk response with or without clonus: abnormal

appear next to the stick figure as well. Arrows pointing upward signify hyperreflexia; conversely, arrows pointing downward signify hyporeflexia.

A superficial reflex should elicit a muscle contraction from the cornea, mucous membrane, or area of the skin that is stimulated. The most frequently tested superficial reflexes are the corneal (which involves CNs V and VII), gag and swallowing (which involve CNs IX and X), and perianal (which involves S3–5). The most frequently tested superficial cutaneous reflexes are upper abdominal (which involves T8–10), lower abdominal (which involves T10–12), cremasteric (which involves L1–2 [males]), and bulbocavernosus (which involves S3–4 [males]) [21]. These reflexes are evaluated by physi-

Table 4-16. Abnormal Cutaneous Reflexes

Reflex	Stimulus	Abnormal Response
Babinski's sign	Stroke lateral plantar surface of foot.	Great toe dorsiflexion with or without splaying of toes
Hoffmann's sign	Snap distal phalanx of index finger.	Clawing of thumb and fingers
Grasp reflex	Touch palmar surface of hand.	Flexion of fingers
Snout reflex	Touch oral region.	Pursing of lips
Sucking reflex	Touch oral region.	Sucking motion of lips

Source: Adapted from JV Hickey. The Clinical Practice of Neurological and Neurosurgical Nursing (3rd ed). Philadelphia: Lippincott, 1992.

cians and are graded as present or absent. Superficial reflexes may be abnormal cutaneous responses or recurrent primitive reflexes (Table 4-16), both of which are suggestive of corticospinal damage or dementia and are graded as present or absent.

Sensation

Sensation testing evaluates the presence or absence of light and deep touch, proprioception, temperature, vibration sense, and superficial and deep pain. For each modality, the neck, trunk, and extremities are tested bilaterally, proceeding in a dermatomal pattern. For more reliable sensation testing results, the patient should look away from the area being tested. Table 4-17 outlines the method of sensation testing by stimulus.

Clinical tip

Before completing the sensory examination, the physical therapist should be sure that the patient can correctly identify stimuli (e.g., that a pinprick feels like a pinprick).

Table 4-17. Sensation Testing

Sensation	Modality and Method
Superficial pain	Touch a pin or pen cap over the extremities or trunk.
Deep pain	Squeeze the patient's forearm bulk and calf bulk.
Light touch	Apply light pressure with the finger, a cotton ball, or wash cloth over the extremities or trunk.
Proprioception	Lightly grasp the distal interphalangeal joint of the patient's finger or great toe, and move the joint slowly up or down. Ask patient to state which direction the finger or toe moved. Test distal to proximal (e.g., toe to ankle to knee).
Vibration	Activate a tuning fork and place on bony prominence. Ask the patient to state when the vibration stops. Proceed distal to proximal.
Temperature	Place test tubes filled with warm or cold water on the area of the patient's body to be tested. Ask the patient to state temperature. (Rarely done in the acute care setting.)
Stereognosis	Place a familiar object in the patient's hand and ask the patient to identify it.
Two-point discrimination	Place two-point caliper tool or drafting compass on area to be tested. Ask the patient to distinguish whether it has one or two points.
Graphesthesia	Trace a letter or number in the patient's open palm and ask the patient to state what was drawn.
Double simultaneous stimulation	Simultaneously touch two areas on the same side of the patient's body. Ask patient to locate and distinguish both points.

Source: Data from KW Lindsay, I Bone, R Callander. Neurology and Neurosurgery Illustrated (2nd ed). Edinburgh: Churchill Livingstone, 1991; S Gilman, SW Newman. Manter and Gatz's Essentials of Clinical Neuroanatomy and Neurophysiology (7th ed). Philadelphia: FA Davis, 1989; and JV Hickey. The Clinical Practice of Neurological and Neurosurgical Nursing (3rd ed). Philadelphia: Lippincott, 1992.

Coordination

Although each lobe of the cerebellum has its own function, coordination tests cannot truly differentiate among them. Coordination tests evaluate the presence of ataxia (general incoordination), dysmetria (overshooting), and dysdiadochokinesia (inability to perform rapid alternating

Table 4-18. Coordination Tests

Test	Method
Upper extremity	
Finger-to-nose	Ask the patient to touch his or her nose. Then ask patient to touch his or her nose and then touch your finger (which should be held an arm's length away). Ask the patient to repeat this rapidly.
Supination and pronation	Ask the patient to rapidly supinate and pronate his or her forearms.
Tapping	Ask the patient to rapidly tap his or her hands on a surface simultaneously, alternately, or both.
Arm bounce	Have the patient flex his or her shoulder to 90 degrees with elbow fully extended and wrist in the neutral position, then apply downward pressure on the arm. (Excessive swinging of the arm indicates a positive test.)
Rebound phenomenon	Ask the patient to flex his or her elbow to approximately 45 degrees. Apply resistance to elbow flexion then suddenly release the resistance. (Striking of the face indicates a positive test.)
Lower extremity	
Heel-to-shin	Ask the patient to move his or her heel down the opposite shin and repeat rapidly.
Tapping	Ask the patient to rapidly tap his or her feet on the floor, simultaneously, alternately, or both.
Romberg test	Ask the patient to stand (heels together) with eyes open. Observe for swaying or loss of balance. Repeat with eyes closed.
Gait	Ask the patient to walk. Observe gait pattern, posture, and balance. Repeat with tandem walking to exaggerate deficits.

Source: Data from KW Lindsay, I Bone, R Callander. Neurology and Neurosurgery Illustrated (2nd ed). Edinburgh: Churchill Livingstone, 1991.

movements) with arm, leg, and trunk movements, as well as with gait [8]. The results of each test are described in terms of the patient's ability to complete the test, accuracy, and presence of tremor (Table 4-18).

Another test is the pronator drift test, which is used to qualify loss of position sense. While the patient is sitting or standing, he or she flexes both shoulders and extends the elbows with the palms upward. The patient is then asked to close his or her eyes. The forearm is observed for (1) pronation or downward drift, which suggests a contralateral corticospinal lesion, or (2) an upward or sideward drift, which suggests loss of position sense [22].

Diagnostic Procedures

There are a multitude of diagnostic tests and procedures used to evaluate, differentiate, and monitor neurologic dysfunction. Each has its own cost, accuracy, advantages, and disadvantages. For the purposes of this text, only the procedures most commonly used in the acute care setting are described.

Cerebral Angiography

Cerebral angiography involves the radiographic visualization (angiogram) of the displacement, patency, stenosis, or vasospasm of intra- or extracranial arteries after the injection of a radiopaque contrast medium via a catheter (usually femoral). It is used to assess aneurysm, arteriovenous malformations (AVMs), or intracranial lesions as a single procedure or in the operating room to check blood flow after surgical procedures (e.g., after an aneurysm clipping) [23].

Clinical tip

Patients are on bed rest for approximately 8 hours after cerebral angiography to ensure proper healing of the catheter insertion site. A sandbag may be placed over the catheter insertion site. Physical therapy intervention may continue if it does not involve the movement of the catheter insertion site (e.g., do not flex the hip if the catheter was inserted in the femoral artery). The therapist should be aware that the patient may experience discomfort at this site even after the 8 hours have passed.

Computed Tomography

In computed tomography (CT), coronal or sagittal views of the head with or without contrast media are used to assess the density, displacement, or abnormality (location, size, and shape) of the cranial vault and fossae, cortical sulci and sylvian fissures, ventricular system, and gray and white matter. It is also used to assess the presence of extraneous abscess, blood, calcification, contusion, cyst, hematoma, hydrocephalus, or tumor. CT of spine or orbits is also available [8, 23, 24].

Digital-Subtraction Angiography

Digital-subtraction angiography (DSA) is the computer-assisted radiographic visualization of the carotids and cranial arteries with a minimal view of background tissues. A picture is taken before the injection of a contrast medium. A second picture is taken after injection and "subtracted" from the first, thus creating a highlight of the vessels. DSA is used to assess aneurysm, AVM, fistula, occlusion, or stenosis. It is also used in the operating room (i.e., television display) to check the integrity of anastomoses or cerebrovascular repairs [24].

Doppler Flowmetry

Doppler flowmetry is the use of ultrasound waves to assess blood flow.

Transcranial Doppler Sonography

Transcranial Doppler (TCD) sonography involves the passage of low-frequency ultrasound waves over thin cranial bones (temporal) or over gaps in bones to determine the velocity of blood flow in the anterior, middle, or posterior cerebral and basilar arteries. It is used to assess the degree of arteriosclerotic disease or vasospasm [8, 23].

Carotid Noninvasives

Carotid noninvasives (CNIs) use the passage of high-frequency ultrasound waves over the common, internal, and external carotid arteries to determine the velocity of blood flow in these vessels. It is used to assess location, presence, and severity of carotid occlusion and stenosis [8, 23].

Electroencephalography

Electroencephalography (EEG) is the recording of electrical brain activity using electrodes affixed to the scalp at rest or sleep, after sleep deprivation, after hyperventilation, or after photic stimulation. Waves may show abnormalities of activity, amplitude, pattern, or speed [23]. EEG is used to assess seizure focus, sleep and metabolic disorder, or dementia.

Electromyography

Electromyography (EMG) is the recording of muscle activity at rest, with movement, and with electrical stimulation with needle electrodes.

It is used to assess peripheral nerve injury and to differentiate neuro-muscular disorders [23].

Evoked Potentials

Evoked potentials (EPs) are electrical responses generated by the stimulation of a sensory organ. A visual evoked response (VER) is measured using electrodes that are placed over the occipital lobe to record occipital cortex activity after a patient is shown flashing lights or a checkerboard pattern. VERs are used to assess optic neuropathies. A brain stem auditory evoked response (BAER) is measured using electrodes that are placed over the vertex to record CN VIII, pons, and midbrain activity after a patient listens to a series of clicking noises through headphones. BAERs are used to assess acoustic tumors or brain stem function (in comatose patients) [8, 23].

Lumbar Puncture

A lumbar puncture (LP) is the collection of CSF from a needle placed into the subarachnoid space below the L1 vertebra, usually between L3 and L4. The patient is placed in a side-lying position with the neck and hips flexed as much as possible. Multiple vials of CSF are collected and tested for color, cytology, chlorine, glucose, protein, and pH. The opening and closing pressures are noted. LP is used to assess autoimmune and infectious processes, and in certain circumstances it is used to verify subarachnoid hemorrhage [8, 23].

Clinical tip

Headache is a common complaint after an LP secondary to meningeal irritation or a drop in CSF pressure. A patient may be placed on bed rest for several hours after an LP to minimize upright positioning, which increases headache. Other short-term complications of LP include backache, bleeding at the needle site, voiding difficulty, and fever.

Magnetic Resonance Imaging and Magnetic Resonance Angiography

Views in any plane of the head taken with magnetic resonance imaging (MRI) or angiography (MRA) are used to assess degenerative diseases, infarction, tumor, hemorrhage, AVMs, and congenital anomalies [8, 23, 24].

Myelography

Myelography uses a CT, fluoroscopy, or x-ray to show how a contrast medium flows through the subarachnoid space and around the vertebral column after the removal of a small amount of CSF and the injection of dye. It is used to assess bone displacement, disc herniation, cord compression, or tumor [8].

Clinical tip

Depending on the type of dye used, a patient may have position restrictions written by a physician after a myelogram. If water-based dye was used, the patient should remain on bed rest with the head of the bed at 30 degrees for approximately 8–24 hours because the dye may cause a seizure if it reaches the cranium. If an oil-based dye was used, the patient may have to remain in bed with the bed flat for 6–24 hours. Additionally, the patient may experience headache, back spasm, fever, or nausea and vomiting regardless of the type of dye used [23].

Positron Emission Tomography

Positron emission tomography (PET) produces three-dimensional cross-section images of brain tissue after the inhalation or injection of nuclide positrons that produce gamma rays and are detected by a scanner. It is used to assess cerebral blood flow and volume, oxygen use, glucose transport, and neurotransmitter metabolism in cerebral trauma, cerebrovascular disease, dementia, or epilepsy [25].

X-Ray

X-rays can provide anterior and lateral views of the skull that are used to assess the presence of calcification, bone erosion, or fracture, especially after trauma or if a tumor is suspected. Anterior, lateral, and posterior views of the cervical, thoracic, and lumbar spine are used to assess the presence of bone erosion, fracture, spondylosis, spur, or stenosis, especially after trauma or if there are motor or sensory deficits [8, 23, 24].

Pathophysiology

Traumatic Head Injury

The medical-surgical treatment of head injury is a complex and challenging task. Head injury, direct or indirect trauma to the skull, brain, or both, typically results in altered consciousness and systemic homeostasis. Traumatic head injury can be described by the following [26, 27]:

1. Location. Head injuries may involve damage to the cranium only, the cranium and brain structures, or to brain structures only. Frequently, head trauma is categorized as (1) closed (protective mechanisms are maintained), (2) open (protective mechanisms are altered), (3) coup (the lesion is deep to the site of impact), (4) contrecoup (the lesion is opposite the site of impact), or (5) coup-contrecoup (a combination of coup and contrecoup).

2. Extent. Head injury may be classified as primary (in reference to the direct biomechanical changes in the brain) or secondary (in reference to the latent intracranial or systemic complications that exacerbate the original injury). The terms *focal* and *diffuse* are often used to describe a specific or gross lesion, respectively.

3. Severity. In addition to diagnostic tests, a head injury may be classified according to cognitive skill deficit and GCS as mild (13–15), moderate (9–12), or severe (3–8), using the GCS scoring system.

4. Mechanism of injury. The two mechanisms responsible for head injury are acceleration-deceleration and rotation forces. These forces may be of low or high velocity and result in the compression, traction, or shearing of brain structures.

Table 4-19 defines the most common types of head injuries and describes the clinical findings and management of each condition.

Spinal Cord Injury

SCI and the resultant para- or quadriplegia is typically due to trauma or less frequently due to impingement of the spinal cord from abscess,

Table 4-19. Clinical Findings and General Management of Head Injuries

Injury	Definition	Clinical Findings	Management
Cerebral concussion	Shaking of the brain secondary to acceleration-deceleration forces, usually as a result of a fall or during sports activity Can be classified as mild or classic Signs and symptoms of cerebral concussion are reversible	Headache, dizziness, irritability, inappropriate laughter, decreased concentration and memory, post-traumatic amnesia, altered gait	Observation
Cerebral contusion	Bruise (small hemorrhage) secondary to acceleration-deceleration forces or beneath a depressed skull fracture most commonly in the frontal or temporal areas	See Cerebral concussion, above	Observation General management
Cerebral laceration	Tear of the cortical surface secondary to acceleration-deceleration forces commonly in occurrence with cerebral contusion over the anterior and middle fossa where there are sharp bony surfaces	Dependent on area involved and degree of mass effect	General management
DAI	Occurs with widespread white matter shearing secondary to high-speed acceleration-deceleration forces, usually as a result of a motor vehicle accident Can be classified as mild, moderate, or severe	Coma, abnormal posturing, and other S/S dependent on area involved and degree of mass effect	General management
EDH	Blood accumulation in the epidural space that compresses deep brain structures	Headache, altered consciousness, abnormal posture, con-	General management

	Description	S/S	Treatment
	secondary to tearing of blood vessels. Associated with cranial fractures, particularly the thin temporal bone and frontal and middle meningeal artery tears	tralateral hemiparesis, dilated ipsilateral pupil, and other S/S dependent on specific location of lesion and degree of mass effect	Hematoma evacuation with vessel ligation
SDH	Blood accumulation in the subdural space that compresses brain structures as a result of traumatic rupture or tear of cerebral arteries, increased intracranial hemorrhage, or continued bleeding of a cerebral contusion. The onset of symptoms may be acute (24–48 hours), subacute (2 days to 2 weeks), or chronic (2 weeks to 3–4 months)	See EDH, above	General management. Small SDH: observation. Large SDH: evacuation
ICH	Blood accumulation in the brain parenchyma secondary to acceleration-deceleration forces, the shearing of cortical blood vessels, or beneath a fracture. May also arise as a complication of hypertension or delayed bleeding with progression of blood into the dural, arachnoid, or ventricular spaces	See EDH, above	General management. Hematoma evacuation (deep lesions are difficult to access)

Note: General management consists of intracranial pressure and temperature control and cardiac, respiratory, and nutritional support.
DAI = diffuse axonal injury; EDH = epidural hematoma; SDH = subdural hematoma; ICH = intracranial hemorrhage; S/S = signs and symptoms.
Source: Data from JV Hickey. The Clinical Practice of Neurological and Neurosurgical Nursing (3rd ed). Philadelphia: Lippincott, 1992; and CM Hudack, BM Gallo. Critical Care Nursing: A Holistic Approach (6th ed). Philadelphia: Lippincott, 1994.

ankylosing spondylitis, or tumor. SCI can be described according to location or mechanism of injury [28, 29]:

1. Location. SCI may involve the cervical, thoracic, or lumbar spines.

2. Mechanism of injury. SCI may result from blunt or penetrating injuries. Blunt forces include (1) forward hyperflexion (with or without axial compression, rotation, or distraction) causing the discontinuity of the posterior spinal ligaments, disc herniation, and vertebral dislocation or fracture or (2) hyperextension causing discontinuity of the anterior spinal ligaments, disc herniation, and vertebral dislocation or fracture. Penetrating forces, such as gunshot or stab wounds, may be (1) low-velocity, in which the spinal cord and protective structures are injured directly, or (2) high-velocity, in which a concussive force injures the spinal cord and the protective structures remain intact.

The severity of SCI is most commonly classified by motor function according to spinal level, or the Frankel Scale Functional Classification [29]. The American Spinal Injury Association has modified the Frankel scale to describe the different grades of SCI according to impairment [30]:

Complete—No sensory or motor function in S4–S5

Incomplete—The preservation of sensory function without motor function below the level of injury

Incomplete—The preservation of motor function below the level of injury. Muscle function below this level is less than fair (3/5).

Incomplete—The preservation of motor function below the level of injury. Muscle function below this level is greater than or equal to fair (3/5).

Normal—Sensory and motor function are intact.

Spinal cord lesions and the abnormal sensory and motor impairments are described as syndromes [28, 29]:

Anterior cord syndrome	Lesion of the anterior third of the spinal cord, with the loss of voluntary motor function and pain and temperature sense

Brown-Séquard's syndrome	Lesion of one half of the spinal cord, with loss of ipsilateral motor function and contralateral light touch, pain, and temperature sense
Cauda equina/conus medullaris syndrome	Lesion between T10 and the coccyx, with the loss of motor, bowel, bladder, and sexual function
Central cord syndrome	Lesion of the central portion of the spinal cord, with decreased upper- and lower-extremity function
Posterior cord syndrome	Lesion of the posterior spinal cord, with the loss of proprioception and vibration sense

The immediate physiologic effect of SCI is spinal shock, the triad of hypotension, bradycardia, and hypothermia secondary to altered sympathetic reflex activity [31]. It is beyond the scope of this book to discuss in detail the physiologic sequelae of SCI. However, other physiologic effects of SCI include autonomic dysreflexia; orthostatic hypotension; impaired respiratory function; bladder, bowel, and sexual dysfunction; malnutrition; stress ulcer; diabetes insipidus; syndrome of inappropriate secretion of antidiuretic hormone; edema; and increased risk of deep venous thrombosis (DVT).

Clinical tip

If during physical therapy intervention, a patient with SCI develops signs and symptoms associated with autonomic dysreflexia, return the patient to a reclined sitting position, and notify the nurse or physician immediately. Signs and symptoms of autonomic dysreflexia include headache, bradycardia, hypertension, and diaphoresis [32].

Cerebrovascular Disease

A patent cerebral vasculature is imperative for the delivery of oxygen to the brain. Alterations of the vascular supply or vascular structures can cause neurologic dysfunction from cerebral ischemia or infarction.

Transient Ischemic Attack

A transient ischemic attack (TIA) is characterized by the sudden onset of focal neurologic deficits such as hemiparesis or altered speech secondary to cerebral ischemia from thrombus or embolus. These deficits last less than 24 hours without residual effects. The management of TIAs involves observation, treatment of causative factor (if possible), anticoagulation, and carotid endarterectomy [33, 34].

Cerebrovascular Accident

A cerebrovascular accident (CVA), otherwise known as a stroke, is characterized by the sudden onset of focal neurologic deficits of more than 24 hours' duration secondary to cerebral insufficiency [33, 34].

The risk factors for CVA include age 65 years or older, hypertension, coronary artery disease, hyperlipidemia, hypercoagulable states, diabetes mellitus, obesity, smoking, and alcohol abuse [35].

Ischemic CVA is the result of cerebral hypoperfusion. An ischemic CVA has a slow onset and is due to thrombotic disease, such as carotid artery stenosis or arteriosclerotic intracranial arteries, or an embolus from the heart in the setting of atrial fibrillation, meningitis, prosthetic valves, patent foramen ovale, or endocarditis. The management of ischemic CVA involves blood pressure control (normal to elevated range), treatment of causative factors (if possible), anticoagulation, corticosteroids, hemodilution, cerebral edema control, and anticonvulsant therapy.

Hemorrhagic CVA involves cerebral hypoperfusion, which is abrupt in onset and is secondary to intraparenchymal hemorrhage associated with hypertension, AVM, trauma, aneurysm, or subarachnoid hemorrhage. The management of hemorrhagic CVA involves blood pressure control (low to normal range), treatment of causative factors (if possible), cerebral edema control, anticoagulation, anticonvulsant therapy, and surgical hematoma evacuation (if appropriate).

The signs and symptoms of CVA depend on the location and the extent of the cerebral ischemia or infarction. General signs and symptoms include contralateral motor and sensory loss, speech and perceptual deficits, altered vision, abnormal muscle tone, headache, nausea, vomiting, and altered affect.

Other terms commonly used to describe CVA include the following:

Completed stroke   A CVA in which the neurologic impairments have fully evolved [36]

Stroke in evolution	A CVA in which the neurologic impairments continue to evolve or fluctuate [36]
Lacunar stroke	A cerebral infarct (less than 1 or 2 cm in diameter) due to the thrombosis of very small cerebral vessels [36]
Watershed stroke	A cerebral infarct between the areas of perfusion of two different arteries, typically between the anterior and middle cerebral arteries [37]

Arteriovenous Malformation

AVM is a malformation in which blood from the arterial system is shunted to the venous system (thereby bypassing the capillaries) through abnormally thin and dilated vessels. An AVM can occur in a variety of locations, shapes, and sizes. The result of the bypass of blood is degeneration of brain parenchyma around the site of the AVM, which creates a chronic ischemic state. Signs and symptoms of AVM include headache, dizziness, fainting, aphasia, bruit, motor and sensory deficits, and the patient's complaint of a swishing noise in the head [33]. Management of AVM includes head CT, EEG, or cerebral angiogram to evaluate the location of the AVM, followed by surgical AVM repair, embolization, or radiation therapy for the nonsurgical candidate.

Cerebral Aneurysm

Cerebral aneurysm is the dilation of a cerebral blood vessel wall due to a smooth muscle defect through which the endothelial layer penetrates. Cerebral aneurysms most commonly occur at arterial bifurcations, in the larger vessels of the anterior circulation, and in the subarachnoid space. Signs and symptoms of cerebral aneurysm include severe headache, stiff neck, photophobia, vomiting, hemiplegia, seizure, and oculomotor (CN III) palsy. Management of cerebral aneurysm involves CT scan or angiogram to evaluate the aneurysm, followed by aneurysm clipping, embolization, or balloon occlusion.

Subarachnoid Hemorrhage

Subarachnoid hemorrhage (SAH) is most commonly the result of aneurysm rupture, or less commonly as a complication of AVM, tumor, infection, or trauma. It is graded from I to V according to the Hunt and Hess scale [33]:

I. Asymptomatic with mild headache, mild nuchal rigidity

II. Moderate to severe headache, nuchal rigidity, with or without neurologic deficit

III. Drowsiness, confusion, with mild focal neurologic deficit

IV. Stupor, hemiparesis

V. Comatose, abnormal posturing

SAH is diagnosed by history, clinical examination, CT scan, LP, or angiogram. The management of SAH depends on its severity and may include surgical aneurysm repair with blood evacuation; ventriculostomy; and supportive measures to maximize neurologic, cardiac, and respiratory status, rehydration, and fluid-electrolyte balance.

Complications of SAH include rebleeding, hydrocephalus, and vasospasm. *Vasospasm is* the spasm of one or more cerebral arteries that occurs 4–12 days after SAH [38]. Diagnosed by either cerebral angiography or CT, the exact etiology of vasospasm is unknown. Vasospasm results in cerebral ischemia distal to the area of spasm. The signs and symptoms of vasospasm are worsening level of consciousness, agitation, decreased strength, altered speech, pupil changes, headache, and vomiting [38].

Ventricular Dysfunction

Hydrocephalus

Hydrocephalus is the acute or gradual accumulation of CSF, causing excessive ventricular dilation and increased ICP. CSF permeates through the ventricular walls into brain tissue secondary to a pressure gradient. There are two types of hydrocephalus:

1. Noncommunicating hydrocephalus, in which there is an obstruction of CSF flow within the ventricular system. There may be thickening of the arachnoid villi or an increased amount or viscosity of CSF. This condition may be congenital or acquired, often as the result of aqueduct stenosis, tumor obstruction, abscess, cyst, or as a complication of neurosurgery [39].

2. Communicating hydrocephalus, in which there is an obstruction in CSF flow as it interfaces with the subarachnoid space. This con-

dition can occur with meningitis, after head injury, with subarachnoid hemorrhage, or as a complication of neurosurgery [2].

Hydrocephalus may be of acute onset characterized by headache, altered consciousness, decreased upward gaze, and papilledema [8]. Management includes treatment of the causative factor if possible, or ventriculoperitoneal (VP) or ventriculoatrial (VA) shunt.

Normal-pressure hydrocephalus (NPH) is hydrocephalus without a rise in ICP as determined by head CT and LP. The hallmark triad of the signs of NPH are altered mental status (confusion), altered gait, and urinary incontinence. NPH is typically gradual and idiopathic. Management of NPH is typically with a VP shunt.

Cerebrospinal Fluid Leak

A CSF leak is the abnormal discharge of CSF from a scalp wound, the nose (rhinorrhea), or the ear (otorrhea) as a result of a meningeal tear. A CSF leak can occur with anterior fossa or petrous skull fractures or, less commonly, as a complication of neurosurgery. With a CSF leak, the patient becomes at risk for meningitis with the altered integrity of the dura. A CSF leak is diagnosed by clinical history, CT cisternography, and testing of fluid from the leak site. If the fluid is CSF (and not another fluid such as mucus), it will test positive for glucose. The patient may also complain of a salty taste in the mouth. Management of CSF leak includes prophylactic antibiotics, dural repair, or VP or VA shunt.

Clinical tip

If it is known that a patient has a CSF leak, the therapist should be aware of vital sign or position restrictions before physical therapy intervention. If a CSF leak increases or a new leak occurs during physical therapy intervention, the therapist should stop the treatment, loosely cover the leaking area, and notify the nurse immediately.

Seizure

A seizure is a phenomenon of excessive cerebral cortex activity with or without loss of consciousness. The signs and symptoms of the seizure depend on the seizure locus on the cortex. Seizures can occur as a complication of CVA, head trauma, meningitis, or surgery. Total body system illnesses, such as a febrile state, drug overdose, hepatic encephalopathy, hypoglycemia, hyponatremia, or uremia are also associated with seizure [40]. Seizures are classified as partial (originating in a focal region of one hemisphere) or generalized (originating in both hemispheres or from a deep midline focus).

Types of partial seizures include the following [40]:

• *Simple partial seizures* are partial seizures without loss of consciousness.

• *Complex partial seizures* involve a brief loss of consciousness marked by motionless staring.

• *Partial seizures with secondary generalization* involve a progression to seizure activity in both hemispheres.

Types of generalized seizures include the following [40]:

• *Tonic seizures* are characterized by sudden flexor or extensor rigidity.

• *Tonic-clonic seizures* are characterized by sudden extensor rigidity followed by flexor jerking. (This type of seizure may be accompanied by incontinence or a crying noise due to rigidity of the truncal muscles.)

• *Clonic seizures* are characterized by jerking muscle movements.

• *Atonic seizures* are characterized by a loss of muscle tone.

• *Absence seizures* are characterized by a very brief period (seconds) of unresponsiveness with blank staring and the inability to complete any activity at the time of the seizure.

• *Myoclonic seizures* are characterized by local or gross rapid jerking movements. (These may be nonepileptic in nature if associated with neurodegenerative disease.)

Signs and symptoms of seizures are of acute onset and with or without any of the following: aura, tremor, paresthesia sensation of fear, gustatory hallucinations, lightheadedness, visual changes, and postictal (following seizure) confusion. Management of seizures involves the treatment of causative factor (if possible) and anticonvulsant therapy.

Syncope

Syncope is the loss of consciousness secondary to cerebral hypoperfusion. Syncope can be any of the following:

- Vasovagal, resulting from blood loss, emotions, fatigue, or pain

- Cardiovascular, resulting from atrial stenosis, aortic aneurysm, cardiac arrest, drug toxicity, dysrhythmias, intracardiac right-to-left shunting, mitral stenosis, pericarditis, physical activity, pulmonary embolism, or pulmonary hypertension

- Cerebrovascular, resulting from TIAs, subclavian steal syndrome (subclavian artery stenosis causing retrograde blood flow in the vertebral artery), or migraine

- Orthostasis

Dementia

Dementia is an alteration of the cerebral cortex that causes abnormal content of cognition. Dementia is acquired and progressive. It is associated with a myriad of conditions, some with additional motor and sensory impairments. It can be associated with alcoholism, Alzheimer's disease, brain tumor, chronic subdural hematoma, meningitis, human immunodeficiency virus infection or acquired immunodeficiency syndrome, Huntington's disease, hepatic disease, hypothyroidism, infection, multiple infarcts, NPH, or Parkinson's disease.

Neuroinfectious Diseases

See Chapter 10 for a description of encephalitis, meningitis, and poliomyelitis.

Neuromuscular Diseases

Amyotrophic Lateral Sclerosis

Amyotrophic lateral sclerosis (ALS), or Lou Gehrig's disease, is the progressive degeneration of upper and lower motor neurons, primarily the motor cells of the anterior horn and the corticospinal tract. The etiology of ALS is unknown. Signs and symptoms of ALS may include hyperreflexia, muscle atrophy, fasciculation, and weakness, which result in dysarthria, dysphagia, respiratory weakness, and immobility. The management of ALS is supportive or palliative depending on the disease state [8].

Guillain-Barré Syndrome

Guillain-Barré syndrome (GBS), or acute inflammatory postinfectious polyneuropathy, is the onset of paresthesia, pain (especially of the lumbar spine), and weakness (proximal followed by distal, including the facial and respiratory musculature), and autonomic dysfunction approximately 1–3 weeks after a viral infection. GBS is diagnosed by history, clinical presentation, CSF sampling (increased protein level), and EMG studies (which show decreased motor and sensory velocities). The management of GBS may consist of pharmacologic therapy (immunosuppressive agents), plasmapheresis, plasma exchange, physical therapy, and the supportive treatment of associated symptoms [8].

Multiple Sclerosis

Multiple sclerosis (MS) is the demyelination of the white matter of the CNS and of the optic nerve, presumably the immune reaction to a virus. MS is categorized by onset and progression as acute remitting-relapsing or chronic progressive. MS typically occurs in 20- to 40-year-olds, in females more than males. It is diagnosed by history (the onset of symptoms must occur and resolve more than once), clinical presentation, CSF sampling (increased myelin protein and IgG levels), and by MRI (which shows the presence of two or more plaques of the CNS). These plaques are located at areas of demyelination where lymphocytic and plasma infiltration and gliosis have occurred. Signs and symptoms of the early stages of MS may include focal weakness, fatigue, diplopia or blurred vision, equilibrium loss (vertigo), and urinary incontinence. Additional signs and symptoms of the latter stages of MS may include ataxia, paresthesias, spasticity, sensory deficits, hyperreflexia, tremor, and nystagmus. The management of MS may include pharmacologic therapy (immunosuppressive agents, corticosteroids, antiviral therapy, muscle relaxants), physical therapy, and the treatment of associated disease manifestations (e.g., bladder dysfunction) [8].

Myasthenia Gravis

Myasthenia gravis (MG) is a disorder of the neuromuscular junction in which there is wide synaptic space and decreased acetylcholine receptors. MG is thought to be an autoimmune reaction characterized by ptosis; diplopia; fatigue; and generalized weakness, including of the ocular, facial, laryngeal, and respiratory muscles. MG is associated with lupus, rheumatoid arthritis, and arrhythmic disorders. Onset typically occurs in young to middle-age adults. The diagnosis of MG is made by history, clinical examination, muscle biopsy, motor-point biopsy, serology tests, and with a strength improvement after anticholinesterase medication. The management of MG may include pharmacologic therapy (anticholinesterase, immunosuppressive agents), plasmapheresis, thymectomy, and ventilatory support if needed [8].

Parkinson's Disease

Parkinson's disease is the idiopathic progressive onset of bradykinesia, altered posture and postural reflexes, resting tremor, and cogwheel rigidity. Other signs and symptoms may include shuffling gait characterized by the inability to start or stop, blank facial expression, drooling, decreased speech volume, and an inability to perform fine motor tasks. Parkinson's disease is diagnosed by history, clinical presentation, and MRI (which shows a light rather than dark substantia nigra). The management of Parkinson's disease mainly includes pharmacologic therapy with antidyskinetic agents (Chapter Appendix Table 4-A.5) and physical therapy. The surgical autotransplantation of adrenal medulla cells into the caudate nucleus is under investigation [8].

General Management

Intracranial and Cerebral Perfusion Pressure

The maintenance of normal ICP or the prompt recognition of elevated ICP is one of the primary goals of the team caring for the postcraniosurgical patient or for the patient with cerebral trauma, neoplasm, or infection.

ICP is the pressure CSF exerts within the ventricles. This pressure (normally 4–15 mm Hg) fluctuates with any systemic condition; body position; or activity that increases cerebral blood flow, blood pressure, or intrathoracic or abdominal pressure or that decreases venous return or increases cerebral metabolism.

The three dynamic variables within the fixed skull are blood, CSF, and brain tissue. As ICP rises, these variables change in an attempt to lower ICP via the following mechanisms: cerebral vasoconstriction, the compression of venous sinuses, decreased CSF production, or the shift of CSF to the subarachnoid space. When these compensations fail, compression of brain structures occurs, and fatal brain herniation will develop if untreated. The signs and symptoms of increased ICP are listed in Table 4-20. The methods of controlling ICP, based on clinical neurologic examination and diagnostic tests, are outlined in Table 4-21.

Cerebral perfusion pressure (CPP), or cerebral blood pressure, is mean arterial pressure minus ICP. It indicates oxygen delivery to the brain. Normal CPP is 70–100 mm Hg. CPPs at or less than 60 mm Hg for a prolonged length of time correlate with ischemia and anoxic brain injury.

Following are terms related to ICP:

Brain herniation   The displacement of brain parenchyma through an anatomic opening; named according to the location of the displaced structure (e.g., transtentorial herniation is the herniation of the cerebral hemispheres, diencephalon, or midbrain beneath the tentorium cerebelli) [26]

Cerebral edema   The presence of fluid in the intracellular space, extracellular space, or both that increases brain bulk and thereby increases ICP; associated with conditions such as head trauma, cerebral ischemia, and cerebral neoplasm [26]

Mass effect   The combination of midline shift, third ventricle compression, and hydrocephalus [8]

Midline shift   The lateral displacement of the falx cerebri secondary to a space-occupying lesion

Space-occupying lesion   A mass lesion, such as a tumor or hematoma, that displaces brain parenchyma and may result in the elevation of ICP and shifting of the brain

Another primary goal of the team is to prevent further neurologic impairment. The main components of management of the patient with neurologic dysfunction in the acute care setting include pharmacologic therapy, surgical and nonsurgical procedures, and physical therapy intervention.

Table 4-20. Early and Late Signs of Increased Intracranial Pressure

Observation	Early	Late
Level of consciousness	Confusion, restlessness, lethargy	Coma
Pupil appearance	Ipsilateral pupil sluggish to light, ovoid in shape, with gradual dilatation	Ipsilateral pupil dilated and fixed or bilateral pupils dilated and fixed (if brain herniation has occurred)
Vision	Blurred vision, diplopia, and decreased visual acuity	Same as early signs but more exaggerated
Motor	Contralateral paresis	Abnormal posturing Bilateral flaccidity if herniation has occurred
Vital signs	Stable blood pressure and heart rate	Increased blood pressure and bradycardia (Cushing's response) Altered respiratory pattern
Additional findings	Headache Seizure Cranial nerve palsy	Headache Vomiting Altered brain stem reflexes

Source: Data from JV Hickey. The Clinical Practice of Neurological and Neurosurgical Nursing (3rd ed). Philadelphia: Lippincott, 1992.

Pharmacologic Therapy

A multitude of pharmacologic agents can be prescribed for the patient with neurologic dysfunction. For the purposes of this handbook, the discussion of medications for this population includes (1) osmotic diuretics, (2) corticosteroids, (3) antiepileptic agents, (4) barbiturates, (5) antidyskinetic/antiparkinsonian agents, and (6) muscle relaxants (Chapter Appendix 4-A). See Chapter Appendix 1-C for a discussion of cardiac medications prescribed for patients with cerebrovascular disease (e.g., beta blockers, calcium channel blockers, nitrates, thrombolytic agents, anticoagulants, loop diuretics, vasodilators, enzyme

Table 4-21. Treatment Options for Elevated Intracranial Pressure

Variable	Treatment
Blood pressure	Antihypertensive agents with beta blockers Sedation
Cerebrospinal fluid drainage	Ventriculostomy to remove cerebrospinal fluid
Positioning	Head of the bed at 30–45 degrees to increase cerebral venous drainage
Ventilation	Hyperventilation to decrease $PaCO_2$
Sedation	Medication during stressful activities
Seizure control	Prophylactic antiseizure medication
Temperature control	Cooling blanket or antipyretic
Diuretics	Medication to minimize cerebral edema

$PaCO_2$ = partial pressure of carbon dioxide.
Source: Data from L Thelan, J Davie, L Urden, M Lough. Critical Care Nursing: Diagnosis and Management (2nd ed). St. Louis: Mosby–Year Book, 1994.

inhibitors, antiarrhythmics), Chapter 5 ("Management") for a discussion of radiation therapy and chemotherapy prescribed for patients with CNS neoplasm, and Appendix VI for a discussion of analgesic medications prescribed for pain control.

Surgical and Nonsurgical Neurologic Procedures

The most common surgical and nonsurgical neurologic procedures are described below (see Chapter 3 for a description of spinal surgical procedures, Chapter 5 for a description of procedures related to cerebral or spinal neoplasm, Appendix IV for a description of ICP monitoring devices, and to Appendix V for general postoperative considerations.)

Aneurysm clipping	The obliteration of an aneurysm with a surgical clip placed at the stem of the aneurysm
Burr hole	A small hole made in the skull with a drill for access to the brain for the placement of ICP

monitoring systems, hematoma evacuation, or stereotactic procedures; a series of burr holes is made before a craniotomy

Craniectomy (bone flap)
The removal of incised bone usually for brain tissue decompression; the bone may be placed in the bone bank or temporarily placed in the subcutaneous tissue of the abdomen (to maintain blood supply)

Cranioplasty
The reconstruction of the skull with a bone graft or acrylic material to restore the protective properties of the scalp and for cosmesis

Craniotomy
An incision through the skull for access to the brain for extensive intracranial neurosurgery, such as aneurysm or AVM repair or tumor removal; craniotomy is named according to the area of the bone affected (e.g., frontal, bifrontal, frontotemporal [pterional], temporal, occipital)

Embolization
The use of arterial catheterization (entrance usually at the femoral artery) to place a material such as a detachable coil, balloon, or sponge to clot off an AVM or aneurysm

Evacuation
The removal of an epidural, subdural, or intraparenchymal hematoma via burr hole or craniotomy

Plasmapheresis
The removal of whole blood followed by the separation of the plasma from the other blood components, followed by the reinfusion of the same blood once the original plasma has been replaced with a synthetic; commonly used with Guillain-Barré syndrome or other polyneuropathies

Shunt placement
The insertion of a shunt system that connects the ventricular system with the right atrium (VA shunt) or peritoneal cavity (VP shunt) to allow the drainage of CSF when ICP rises

Stereotaxis
The use of a stereotactic frame (a frame that temporarily attaches to the patient's head) in conjunction with head CT results to specifi-

cally localize a pretargeted site as in tumor biopsy; a burr hole is then made for access to the brain

---

Clinical tip

The physical therapist should be aware of the location of a craniectomy because the patient should not have direct pressure applied to that area. Look for signs posted at the patient's bedside that communicate positioning restrictions.

Physical Therapy Intervention

Goals

The primary physical therapy goals in treating patients with primary neurologic pathology in the acute care setting include maximizing independence and promoting safety with gross functional activity.

Basic Concepts for the Treatment of Patients with Neurologic Dysfunction

- A basic understanding of neurologic pathophysiology is necessary to create appropriate functional goals for the patient. The therapist must appreciate the difference between reversible and irreversible and between nonprogressive and progressive disease states.

- A basic knowledge of the factors that affect ICP and the ability to modify treatment techniques or conditions during the initial postoperative mobilization of the intracranial surgical patient are necessary for patient safety.

- There are a variety of therapeutic techniques and motor control theories for the treatment of the patient with neurologic dysfunction. Do not hesitate to experiment with or combine techniques from different schools of thought.

- Be persistent with patients who do not readily respond to your typical treatment techniques because these patients most likely present with perceptual impairments superimposed on motor and sensory deficits.

- Recognize that it is rarely possible to fix all of the patient's impairments at once. Teaching compensatory techniques is acceptable.

References

1. Marieb EN. Human Anatomy and Physiology. Redwood City, CA: Benjamin-Cummings, 1989;172.
2. Moore KL. The Head. In KL Moore (ed), Clinically Oriented Anatomy (2nd ed). Baltimore: Williams & Wilkins, 1985;794.
3. Westmoreland BF, Benarroch EE, Daube JR, et al. Medical Neurosciences: An Approach to Anatomy, Pathology, and Physiology by Systems and Levels (3rd ed). New York: Little, Brown, 1986;107.
4. Thelan L, Davie J, Urden L, Lough M. Critical Care Nursing: Diagnosis and Management (2nd ed). St. Louis: Mosby–Year Book, 1994;477.
5. Marieb EN. Human Anatomy and Physiology. Redwood City, CA: Benjamin-Cummings, 1989;375.
6. Westmoreland BF, Benarroch EE, Daube JR, et al. Medical Neurosciences: An Approach to Anatomy, Pathology, and Physiology by Systems and Levels (3rd ed). New York: Little, Brown, 1986;273.
7. Goldberg S. The Four-Minute Neurological Exam. Miami: MedMaster, 1992;20.
8. Lindsay KW, Bone I, Callander R. Neurology and Neurosurgery Illustrated (2nd ed). Edinburgh: Churchill Livingstone, 1991.
9. Plum F, Posner J. The Diagnosis of Stupor and Coma (3rd ed). Philadelphia: FA Davis, 1980;1.
10. Jennett B, Teasdale G. Management of Head Injuries. Philadelphia: FA Davis, 1981;77.
11. Strub RL, Black FW. Mental Status Examination in Neurology (2nd ed). Philadelphia: FA Davis, 1985;9.
12. Love RJ, Webb WG. Neurology for the Speech-Language Pathologist (2nd ed). Boston: Butterworth–Heinemann, 1992;183.
13. Specter RM. The Pupils. In HK Walker, WD Hall, JW Hurst (eds), Clinical Methods: The History, Physical, and Laboratory Examinations (3rd ed). Boston: Butterworth, 1990;300.
14. Thelan L, Davie J, Urden L, Lough M. Critical Care Nursing: Diagnosis and Management (2nd ed). St. Louis: Mosby–Year Book, 1994;504.
15. Kisner C, Colby LA. Therapeutic Exercise: Foundations and Techniques (2nd ed). Philadelphia: FA Davis, 1985;3.
16. Crutchfield CA. Neuromuscular Causes of Movement Dysfunction and Physical Disability. In RM Scolly, MR Barnes (eds), Physical Therapy. Philadelphia: Lippincott, 1989;174.
17. Landau WM. Muscle Tone: Hypertonus, Spasticity, Rigidity. In G Adelman (ed), Encyclopedia of Neuroscience (Vol II). Boston: Birkhäuser Boston, 1987;721.
18. Schneider FJ. Traumatic Spinal Cord Injury. In DA Umphred (ed), Neurological Rehabilitation (2nd ed). St. Louis: Mosby, 1990;423.

19. Charness A. Gathering the Pieces: Evaluation. In A Charness (ed), Stroke/Head Injury: A Guide to Functional Outcomes in Physical Therapy Management. Rockville, MD: Aspen, 1986;1.
20. Hickey JV. Assessment of Neurological Signs. In JV Hickey (ed), The Clinical Practice of Neurological and Neurosurgical Nursing (3rd ed). Philadelphia: Lippincott, 1992;113.
21. Hickey JV. The Neurological Physical Examination. In JV Hickey (ed), The Clinical Practice of Neurological and Neurosurgical Nursing (3rd ed). Philadelphia: Lippincott, 1992;59.
22. Bates B. The Nervous System. In B Bates (ed), A Guide to Physical Examination and History Taking (6th ed). Philadelphia: Lippincott, 1995;491.
23. Hickey JV. Diagnostic Evaluation. In JV Hickey (ed), The Clinical Practice of Neurological and Neurosurgical Nursing (3rd ed). Philadelphia: Lippincott, 1992;89.
24. Thelan L, Davie J, Urden L, Lough M. Critical Care Nursing: Diagnosis and Management (2nd ed). St. Louis: Mosby–Year Book, 1994;515.
25. Davis KR, Martin JB. Imaging of the Nervous System. In KJ Isselbacher, E Braunwald, JD Wilson et al. (eds), Harrison's Principles of Internal Medicine (13th ed). New York: McGraw-Hill, 1994;2212.
26. Hickey JV. Craniocerebral Trauma. In JV Hickey (ed), The Clinical Practice of Neurological and Neurosurgical Nursing (3rd ed). Philadelphia: Lippincott, 1992;351.
27. Hudak CM, Gallo BM. Head Injury. In CM Hudak, BM Gallo (eds), Critical Care Nursing: A Holistic Approach (6th ed). Philadelphia: Lippincott, 1994;705.
28. Zejdlik CP. Physiological Consequences and Assessment of Injury to the Spine and Spinal Cord. In CP Zejdlik (ed), Management of Spinal Cord Injury (2nd ed). Boston: Jones & Bartlett, 1992;53.
29. Buchanan LE. An Overview. LE Buchanan, DA Nawoczenski (eds), Spinal Cord Injury Concepts and Management Approaches. Baltimore: Williams & Wilkins, 1987;3.
30. American Spinal Injury Association. Standards for Neurological Functional Classifications of Spinal Cord Injury. 1992.
31. Zejdlik CP. Critical Care: A Rehabilitative Focus. In CP Zejdlik (ed), Management of Spinal Cord Injury (2nd ed). Boston: Jones & Bartlett, 1992;105.
32. Zejdlik CP. Regulatory Cardiovascular Function and Body Temperature. In CP Zejdlik (ed), Management of Spinal Cord Injury (2nd ed). Boston: Jones & Bartlett, 1992;305.
33. Thelan L, Davie J, Urden L, Lough M. Critical Care Nursing: Diagnosis and Management (2nd ed). St. Louis: Mosby–Year Book, 1994;522.
34. Hudak CM, Gallo BM. Common Neurologic Disorders. In CM Hudak, BM Gallo (eds), Critical Care Nursing: A Holistic Approach (6th ed). Philadelphia: Lippincott, 1994;729.
35. Gilroy J. Clinical Applications and Introduction to Cerebrovascular Anatomy, Physiology, and Pathology. In CL Rumbaugh, A Wang, FY Tsai (eds), Cerebrovascular Disease: Imaging and Interventional Treatment Options. New York: Igaku-Shoin Medical Publishers, 1995;3.

36. Kistler JP, Ropper AA, Martin JB. Cerebrovascular Diseases. In JD Wilson, E Braunwald, KJ Isselbacher et al. (eds), Harrison's Principles of Internal Medicine (12th ed). New York: McGraw-Hill, 1991;1977.

37. Ramsey RG. Neuroradiology—Which Tests to Order? In WJ Weiner, CG Goetz (eds), Neurology for the Non-Neurologist (2nd ed). Philadelphia: Lippincott, 1989;25.

38. Armstrong SL. Cerebral vasospasm: early detection and intervention. Crit Care Nurse 1994;14:33.

39. Greenberg DA, Aminoff MJ, Simon RP. Disorders of Cognitive Function: Dementia and Amnestic Syndromes. In DA Greenberg, MJ Aminoff, RP Simon (eds), Clinical Neurology (2nd ed). East Norwalk, CT: Appleton & Lange, 1993;48.

40. Drury IJ, Gelb DJ. Seizures. In DJ Gelb (ed), Introduction to Clinical Neurology. Boston: Butterworth–Heinemann, 1995;123.

Appendix 4-A:
Nervous System Medications

Table 4-A.1. Osmotic Diuretics

Purpose
  To decrease cerebral edema and decrease interstitial pressure
Generic name (brand name)
  Mannitol (Osmitrol)
  Glycerin (Glyrol, Osmoglyn)
  Urea (Carbamide, Carmol, Ureacin, Ureaphil)
Mechanisms of action
  Increase plasma osmolarity and induce the diffusion of water into the
    extravascular spaces and plasma
General side effects
  Confusion, headache, nausea, vomiting, blurred vision, fever, hyper- or
    hypotension, tachycardia, fluid electrolyte imbalance

Source: Data from MT Shannon, BA Wilson, CL Stang. Govoni & Hayes Drugs and
Nursing Implications (8th ed). East Norwalk, CT: Appleton & Lange, 1995.

Table 4-A.2.   Corticosteroids

Purpose
    To decrease cerebral edema and/or to decrease inflammation in neoplastic
        or inflammatory diseases
Generic name (brand name)
    Dexamethasone (Aeroseb-Dex, Decaderm, Decadron, Decaspray, Dexameth,
        Dexamethasone Intensol, Dexasone, Dexone, Hexadrol, Maxidex,
        Mymethasone)
    Dexamethasone acetate (Dalalone DP, Dalalone-LA, Dexone LA, Solurex)
    Methylprednisolone (Medrol, depMedalone, Depoject, Depo-Medrol,
        Depopred, Duralone, Med-Depo, Medralone, Medrone, M-Prednisol,
        Pre-Dep, Rep-Pred, A-Methapred, Solu-Medrol)
    Prednisone (Deltasone, Meticorten, Orasone, Panasol, Prednicen-M,
        Sterapred)
Mechanism of action
    Prevent the accumulation of inflammatory cells at the infectious site
    Inhibit lysosomal enzyme release, chemical mediators of inflammatory
        response, and phagocytosis
    Reduce capillary dilation and permeability
General side effects
    Headache, vertigo, euphoria, insomnia, seizure, CHF, edema, diaphoresis,
        cushingoid features, hyperglycemia, osteoporosis, muscle weakness,
        decreased wound healing

CHF = congestive heart failure.
Source: Data from MT Shannon, BA Wilson, CL Stang. Govoni & Hayes Drugs and
Nursing Implications (8th ed). East Norwalk, CT: Appleton & Lange, 1995.

Table 4-A.3. Antiepileptic Agents

Purpose
  To decrease seizure activity
Generic name (brand name)
  Carbamazepine (Epitol, Tegretol)
  Clonazepam (Klonopin, Rivotril)
  Diazepam (E-Pam, Meval, Valium, Valrelease)
  Ethosuximide (Zarontin)
  Methsuximide (Celontin)
  Phensuximide (Milontin)
  Phenytoin (Dilantin-125, Dilantin-30, Dilantin Kapseals, Dilantin,
    Diphenylan Sodium)
  Primidone (Mysoline)
  Valproic acid (Depakene, Depakote, Depakote Sprinkle, Epival)
Mechanism of action
  Exact mechanism of action is unclear; however, electrical impulses from
    the cerebral motor cortex are decreased in frequency and voltage
General side effects
  Confusion, agitation, fatigue, dizziness, vertigo, headache, visual halluci-
    nation, diplopia, hyperreflexia, tremor, hypo- or hypertension,
    arrhythmia, CHF, edema, nausea, vomiting, urinary frequency or
    retention

CHF = congestive heart failure.
Source: Data from MT Shannon, BA Wilson, CL Stang. Govoni & Hayes Drugs and
Nursing Implications (8th ed). East Norwalk, CT: Appleton & Lange, 1995.

Table 4-A.4. Barbiturates

Purpose
  To decrease previously uncontrollable intracranial pressures or stop previously uncontrollable seizure activity (through the induction of sedation or coma)
Generic name (brand name)
  Mephobarbital (Mebaral, Methylphenobarbitol)
  Pentobarbital (Nembutal, Nembutal Sodium)
  Phenobarbital (Barbita, Gardenal, Luminal, Solfoton, Luminal Sodium)
  Secobarbital (Seconal, Seconal Sodium)
Mechanism of action
  Inhibit the reticular activating system and alter the electrical transmission of impulses of the cerebral cortex
General side effects
  Confusion, somnolence, depression, dizziness, headache, nystagmus, nausea, vomiting, diarrhea, bradycardia, hypotension, laryngo- or bronchospasm, hypoventilation, apnea, hypocalcemia, ataxia

---

Source: Data from MT Shannon, BA Wilson, CL Stang. Govoni & Hayes Drugs and Nursing Implications (8th ed). East Norwalk, CT: Appleton & Lange, 1995; and BA Rose. Neurologic therapies in critical care. Crit Care Nurs 1993;5:237.

Table 4-A.5. Antidyskinetic/Antiparkinsonism Agents

Purpose
  To decrease bradykinesia, rigidity, and tremor (as in parkinsonian disorders)
Generic name (brand name)
  Amantadine (Symmetrel)
  Benztropine (Cogentin)
  Biperiden (Akineton)
  Biperiden (Akineton)
  Bromocriptine (Parlodel)
  Carbidopa-levodopa (Sinemet)
  Ethopropazine (Parsidol)
  Levodopa or L-dopa (Dopar, Larodopa)
  Procyclidine (Kemadrin)
  Selegiline or L-deprenyl (Eldepryl)
  Trihexyphenidyl (Artane, Trihexy)
Mechanism of action
  Block cerebral cholinergic receptors or increase amount of dopamine in
    the brain
General side effects
  Confusion, restlessness, insomnia, blurred vision, diplopia, headache,
    tachycardia, palpitations, orthostatic hypotension, hypertension, flush-
    ing, sweating, rhinorrhea, urinary incontinence, weight loss or gain,
    anemia, decreased hematocrit and hemoglobin

Source: Data from MT Shannon, BA Wilson, CL Stang. Govoni & Hayes Drugs and
Nursing Implications (8th ed). Norwalk, CT: Appleton & Lange, 1995; and JB Clark,
SF Queener, VB Karb. Drugs for Parkinson's Disease and Alzheimer's Disease. In JB
Clark, SF Queener, VB Karb (eds), Pharmacologic Basis of Nursing Practice (5th ed).
St. Louis: Mosby–Year Book, 1997;696.

Table 4-A.6. Muscle Relaxants

Purpose
  To decrease muscle spasticity

Generic name (brand name)
  Baclofen (Lioresal, Lioresal DS)
  Dantrolene (Dantrium)
  Diazepam (E-Pam, Meval, Valium, Valrelease)

Mechanism of action
  Depress mono- and polysynaptic afferent spinal reflex activity or alter
    calcium ion activity within muscle

General side effects
  Confusion, drowsiness, fatigue, weakness, insomnia, hypotension,
    diplopia, nausea, vomiting, urinary frequency, hyperglycemia, ataxia

---

Source: Data from MT Shannon, BA Wilson, CL Stang. Govoni & Hayes Drugs and
Nursing Implications (8th ed). East Norwalk, CT: Appleton & Lange, 1995; and JB
Clark, SF Queener, VB Karb. Centrally Acting Skeletal Muscle Relaxants. In JB Clark,
SF Queener, VB Karb (eds), Pharmacologic Basis of Nursing Practice (5th ed). St.
Louis: Mosby–Year Book, 1997;705.

5

Oncology

Timothy J. Troiano

Introduction

The physical therapist requires an understanding of underlying cancer pathology, as well as the side effects, considerations, and precautions related to cancer care to enhance clinical decision making and enable him or her to safely and effectively treat the patient with cancer. This knowledge will also assist the physical therapist with the early detection of previously undiagnosed cancer. The objectives for this chapter are the following:

1. To provide an understanding of the clinical assessment of a patient with cancer, including staging and classification

2. To provide an understanding of the various medical and surgical methods of managing patients with cancer

3. To provide a better understanding of a variety of the different body system cancers

4. To provide evaluation and treatment considerations for the physical therapist

A multidisciplinary team is best suited to manage a patient with cancer. This oncology team may include the medical oncologist, surgeon, radiation oncologist, nurse, nurse practitioner, physical therapist, occupational therapist, nutritionist, and social worker. As a member of the this team, the physical therapist can communicate valuable information regarding the functional mobility and activity tolerance of a patient during various stages of cancer care.

Neoplasms

Normal cells have the ability to differentiate and adapt their structure and function according to the specific needs of the tissues [1]. Malignant neoplasms, or malignant tumors, lose this ability and instead grow uncontrollably, invading normal tissues as well as causing destruction to surrounding tissues and organs. Malignant neoplasms may spread, or metastasize, to other areas of the body through the cardiovascular or lymphatic system.

Neoplasms may also be benign and consist of the abnormal growth of the same type of cell. Benign tumors do not metastasize to or invade surrounding tissue. Benign neoplasms may still be significant, however, because of their proximity to vital organs or organ systems and the potential of compressing these structures. Tables 5-1 and 5-2 describe tumor classification and characteristics.

Clinical Assessment

Screening for Risk Factors

Suspicion of cancer can occur for various reasons and in various circumstances. For example, risk factors or incidental findings indicative of cancer (e.g., detecting a mass during palpation or if the patient reports blood in his or her sputum) may be discovered during a physical examination, diagnostic testing for other complaints, or routine care. Patients may also exhibit warning signs (Table 5-3), identifiable symptoms of cancer, or both. Common risk factors for selected cancer sites are listed in Table 5-4; Table 5-5 describes occupational exposures that can increase the risk of cancer.

Additional signs and symptoms that may indicate cancer are the following:

- Fever
- Weight loss of more than 10 lbs

Table 5-1. Classification of Benign and Malignant Tumors

Tissue of Origin	Benign Tumor	Malignant Tumor
Epithelial		
Surface epithelium	Papilloma	Carcinoma
Epithelial lining of glands or ducts	Adenoma	Adenocarcinoma
Connective tissue and muscle		
Fibrous tissue	Fibroma	Fibrosarcoma
Cartilage	Chondroma	Chondrosarcoma
Bone	Osteoma	Osteosarcoma
Smooth muscle	Leiomyoma	Leiomyosarcoma
Striated muscle	Rhabdomyoma	Rhabdomyosarcoma
Nerve tissue		
Glial	—	Glioma
Meninges	Meningioma	Meningeal sarcoma
Retina	—	Retinoblastoma

Source: Reprinted with permission from S Baird (ed). A Cancer Source Book for Nurses (6th ed). Atlanta: American Cancer Society, 1991;28.

Table 5-2. Characteristics of Benign and Malignant Neoplasms

Benign	Malignant
Encapsulated	Nonencapsulated
Noninvasive	Invasive
Highly differentiated	Poorly differentiated
Mitoses rare	Mitoses relatively common
Slow growth	Rapid growth
Little or no anaplasia	Anaplastic to varying degrees
No metastasis	Metastasis

Source: Reprinted with permission from S Baird (ed). A Cancer Source Book for Nurses (6th ed). Atlanta: American Cancer Society, 1991;23.

Table 5-3. Seven Warning Signs of Cancer

1. Change in bowel or bladder habits
2. A sore that does not heal
3. Unusual bleeding or discharge
4. Thickening or lump in breast or elsewhere
5. Indigestion or difficulty swallowing
6. Obvious change in a wart or mole
7. Nagging cough or hoarseness

Source: Reprinted with permission from S Baird (ed). A Cancer Source Book for Nurses (6th ed). Atlanta: American Cancer Society, 1991;43.

Table 5-4. Risk Factors for Selected Cancer Sites

Cancer Site	High-Risk Factors
Lung	Heavy smoker over age 50
	Smoked a pack a day for 20 years (20 pack years)
	Started smoking at age 15 or before
	Smoker working with or near asbestos
Breast	Lump in breast or nipple discharge
	History of breast cancer in other breast or benign breast disease
	Family history of breast cancer
	Diet high in fat
	Nulliparous or first child after age 30
	Early menarche or menopause
Colon-rectum	History of rectal polyps or colonic adenomatosis
	Family history of rectal polyps
	Ulcerative colitis or Crohn's disease
	Obesity
	Increasing age
Uterine-endometrial	Unusual vaginal bleeding or discharge
	History of menstrual irregularity
	Late menopause (after age 55)
	Nulliparity
	Infertility through anovulation
	Diabetes, hypertension, and obesity
	Age 50–64

Cancer Site	High-Risk Factors
Skin	Excessive exposure to the sun
	Fair complexion that burns easily
	Presence of congenital moles or history of dysplastic nevi or cutaneous melanoma
	Family history of melanoma
Oral	Heavy smoker and alcohol drinker
	Poor oral hygiene
	Long-term exposure to the sun, particularly to the lips
Ovary	History of ovarian cancer among close relatives
	Nulliparity or delayed age at first pregnancy
	Age 50–59
Prostate	Increasing age
	Occupations relating to the use of cadmium
Stomach	History of stomach cancer among close relatives
	Diet heavy in smoked, pickled, or salted foods

Source: Reprinted with permission from S Baird (ed). A Cancer Source Book for Nurses (6th ed). Atlanta: American Cancer Society, 1991;32.

- Fatigue

- Pain

- Paraneoplastic symptoms (effects not related to the direct involvement of the cancer but due to systemic hormonal effects. These symptoms are associated with Cushing's disease, hypercalcemia, dermatomyositis, Eaton-Lambert syndrome, cerebellar degeneration, hypertrophic pulmonary osteoarthroplasty, and cachexia [2])

With any of the aforementioned signs and symptoms, definitive workup and diagnosis are indicated for early detection and intervention.

Patients with a known history of cancer should also be assessed for potential recurrence of the cancer. The clinician should have a higher suspicion of abnormal symptoms related to cancer in patients who have a history of cancer.

Table 5-5. Occupational Exposures That Increase the Risk for Cancer

Cancer Sites	Causal Agents	Work or Exposure
Lung	Bichloromethyl ether	Ion-exchange resin producers
	Chromium	Ore and pigment manufacturers
	Mustard gas	Poison gas producers
Lung, pleura	Asbestos	Asbestos miners, insulation, shipyard workers
Lung and skin	Arsenic	Smelter and pesticide workers
	Polycyclic hydrocarbons	Mineral oil and tar workers
Lung and nasal	Nickel	Nickel refiners
Skin	Ultraviolet light	Outdoor workers, fishermen
Liver	Vinyl chloride	Vinyl chloride workers
	Alcohol	Brewery workers
Bladder	Aromatic amines	Dye and rubber workers
Leukemia	Benzene	Glue and varnish workers
Nasal	Isopropyl alcohol	Isopropyl alcohol manufacturers
	Wood dust	Furniture workers
Multiple sites	Ionizing radiation	Radium dial painters

Source: Reprinted with permission from S Baird (ed). A Cancer Source Book for Nurses (6th ed). Atlanta: American Cancer Society, 1991;37.

Although the physical therapist will probably not play a significant role in the screening of cancer in the acute care setting, knowledge of the risk factors and warning signs may help identify symptoms that could affect physical therapy interventions and require further medical attention.

Diagnosis

The diagnosis of cancer can be made during any stage of disease progression. Signs and symptoms consistent with cancer are evaluated with medical testing and procedures to determine if a malignancy is present. Tables 5-6 and 5-7 list the procedures performed in the differential diagnosis of cancer. These procedures consist of either direct sampling

Table 5-6. Diagnostic Tests for Cancer

Type	Description
Biopsy	A sample of tumor cells is taken with aspiration, needle, incisional, and excisional procedures, which are described in Table 5-7. The tissue sample is assessed by the pathologist to identify the type of cancer cell through histology. The procedure may be guided by computed tomography scan or ultrasound.
Blood tests	Various blood tests are conducted. Abnormal values or cytologic tumor markers can be identified with a blood test [2]. Normal values of common blood tests are noted below [16].
Platelet counts	150,000–400,000 count/µl [5]
Hematocrit	Females: 37–47% Males: 40–50%
Hemoglobin	Females: 12–16 g/100 ml Males: 14–18 g/100 ml
Blood glucose	80–120 mg/dl
Leukocytes	5,000–10,000/µl
Urinalysis	Test is used to detect blood, cancer cells in urine.
Stool guaiac	Sample is used to detect blood in small quantities in the stool. Samples may be taken during digital rectal examination or after a bowel movement.
Sigmoidoscopy	The sigmoid colon is examined with a sigmoidoscope.
Colonoscopy	The upper portion of the rectum is examined with a colonoscope.
Mammography	A radiographic method is used to look for a mass in breast tissue.
Radiograph	The x-ray is used to detect tumors of bone or lung.
Magnetic resonance imaging	This noninvasive nuclear imaging technique is used to assess lesions suspected of being cancerous.
Computed tomography scan	This radiologic imaging technique is used to locate the site of cancer and determine its size.
Bone scan	This radiographic method is used to assess for tumor or metastatic growth in bone.
Sputum cytology	A sputum specimen is inspected for cancerous cells.

Table 5-6. *Continued*

Type	Description
Bronchoscopy	A tissue or sputum sample can be taken by rigid or flexible bronchoscopy. (Greater detail of this procedure is discussed in "Flexible Bronchoscopy" in Chapter 2.)

of tissues and fluids (e.g., biopsy or sputum cytology) or direct imaging and observation of suspected cancer sites (e.g., mammography, radiographs, computed tomography [CT], magnetic resonance imaging [MRI], bone scan, or bronchoscopy).

Staging and Classification

After the diagnosis of cancer is established, anatomic staging is performed to describe the location and size of the primary site of the tumor, the extent of lymph node involvement, and the presence or absence of metastasis. Staging helps to determine treatment options, predict life expectancy, and determine prognosis for complete resolution.

Tumors are classified according to the American Joint Committee on Cancer using the TNM Classification System (T stands for tumor, N stands for node, and M stands for metastasis). This system is based on criteria for classification by specific anatomic sites (Table 5-8).

Staging of cancer is determined and noted as stages 0–IV. This system is used to describe the extent of the disease [3].

Stage 0		Cancer in situ
Stage I	(T2, N0, M0)	Cancer limited to original organ
Stage II	(T2, N1, M0)	Cancer has spread to the surrounding tissue in the same anatomic region
Stage III	(T3, N2, M0)	High probability of metastatic disease
Stage IV	(T4, N3, M1)	Metastatic spread to other regions

Table 5-7. Biopsy Procedures Used in the Diagnosis of Cancer

Type of Biopsy	Definition	Note
Aspiration	Aspiration of cells and tissue fragments through a needle that has been guided into suspected malignant tissue	Cytologic analysis can provide a tentative diagnosis. Because a tumor can be missed, only a positive test is diagnostically significant.
Needle	Obtaining a core of tissue through a specially designed needle introduced into suspected malignant tissues	This is sufficient for the diagnosis of most tumors. Differentiating benign and reparative lesions from malignancies is often difficult with soft tissue and bony sarcomas. Because the tumor can be missed, only a positive test is diagnostically significant.
Incisional	Removal of a small wedge of tissue from a larger tumor mass	This is the preferred method for diagnosing soft tissue and bony sarcomas.
Excisional	Excision of the entire suspected tumor tissue	This is the procedure of choice for small, accessible tumors.

Source: Reprinted with permission from S Baird (ed). A Cancer Source Book for Nurses (6th ed). Atlanta: American Cancer Society, 1991;58.

Table 5-8. TNM Clinical Classification System

Primary tumor (T)

   TX: Cannot be assessed

   T0: No evidence of a primary tumor

   Tis: Carcinoma in situ

   T1, T2, T3, and T4: Increasing size, local extent, or both, of primary tumor

Regional lymph nodes (N)

   NX: Cannot be assessed

   N0: No metastasis

   N1, N2, and N3: Increasing involvement of regional lymph nodes

Metastasis (M)

   MX: Cannot be assessed

   M0: No distant metastasis

   M1: Distant metastasis

Source: Data from American Joint Committee on Cancer. Manual for Staging of Cancer (4th ed). Philadelphia: Lippincott, 1992;3–9.

Clinical tip

Knowing the stage of cancer that a patient is in helps the physical therapist modify treatment parameters and establish realistic goals.

Physical Performance Status

A patient's physical performance status can also be used to determine the appropriateness and tolerance of cancer treatment. Different methods may be used to assess a patient's physical capacity or performance. Methods described in Tables 5-9 through 5-12 include the World Health Organization scale, Karnofsky Performance Status scale, Eastern Cooperative Oncology Group scale, and the American Joint Committee on Cancer scale [4]. Graded exercise tolerance tests (maximal or submaximal) may also be conducted to determine exercise capacity. These tests are discussed in "Exercise Testing" in Chapter 1. The 6- or 12-minute walk test can also be used to determine exercise capacity and is easily conducted (Appendix IX).

Table 5-9. World Health Organization Performance Status Scale

Score	Status
0	Fully active, able to carry out all predisease activities without restriction
1	Restricted in strenuous activity but ambulatory and able to carry out light work or pursue sedentary occupation
2	Ambulatory and capable of all self-care but unable to carry out any light work; up and about more than 50% of waking hours
3	Capable of only limited self-care; confined to bed or chair more than 50% of waking hours
4	Completely disabled; unable to carry out any self-care and confined totally to bed or chair

Source: Data from SS O'Mary. Diagnostic Evaluation, Classification, and Staging. In SL Groenwald, MH Frogge, M Goodman, CH Yarbro (eds), Cancer Nursing: Principles and Practice. Boston: Jones & Bartlett, 1993.

Table 5-10. Karnofsky Performance Status Scale

Score	Status
100%	Normal; no complaints; no evidence of disease
90%	Able to carry on normal activity; minor signs or symptoms of disease
80%	Normal activity with effort; some signs or symptoms of disease
70%	Cares for self; unable to carry on normal activity or to do active work
60%	Requires occasional assistance but able to care for most needs
50%	Requires considerable assistance and frequent medical care
40%	Disabled; requires special care and assistance
30%	Severely disabled; hospitalization indicated, although death not imminent
20%	Very sick; hospitalization necessary
10%	Moribund; fatal processes progressing rapidly
0%	Dead

Source: Data from SS O'Mary. Diagnostic Evaluation, Classification, and Staging. In SL Groenwald, MH Frogge, M Goodman, CH Yarbro (eds), Cancer Nursing: Principles and Practice. Boston: Jones & Bartlett, 1993.

Table 5-11. Eastern Cooperative Oncology Group Performance Status Scale

Score	Status
0	Asymptomatic
1	Symptomatic; fully ambulatory
2	Symptomatic; in bed less than 50% of day
3	Symptomatic; in bed more than 50% of day but not bedridden
4	Bedridden

Source: Data from SS O'Mary. Diagnostic Evaluation, Classification, and Staging. In SL Groenwald, MH Frogge, M Goodman, CH Yarbro (eds), Cancer Nursing: Principles and Practice. Boston: Jones & Bartlett, 1993.

Table 5-12. American Joint Committee on Cancer Performance Status Scale

Score	Status
H0	Normal activity
H1	Symptomatic and ambulatory; cares for self
H2	Ambulatory more than 50% of time; occasionally needs assistance
H3	Ambulatory 50% or less of time; nursing care needed
H4	Bedridden; may need hospitalization

Source: Data from SS O'Mary. Diagnostic Evaluation, Classification, and Staging. In SL Groenwald, MH Frogge, M Goodman, CH Yarbro (eds), Cancer Nursing: Principles and Practice. Boston: Jones & Bartlett, 1993.

Cancers of the Body Systems

Cancer can affect or invade any organ or tissue in the human body. The following is a description of various cancers in each body system.

Thoracic Cancer

Cancer can invade any structure within the thorax. Table 5-13 describes thoracic cancer sites and surgical procedures used in their management. Lung and esophageal cancer are commonly encountered diagnoses in the acute care setting and are described below.

Table 5-13. Surgical Interventions for Thoracic Cancers

Area Involved	Surgical Procedure	Excision of
Hilar and mediastinal lymph nodes	Lymphadenectomy	Lymph node or multiple nodes
Pleura	Pleurectomy	Portion of pleura
Rib	Rib resection	Portion of rib
Trachea and bronchi	Tracheal repair and reconstruction	Trachea and/or carina
	Sleeve resection	Portion of main stem bronchus
Lung	Pneumonectomy	Entire single lung
	Lobectomy	Single or multiple lobes of the lung
	Wedge resection	Wedge-shaped segment of lung
Esophagus	Esophagectomy	Portion of esophagus
Esophagus and stomach	Esophagogastrectomy	All or a portion of esophagus and stomach

The common types of lung cancer are squamous cell carcinoma, adenocarcinoma, small cell carcinoma, and large cell carcinoma [1, 2]. Symptoms associated with these include chronic cough, dyspnea, adventitious breath sounds (wheezing, crackles), chest pain, and hemoptysis [1].

The common types of cancer of the esophagus are squamous cell cancer, which affects the upper and middle one-third of the esophagus, and adenocarcinoma, which affects the lower segment of the esophagus [1, 2]. Signs and symptoms associated with cancers of the esophagus are difficulty swallowing, weight loss, and indigestion [1].

Clinical tip

• Thoracic surgery may involve a large incision on the thoracic wall or thoracotomy. Deep-breathing exercises, including lateral costal expansion, along with mucus clearance techniques while splinting the incision and range-of-motion exercises of the upper extremity on the side of the incision, are important to restore mobility and prevent postoperative complications. Assessment regarding continued physical therapy after discharge from the hospital should be made, with subsequent home exercise instruction, referral to home care or outpatient physical therapy, or both.

• Patients may have chest tubes in place immediately after surgery. Patients may be able to ambulate while the chest tubes are in place by placing the chest tubes on a portable suctioning device or extending the length of tubing if portable suction is not available. If the patient is not on suction, the chest tube drainage system can be transported during functional mobility (see Appendix IV-C).

• Oxygen supplementation may be required in post-thoracic surgical patients. Oxyhemoglobin saturation (SaO_2) should be monitored to ensure adequate oxygenation, especially when increasing activity levels.

• Caution must be taken when positioning patients after pneumonectomy. Placing patients with the existing lung in the dependent position may adversely affect ventilation, perfusion, and ultimately oxygenation. Positioning guidelines should be stated by the surgeon [5].

Musculoskeletal Cancers

Tumors of bone are most commonly discovered after an injury or fracture. Some tumors in the bone or muscle may arise from other primary sites. Common primary tumors that metastasize to bone include breast, lung, prostate, kidney, and thyroid [1]. Treatment of musculoskeletal tumors can include radiation, chemotherapy, amputation, arthroplasty (joint replacement), and reconstruction using an allograft (cadaver bone). Types of primary orthopedic cancers are described in Table 5-14.

Surgical intervention can be used for a patient with a bone metastasis because of the risk of pathologic fracture. These procedures may include the use of intramedullary rods, plates, and prosthetic devices (e.g., total joint arthroplasty) and are described in Chapter 3 in the discussion of equipment and fractures.

Table 5-14. Orthopedic Cancers

Type of Tumor	Common Age Group	Common Site of Tumors
Osteosarcoma	Young children and young adults	Distal femur, proximal tibia Commonly metastasize to lung
Chondrosarcoma	Adults	Pelvis or femur
Fibrosarcoma	Adults	Femur or tibia
Ewing's sarcoma (rhabdomyo-sarcoma)	Children and adolescents	Trunk, pelvis, and long bones

Source: Data from S Baird (ed). A Cancer Source Book for Nurses (6th ed). Atlanta: American Cancer Society, 1991.

Clinical tip

Patients commonly experience fractures due to metastatic disease in the vertebrae, proximal humerus, and femur [6]. Therefore, patients should be instructed in safety management to avoid falls or trauma to involved areas.

Breast Cancer

Breast cancer, although more prevalent in females, is also diagnosed in males to a lesser extent. It may be discovered during routine breast examinations or mammography. Common surgical procedures for the treatment of breast cancer are listed in Table 5-15.

Clinical tip

• Postoperatively, the physical therapist should assess the neck and shoulder regions, as these may be most affected during surgical interventions for breast cancer.

• Patients may exhibit postoperative pain, lymph edema, or nerve injury due to trauma or traction during the operative procedure.

Table 5-15. Surgical Interventions for Breast Cancer

Surgical Intervention	Tissues Involved
Radical mastectomy	Removal of breast tissue, skin, pectoralis major and minor, rib and lymph nodes
Modified radical mastectomy	Removal of breast, skin, and sampling of axillary lymph nodes
Simple or total mastectomy	Removal of breast, then in a another procedure a sampling of the axillary lymph nodes
Partial mastectomy	Removal of tumor and surrounding wedge of tissue
Lumpectomy or local wide excision	Removal of tumor and axillary lymph nodes resected in separate procedure
Reconstruction	
Implants	Silicone or saline implanted surgically beneath the skin or muscle
Muscle flap transfer	Muscle from stomach or back including layers of skin fat and fascia transferred to create a breast (The transverse rectus abdominal or latissimus dorsi may be used.)

• Postoperative drains may be in place immediately after surgery, and the physical therapist should take care to avoid manipulating the drain.

• Incisions, resulting from muscle transfer flaps involving the rectus abdominis, pectoralis, or latissimus dorsi, should be supported when the patient coughs.

• The physical therapist should instruct the patient in the log-roll technique, which is used to minimize contraction of the abdominal muscles while the patient is getting out of bed.

• The therapist should also instruct the patient to minimize contraction of the shoulder musculature during transfers.

• The physical therapist should check the physician's orders regarding upper-extremity range-of-motion restrictions, especially with muscle transfers. The therapist must know what muscles were resected or transferred during the procedure, the location of the incision, and if there was any nerve involvement before mobilization.

• Lymphedema may need to be controlled with massage, elevation, exercise, elastic garments, or compression pneumatic pumps, especially when surgery involves lymph nodes that are near the extremities. Circumferential or water displacement measurements of the involved upper extremity may be taken to record girth changes and to compare with the noninvolved extremity.

• The physical therapist should consider the impact of reconstructive breast surgery on the patient's sexuality, body image, and psychological state [1].

Gastrointestinal and Genitourinary Cancers

Gastrointestinal cancers can involve the esophagus, stomach, colon, rectum, liver, and pancreas. Esophageal tumors are discussed in "Thoracic Oncology" (see also Table 5-13). Genitourinary cancers can involve the uterus, ovaries, kidney, testicles, bladder, and prostate. Surgical procedures used to treat genitourinary cancers are listed in Table 5-16; surgical procedures used to treat gastrointestinal cancers are described in Table 5-17.

Clinical tip

• Patients with genitourinary cancer may experience incontinence. Bladder control training, pelvic floor exercises, and biofeedback or electrical stimulation may be necessary to restore control of urinary flow.

• Patients with gastrointestinal cancer may also experience incontinence. Both bowel and bladder incontinence can lead to areas of dampened skin, which are prone to breakdown.

Table 5-16. Surgical Interventions for Genitourinary System Cancers

Area Involved	Surgical Intervention	Excision
Uterus	Hysterectomy	Uterus through abdominal wall or vagina
	Total abdominal hysterectomy	Body of uterus and cervix through abdominal wall
	Subtotal abdominal hysterectomy	Uterus (cervix remains)
Ovary	Oophorectomy	One ovary
Ovaries and oviducts	Bilateral salpingo-oophorectomy	Both ovaries and oviducts
Prostate	Radical prostatectomy	Entire prostate
Testes	Orchiectomy	One or both testes

Therefore, physical therapists should be careful to minimize shearing forces in these areas during mobility.

Leukemia and Lymphoma

Cancers may not be located in one tumor site but be widespread in the blood, bone marrow, or lymph system. Leukemias (including acute myelogenous, acute lymphoblastic, chronic myelogenous, and chronic lymphocytic) involve abnormal growth of lymphocytes (white blood cells) [7]. Patients with leukemia may present with any of the following signs or symptoms: general fatigue, weight loss, loss of appetite, infections, bruising, dyspnea, palpitations, tachycardia, malaise, pallor, abdominal discomfort, headache, lethargy, excessive bleeding, fever, chills, neurologic changes, and bone or joint pain [7].

Treatment of these leukemias may include chemotherapy, radiation, hormone therapy, and bone marrow transplantation [7].

Lymphoma, which usually originates in the lymph nodes or bone marrow, includes Hodgkin's lymphoma and non-Hodgkin's lymphoma. These cancers can spread to other lymph nodes and other body organs. Signs and symptoms may include enlargement of a lymph node, cough,

Table 5-17. Surgical Interventions for Gastrointestinal System Cancers

Area Involved	Surgical Intervention	Excision
Stomach	Subtotal gastrectomy	Portion of the stomach
	Near-total gastrectomy	Body of the stomach
	Total gastrectomy	Entire stomach
	Gastroduodenostomy (Billroth I)	Portion of the stomach and duodenum
	Gastrojejunostomy (Billroth II)	Portion of the stomach and jejunum
Colon	Hemicolectomy	Portion of the colon, less than one-half
	Colectomy	All or a portion of the colon
Rectum	Anterior or low-anterior resection	Upper third of rectum
	Abdominal perineal resection	Middle and lower third of rectum
Pancreas	Pancreatoduodenectomy (Whipple procedure)	Duodenum and proximal pancreas
	Total pancreatectomy	Complete pancreas
Liver	Segmental resection	Complete segment of liver
	Subsegmental resection	Portion of a segment of liver

Source: Data from American Cancer Society. Cancer Manual (8th ed). Boston: American Cancer Society, 1990; and S Baird. A Cancer Source Book for Nurses (6th ed). Atlanta: American Cancer Society, 1991.

and dyspnea. Treatments may include chemotherapy, radiation therapy, and bone marrow transplant [7].

Two other forms of lymphoma are lymphangioma and lymphangiosarcoma. Lymphangioma is a benign tumor of the lymphatic system that occurs during embryonic development and grows in proportion to the growth of the child. Treatment usually consists of aspiration of cysts that form, surgical excision of the tumors, or both [8].

Lymphangiosarcoma is a highly malignant tumor of the lymphatic system that is almost always associated with postmastectomy lymphedema. The lesions are nodular, with a reddish-purple color. Traditional management has consisted of radical amputation of involved extremities, as other oncologic therapies have shown inconsistent success with this tumor. Overall, prognosis is poor [8].

Associated with lymphatic tumors and cancer management procedures is lymphedema, the accumulation of protein-rich interstitial fluid that results from lymphatic dysfunction, usually obstruction, and if allowed to progress, leads to subcutaneous fibrosis that will further limit lymphatic absorption and flow. Lymphedema can be categorized as primary or secondary. Primary lymphedema results from a congenital defect in the anatomy or physiology of the lymphatic system. Secondary lymphedema results from an acquired obstruction to the lymphatic system from surgery, trauma, irradiation, infection (lymphangitis), inflammation, or tumor invasion.

Clinical presentation of either primary or secondary lymphedema is an initially soft and pitting edema in dependent extremities that can progress to firm, nonpitting edema (from protein accumulation in the interstitial spaces) that is nonresponsive to treatment [8].

Management of lymphedema consists of edema control by extremity elevation, compression stockings (elastic or pneumatic), active exercises of the extremities, diuretic administration, and surgical excision of fibrous areas with subsequent skin grafting or surgical relocation of lymphatic vessels to enhance lymphatic drainage and flow [8].

Clinical tip

- Platelet counts and hematocrit should be assessed to determine a safe level of activity or exercise. See "Bone Marrow Transplant" for specific guidelines.

- Use caution when exercising patients with a fever. Elevated body temperature may increase pulse and respiratory rate. Physical therapy intervention may need to be delayed until the fever is reduced.

Head, Neck, and Facial Tumors

Head, neck, and facial cancers include processes in the paranasal sinuses, nasal and oral cavities, salivary glands, pharynx, and larynx. Environmental factors and personal habits (e.g., tobacco use) are often closely associated with the development of cancer in this region [9].

Physical therapy intervention may be indicated after the treatment of head, neck, and facial tumors. Surgical procedures include radical neck dissection, laryngectomy, and reconstructive surgery. Radical neck dissections may include removal or partial removal of the larynx; tonsils; lip; tongue; thyroid gland; parotid gland; cervical musculature, including the sternocleidomastoid, platysma, omohyoid, and floor of the mouth; internal and external jugular veins; and lymph nodes [10]. Reconstructive surgery may include a skin flap, muscle flap, or both to cover resected areas of the neck and face. The pectoralis or trapezius muscle is used during muscle flap reconstructive procedures. A facial prosthesis is sometimes used to help the patient attain adequate cosmesis and speaking and swallowing function.

Clinical tip

• Postoperatively, impairment of the respiratory system should be considered in patients with head, neck, and facial tumors because of possible obstruction of the airway or difficulty managing oral secretions. A common associated factor in patients with oral cancer is the use of tobacco (both chewing and smoking); therefore, possible underlying lung disease must also be considered. During physical therapy assessment, the patient should be assessed for adventitious breath sounds and effectiveness of airway clearance. Oral secretions should be cleared effectively before assessing breath sounds. Proper positioning is important to prevent aspiration and excessive edema that may occur after surgery of the face, neck, and head. Patients may also require a tracheostomy, artificial airway, or both to manage the airway and secretions.

• Physical therapy treatment to restore posture and neck, shoulder, scapulothoracic, and temporomandibular motion is emphasized. After a surgical procedure, activity and range-of-motion restrictions should be determined by the physician, especially after skin and muscle flap reconstructions.

• When treating patients with head, neck, and facial cancers, it is important to consider the potential difficulties with speech, chewing, or swallowing and loss of sensations, including smell, taste, hearing, and sight.

- Because the patient may have difficulty with communicating and swallowing, referring the patient to a speech therapist and registered dietitian may be necessary.

Neurologic Cancers

Tumors of the nervous system can invade the brain, spinal cord, and peripheral nerves. Brain tumors can occur in astrocytes (astrocytoma), meninges (meningeal sarcoma), or the nerve cells (neuroblastoma), or they can be the result of cancer that has metastasized to the brain [1]. Symptoms related to cancers of the nervous system depend on the size of the tumor and the area of the nervous system involved. Neurologic symptoms can persist after tumor excision due to destruction of neurologic tissues. Changes in neurologic status due to compression of tissues within the nervous system can indicate further spread of the tumor or may be related to edema of brain tissue. Patient considerations include cognitive deficits, skin care, bowel and bladder control problems, sexual dysfunction, and the need for assistive devices and positioning devices. After resection of a brain tumor, patients may demonstrate many neurologic sequelae, including hemiplegia or ataxia. Radiation therapy to structures of the nervous system may also cause transient neurologic symptoms.

Clinical tip

The therapist should assess the patient's need for skin care, splinting, positioning, assistance in activities of daily living, cognitive training, gait training, balance, assistive devices, and special equipment. See Chapter 4 for further treatment considerations.

Skin Cancer

The physical therapist may identify suspicious lesions during evaluation or treatment, and these should be reported to the medical doctor. Suspicious lesions are characterized by (1) irregular or asymmetric borders; (2) uneven coloring; (3) nodules or ulceration; (4) bleeding or crusting; and (5) change in color, size, or thickness. Cancers of the skin include basal cell cancer, squamous cell cancer, malignant melanoma, and Kaposi's sarcoma.

Basal cell carcinoma is the most common skin cancer [1]. It is usually found in areas exposed to the sun, including the face, ears, neck, scalp, shoulders, and back. Risk factors include chronic exposure to the sun, light eyes, and fair skin. Diagnosis is made with a biopsy or a tissue sample. The following are five warning signs of basal cell carcinoma the physical therapist should look for when working with patients [11]:

• Open sore that bleeds, oozes, or crusts and remains open for 3 or more weeks

• Reddish patch or irritated area, which may crust, itch, or hurt

• Smooth growth with an elevated, rolled border and an indentation in the center; tiny vessels may develop on the surface

• Shiny bump or nodule that is pearly or translucent and is often pink (can be tan, black, or brown in dark-haired individuals)

• Scar-like area that is white, yellow, or waxy, with poorly defined borders and shiny, taut skin

Squamous cell cancer usually occurs in areas exposed to the sun or ultraviolet radiation. Lesions may be elevated and appear scaly or keratotic (horny growth) [1]. Squamous cell lesions can metastasize to the lymph nodes, lungs, bone, and brain.

Malignant melanoma is a neoplasm that arises from the melanocytes. Risk factors include previous history or family history of melanoma, immunosuppression, and a history of blistering sunburns before age 20. Malignant melanoma can metastasize to the lymph nodes, lung, brain, liver, bone, and other areas of the skin [1]. Moles or pigmented spots exhibiting the following signs (called the ABCD rule) may indicate malignant melanoma [1]:

A = *A*symmetry

B = Irregular *b*order

C = Varied *c*olor

D = *D*iameter of more than 6 mm

Kaposi's sarcoma is another form of skin cancer that may present as dark blue or reddish-purple spots on the arms or legs. It may also present on the trunk, head, and neck. Patients may present with edema, diarrhea, dyspnea, orthopnea, cough, fever, weight loss, malaise, and anorexia due to lesions on organs other than the skin [1]. It has a higher incidence in those with immunosuppression, such as individuals with acquired immunodeficiency syndrome and transplant recipients taking immunosuppressive medications.

Clinical tip

• After resection of skin lesions, proper positioning is important to prevent skin breakdown.

• The physical therapist should assess the need for positioning and splinting devices.

• The physical therapist should determine the location of the lesion and the need for range-of-motion exercises to prevent contractures. If the lesion involves an area that will be stressed (e.g., joints), the physical therapist should check the physician's orders for precautions limiting motion.

• Wound management may be important in an individual who does not heal well after a procedure. Modalities such as a sterile whirlpool may be used (see Chapter 7).

Management

The primary methods of managing cancer involve either removing (surgically) or destroying (radiation) the cancerous area, preventing or treating the systemic spread of cancer (chemotherapy), or all three.

Surgical Procedures

Surgical intervention is determined by the size, location, and type of cancer, as well as the patient's age, general health, and performance status. The following are the types of general surgical procedures for resecting or excising a neoplasm:

• Exploratory surgery involves removing regions of the tumor to explore for staging and to determine further treatment.

- Excisional surgery involves removing malignant cells and the surrounding margin of normal tissue. Tissue cells are sent to pathology to determine the type of cancer cell and to determine if the entire growth was removed by detecting clean margins with normal cells.

- Electrosurgery involves cauterizing cancerous tissue with a curette and electric needle.

- Cryosurgery involves freezing malignant cells with liquid nitrogen so that they can be completely removed.

- Debulking is an incomplete resection used to reduce the size of the tumor.

- Laser surgery involves destroying malignant cells with a laser beam.

- Mohs surgery is a microscopically controlled surgery in which layers of the tumor are removed and inspected microscopically until all layers have been removed [12].

- Lymph node surgery involves resection of malignant lymph nodes to help control the spread of cancer.

- Brachytherapy, or implantation of radioactive material, may be completed during a surgical procedure [1].

- Skin grafting may be indicated in large resections of tumors to replace areas of skin removed during resection of a neoplasm with donor skin.

- Reconstructive surgery is the surgical repair of a region with a flap of skin, fascia, muscle, and vessels. It aids in a more cosmetic and functional result of surgical repair.

Clinical tip

- If possible, the physical therapist should perform pre-operative assessment and teaching to determine if any conditions exist that may limit the patient's progression. Range-of-motion, strength, functional mobility, and endurance baselines should be established. Preoperative assessment also assists the physical therapist in informing the patient of physical therapy expectations postoperatively. Instruction regarding crutch training, preprosthetic training, or proper breathing exercises and mucus clearance techniques that will be used postoperatively may also be beneficial.

- The physical therapist should conduct postoperative assessment of the areas involved in the surgery and determine the exact structures involved to determine appropriate mobilization techniques and therapeutic exercise programs.

- The physical therapist should familiarize himself or herself with mobility restrictions set by the surgeon. These restrictions should be documented in the physician order book and discussed during patient care rounds.

- Restriction in range of motion or splinting before mobilization may also be necessary. Activity and range-of-motion restrictions should be clearly communicated to the patient, family members, nurses, and other health care providers.

- Postsurgical pain control will be a necessary priority to enable early mobilization (if appropriate) to prevent complications and ensure early return to function.

Chemotherapy

Chemotherapy uses toxic chemicals to destroy cancerous cells while attempting to preserve normal cells as much as possible. These agents affect synthesis and function of DNA and RNA. The overall purpose of chemotherapy is to treat metastatic disease and reduce the size of the tumor for surgical resection or palliative care. Patients may receive single agents or a combination of agents. Chemotherapy can be performed both preoperatively and postoperatively. Various classes of chemotherapy agents are described in Chapter Appendix 5-A. Antimetabolite, alkylating, plant alkaloid, and antibiotic agents are used to kill cancer cells by retarding growth and reducing the size of the tumor. Cytokines inhibit mitotic division of cells, and hormones are used to block hormone function and prohibit tumor growth [12].

Clinical tip

• Rehabilitation should be delayed or modified until the side effects from chemotherapy are minimized or alleviated. Patients should be aware of the possible side effects and understand the need for modification or delay of rehabilitation efforts. Patients should be given emotional support and encouragement when they are unable to achieve the goals they have initially set. Intervention may be coordinated around the patient's medication schedule.

• Vital signs should always be monitored, especially when patients are taking the more toxic chemotherapy agents that affect the heart, lungs, and the central nervous system.

• Laboratory data should be reviewed to determine if it is safe for the patient to engage in resistive or aerobic exercise. These restrictions are discussed further in "Bone Marrow Transplant."

• Chemotherapy agents will affect the patient's nutritional status and can inhibit the patient's progression in strength and conditioning programs. Proper nutritional support should be provided and directed by a nutritionist. Consulting with the nutritionist may be beneficial when planning the appropriate activity level based on a patient's caloric intake.

• Patients undergoing chemotherapy may be on neutropenic precautions. (A neutrophil is a type of leukocyte or white blood cell; neutropenia is an abnormally low neutrophil count.) Fever that occurs after chemotherapy treatment is a sign of neutropenia. Patients with neutropenia are at risk for infections and sepsis [2]. Follow the institution's guidelines for precautions when treating these patients to help reduce the risk of infections. Treatment may also need to be discontinued until an acceptable neutrophil count is achieved.

• Patients may be taking antiemetics, which help to control nausea and vomiting after chemotherapy. The physical therapist should alert the physician when nausea and vomiting limit the patient's ability to participate in physical therapy so that the antiemetic regimen may be modified or enhanced. Antiemetics are listed in Chapter Appendix 5-B.

Radiation Therapy

High-ionizing radiation is used to destroy or prevent cancer cells from growing further while minimizing the damage to surrounding healthy tissues. Radiation therapy reduces the size of a tumor to allow for resection surgically, to relieve compression on structures surrounding the tumor, and to relieve pain (by relieving compression on pain-sensitive structures). Reducing the size of a tumor with radiation therapy may also help to reduce the need for a large resection, amputation, or complete mastectomy [2]. A radiation oncologist directs the radiation therapy procedure. Radiation therapy is indicated for basal cell cancer; Hodgkin's disease; non-Hodgkin's lymphoma; and cancers of the larynx, thyroid, lung, breast, prostate, bladder, cervix, brain, head, and neck [1]. The following are terms used to describe radiation therapy:

- *Radiation dosages* are measured in Grays (Gy), which are equal to 100 rads.

- *Fractions* are smaller doses of radiation given over a period of weeks or days. This prevents administering a lethal dose of radiation.

The following are methods of administering radiation therapy:

- Teletherapy uses an external beam that is focused on the tumor to reduce its size.

- Brachytherapy is the internal implantation of radioactive material into a tumor or body cavity to reduce the size of the tumor.

- Intraoperative or intracavitary radiation therapy reduces the size of the tumor and kills cancerous cells surrounding the tumor by using a high dose of radiation via external beam during the operative procedure.

- Palliative care involves reducing the size of the tumor with radiation for symptom control rather than for a cure of the cancer.

Common side effects of radiation therapy include skin reactions, slow healing of lesions, limb edema, contractures, fibrosis, alopecia, neuropathy, headaches, cerebral edema, seizures, visual disturbances, bone marrow suppression, cough, pneumonitis, fibrosis, esophagitis, nausea, vomiting, diarrhea, cystitis, and urinary frequency [1, 2].

Clinical tip

• After radiation treatment, the physical therapist should carefully monitor the patient for signs of neuropathy that may become evident during functional mobility.

• Significant fibrosis of tissues that have been irradiated may occur. Early use of range-of-motion and mobility techniques can help prevent contractures. Healing is usually slower in irradiated tissues, and the time frame to achieve goals may need to be modified after radiation.

• The physical therapist should educate patients on the effects of radiation (e.g., slower healing in irradiated tissues) so that they will have more realistic expectations regarding rehabilitation.

• Edema of tissues is a common side effect and should be managed soon after radiation therapy to prevent range-of-motion and functional mobility limitations.

• The side effects of radiation involving the surrounding tissue can last up to 1 year after radiation treatment. It is therefore important to continue range-of-motion exercises to prevent contractures caused by the fibrosis of these tissues.

• The physical therapist should not perform deep massage or apply creams during radiation treatment (doing so may be contraindicated for 6 months to a year) unless such techniques are cleared with the physician.

• The physical therapist should not apply superficial heat for 6 months to a year, and deep heat should never be used in the irradiated area [1, 13, 14].

• Physical therapy intervention may be discontinued during brachytherapy. The physical therapist should anticipate restricted range of motion at the site of treatment.

- As previously discussed in "Chemotherapy," a patient may be prescribed antiemetics after radiation treatment to control nausea and vomiting. Notify the physician if antiemetic therapy is insufficient to control the patient's nausea or vomiting during physical therapy sessions (see Chapter Appendix 5-B).

Bone Marrow Transplant

Bone marrow transplantation is the process of removing diseased marrow and replacing it with either the healthy marrow of a donor or stored autologous marrow. Bone marrow transplantation is used to treat leukemias (non-Hodgkin's lymphoma, Hodgkin's disease, myelodysplastic syndrome) and aplastic anemia [1]. High-dose radiation, chemotherapy, and steroids are used to destroy the diseased marrow. Donor marrow is usually harvested by aspiration from the pelvis (ilium) or sometimes the sternum. The harvested bone marrow is infused into the recipient through an intravenous catheter. The following are the types of bone marrow transplants:

- Allogeneic bone marrow transplants come from a matched donor.

- Syngeneic bone marrow transplants come from an identical twin.

- Autologous bone marrow transplants come from the patient's native marrow. The marrow is treated to destroy the disease before transplantation. Healthy native marrow that was stored during remission of the disease may also be used.

During recovery from bone marrow transplant, physical therapy is often indicated to assist patients in returning to functional activities. Because of complications and side effects of the bone marrow transplant, as well as high-dose radiation and chemotherapy, close supervision of activities are important to safely progress patients. These complications and side effects may place certain restrictions on functional activities and exercise. As with any transplant, rejection of bone marrow is a possible side effect that can have lethal complications.

The physical therapist should always check with the physician or refer to the institution's guidelines before initiating physical therapy, since institutions can vary in their activity and exercise restrictions. Certain laboratory values (listed below) determine what physical activities can be safely performed, and each institution develops its own acceptable ranges of laboratory values that are considered safe to allow exercise. The following are general guidelines of laboratory values for exercise therapy after bone marrow transplant:

1. Platelet counts [6, 15]

   Normal range:
   150,000–400,000 µl (It is safe for the patient to carry on a regular exercise program.)

   Abnormal ranges:
   Less than 50,0000/µl (The patient should avoid resistive exercise and prolonged stretching [6, 7, 12].)
   Less than 25,000/µl (The physical therapist should restrict the patient's activity because the patient may be at significant risk for bleeding [1, 2, 6, 7, 15].)

2. Hematocrit [16]

   Normal values (females: 37–47%; males: 40–54%):
   It is safe for the patient to carry on a regular exercise program.

   Abnormal values:
   With less-than-normal values, the physical therapist should observe for changes in the patient's heart rate, blood pressure, and respiratory rate, especially with exercise and modify the program or discontinue as appropriate.

3. SaO_2

   Normal range (95–100%):
   During exercise, SaO_2 should be maintained at greater than 90%.)

   Abnormal range:
   If SaO_2 is below normal, supplemental oxygen may need to be provided.

Patients may experience complications after bone marrow transplantation due to immunosuppression, including intracranial bleeding, infections, veno-occlusive disease, lung infections, mucositis, and graft-versus-host disease. Prolonged bed rest after bone marrow transplantation can also cause deconditioning, weakness, and skin sores.

Clinical tip

• After the bone marrow aspiration procedure, activity is usually resumed within a few hours. Discomfort in the region is normal. Instructions are provided to the patient to avoid straining the area until it has healed and to monitor for signs of bleeding at the donor site [5].

• After bone marrow transplantation, the patient may be neutropenic and infection control precautions should be observed.

Immunotherapy and Hormonal Therapy

Immunotherapy is the treatment of cancer by enhancing the patient's immune system to destroy cancer cells [2]. This mode of treatment uses biological response modifiers, including alpha interferon. The routes of administration and common side effects of alpha interferon are listed in Chapter Appendix 5-A.

Treatment of cancer can also be combined with hormonal therapy, which may include medically or surgically eliminating the hormone source of cancer (such as with orchiectomy, oorphorectomy, or adrenalectomy) or pharmacologically changing hormone levels [2]. Corticosteroids are a form of hormonal therapy used to reduce pain and to reduce intracranial and spinal cord compression around tumor sites. Hormonal agents are listed in Chapter Appendix 5-A.

Medications

Medications used in cancer care include chemotherapy, antiemetics, hormones, and pain control agents. Chemotherapy agents are discussed in "Chemotherapy" (see also Chapter Appendix 5-A).

As mentioned previously, antiemetics may be prescribed after radiation or chemotherapy for nausea and vomiting. Controlling nausea and vomiting is important to ensure the patient's participation in physical therapy.

Hormones are used to inhibit the growth of a neoplasm and may be combined with chemotherapy agents. Chapter Appendix 5-A describes hormones commonly used in cancer care. Pharmacologic pain control can be attained with many choices of medications. These medications include both narcotics and non-narcotics. Non-narcotics include aspirin, acetaminophen, and nonsteroidal anti-inflammatory drugs. Aspirin increases the risk of bleeding and therefore may be contraindicated in patients with a low platelet count. Patients should be referred to the physician for guidance. Narcotics include opioids and suppress the central nervous system. Patients taking narcotics should be monitored for sedation and suppression of the respiratory system and may experience constipation, which can inhibit participation in physical therapy treatment.

Pain Management

To increase patient participation in rehabilitation, effective pain management is vital. Pain management helps to improve the patient's quality of life, ensure compliance with treatment programs, and prevent postoperative complications. The physical therapist may help determine whether the patient's pain is a result of cancer or if it is unrelated to the cancer (e.g., due to postural dysfunction, previous musculoskeletal dysfunction, or cardiac or gastrointestinal complications). The physical therapist can also identify when pain is limiting a patient's tolerance to functional activities and postoperative care and communicate the need for adequate pain control to the oncology team.

The oncology team can use multiple modalities to control pain in cancer patients, including the following:

- Radiation therapy involves reducing the size of a lesion in a pain-sensitive structure (see "Radiation Therapy").

- Behavioral therapy involves techniques such as behavior modification, relaxation, biofeedback, and imagery to reduce symptoms and manage pain.

- Pharmacologic management is used to control symptoms of pain.

- Transcutaneous electrical nerve stimulation may inhibit pain transmission at the cutaneous or spinal level.

- Electrodes are implanted in the spinal cord to inhibit pain (nerves are stimulated to block the transmission of pain).

- Surgical therapy involves the decompression or resection of the tumor to reduce pressure on pain-sensitive structures.

- The patient may use patient-controlled analgesia (see Appendix VI).

Clinical tip

- Patient participation can be optimized in the acute care setting when patient-controlled analgesia is used while the patient undergoes physical therapy.

- Coordination of pain control medications and physical therapy intervention may allow for more effective patient participation if symptoms of pain are better controlled.

- Patients experiencing pain may remain in one position. Repositioning may help precent contractures and skin breakdown.

General Physical Therapy Guidelines for Cancer Care

The following are general goals and guidelines for the physical therapist working with the patient who has cancer. These guidelines should be adapted to a patient's specific needs.

The primary goals in this patient population are similar to those of other patients in the acute care setting; however, because of the systemic nature of cancer, the time frames for achieving goals will most likely be longer. These goals are to (1) optimize functional mobility, (2) maximize activity tolerance and endurance, (3) prevent joint contracture and skin breakdown, (4) prevent or reduce limb edema, and (5) prevent postoperative pulmonary complications.

General guidelines include, but are not limited to, the following:

- Patients may be placed on bed rest while receiving cancer treatment or postoperatively and will be at risk for developing pulmonary complications, deconditioning, and skin breakdown. Deep-breathing exercises, frequent position changes and an exercise program that can be performed in bed will be beneficial in counteracting these complications.

• Patients who have metastatic processes, especially to bone, are at high risk for pathologic fracture. Patient and family education regarding safety management, postural awareness, and body mechanics during activities of daily living should be provided. An assessment of the appropriate assistive devices, prosthetics, and required orthotics should also be performed. Decreased sensation requires special attention when prescribing and fitting adaptive devices.

• Metastatic processes should also be considered when prescribing resistive exercises to patients, as the muscle action on the frail bone may be enough to cause fracture.

• Pulmonary hygiene is indicated for most patients who undergo surgical procedures. Care should be taken with patients who have metastatic processes during the performance of manual techniques.

• If a patient is placed on isolation precautions, exercise equipment such as stationary bicycles or upper-extremity ergometers (after being thoroughly cleaned with sterile solutions) should be placed in his or her room. Assessment is necessary for the appropriateness of this equipment, along with the safety of independent use.

• When performing mobility or exercise treatments, care should be taken to avoid bruising or bleeding into joint spaces when patients have low platelet counts.

• Emotional support for both the patient and family is at times the most appreciated and effective method in helping to accomplish the physical therapy goals.

• Timely communication with the oncology team is essential for safe and effective care.

Discharge Planning

Patients may be discharged with continued physical therapy care (including inpatient rehabilitation and home care), inpatient or home hospice care, or outpatient care. Discharge plans are based on the need for further medical care, the patient's physical capacity, and family support. The physical therapy assessment of physical capacity and functional mobility is important in determining the discharge plan.

It is important for the physical therapist to educate the patient and family before the patient is discharged from the hospital. The physical therapist should communicate specific precautions and potential signs and symptoms the patient should anticipate and ways to manage these. The physical therapist should assess for appropriate assistive devices, special equipment, or home modifications as identified by speaking with the patient and family. When developing a discharge plan for a patient with cancer, the physical therapist should consider prognosis, functional abilities, family support, and patient goals. Professional assessment and recommendations facilitate the transition from the hospital to the home or rehabilitation center.

References

1. Baird S. A Cancer Source Book for Nurses (6th ed). Atlanta: American Cancer Society, 1991.
2. American Cancer Society. Cancer Manual (8th ed). Boston: American Cancer Society, 1990;292.
3. American Joint Committee on Cancer. Manual for Staging of Cancer (4th ed). Philadelphia: Lippincott, 1992;3.
4. O'Mary SS. Diagnostic Evaluation, Classification, and Staging. In SL Groenwald, MH Frogge, M Goodman, CH Yarbro (eds), Cancer Nursing: Principles and Practice. Boston: Jones & Bartlett, 1993;170.
5. Burrell LO. Adult Nursing in Hospital and Community Settings. East Norwalk, CT: Appleton & Lange, 1992;558, 816.
6. Hicks JE. Exercise for Cancer Patients. In JV Basmajian, SL Wolf (eds), Therapeutic Exercise. Baltimore: Williams & Wilkins, 1990;351.
7. McGarvey CL III. Physical Therapy for the Cancer Patient. New York: Churchill Livingstone, 1990;85.
8. Moore WS. Vascular Surgery: A Comprehensive Review (4th ed). Philadelphia: Saunders, 1993;90.
9. Reese JL. Head and Neck Cancers. In R McCorkle, M Grant, M Frank-Stromberg, S Baird (eds), Cancer Nursing: A Comprehensive Textbook (2nd ed). Philadelphia: Saunders, 1996;567.
10. Haskell CM. Cancer Treatment (4th ed). Philadelphia: Saunders, 1995;343, 457.
11. Robins P, Kopf A. Squamous Cell Carcinoma [pamphlet]. New York: Skin Cancer Foundation, 1990;1.
12. Moreau D. Nursing '96 Drug Handbook. Springhouse, PA: Springhouse, 1996;657, 944.
13. Interdisciplinary care of the patient with cancer in a community hospital. Clinical Management 1982;2;11.
14. National Institutes of Health. Radiation Therapy and You. Washington, DC: National Institutes of Health, 1993;13.
15. Sayre RS, Marcoux BC. Exercise and autologous bone marrow transplants. Clin Manage 1992;12:81.
16. Taber's Cyclopedic Medical Dictionary (15th ed). Philadelphia: FA Davis, 1985.

Appendix 5-A: Antineoplastic Agents

Table 5-A.1. Alkylating Agents*

Alkylating Agents (Generic Name [Brand Name])	Side Effects
Busulfan (Myleran)	Myelosuppression, pulmonary fibrosis, anemia, leukopenia, thrombocytopenia, fatigue, weight loss
Carboplatin (Paraplatin)	Myelosuppression, nausea, vomiting, neurotoxicity
Carmustine (BiCNU)	Nausea; vomiting; pain; tissue necrosis; pulmonary, renal, and hepatotoxicity
Chlorambucil (Leukeran)	Nausea, vomiting, stomatitis, thrombocytopenia, myelosuppression, neutropenia, anemia, interstitial pneumonitis, exfoliative dermatitis, hyperuricemia
Cisplatin (Platinol)	Peripheral neuritis, tinnitus, nausea, vomiting, leukopenia, thrombocytopenia, anemia, renal toxicity
Cyclophosphamide (Cytoxan, Neosar)	Cardiotoxicity, leukopenia, thrombocytopenia, anemia, pulmonary fibrosis
Dacarbazine (DTIC-Dome)	Nausea, leukopenia, thrombocytopenia, fever, malaise

Table 5-A.1. *Continued*

Alkylating Agents (Generic Name [Brand Name])	Side Effects
Ifosfamide (IFEX)	Lethargy, somnolence, confusion, depressive psychosis, ataxia, coma, seizures, nausea, vomiting, hemorrhagic cystitis, hematuria, leukopenia, thrombocytopenia, myelosuppression, alopecia
Lomustine (CeeNU)	Nausea, vomiting, anemia, leukopenia, thrombocytopenia
Mechlorethamine (Mustargen, Nitrogen Mustard)	Headache, weakness, tinnitus, nausea, vomiting, myelosuppression, metallic taste in the mouth
Melphalan (Alkeran)	Thrombocytopenia, agranulocytosis, pneumonitis, pulmonary fibrosis, anaphylaxis
Streptozocin (Zanosar)	Nausea, vomiting, diarrhea, anemia, leukopenia, thrombocytopenia, anemia, hyperglycemia
Thiotepa (Thiotepa)	Headache, dizziness, nausea, leukopenia, thrombocytopenia, anemia
Uracil Mustard (Uracil Mustard)	Irritability, nervousness, nausea, thrombocytopenia, anemia, hyperpigmentation of skin

*Alkylating agents inhibit DNA function and replication; side effects are caused by these effects on normal cells.
Source: Data from C Ciccone. Cancer Chemotherapy. Philadelphia: FA Davis, 1996; and D Moreau. Nursing '96 Drug Handbook. Springhouse, PA: Springhouse, 1996.

Table 5-A.2. Antimetabolite Agents*

Antimetabolite Agent (Generic Name [Brand name])	Side Effects
Cladribine (2-Chlorodeoxyadenosine)	Neutropenia, anemia, leukopenia, nausea, rash, chills, diaphoresis, arthralgia, myalgia, malaise
Cytarabine (Cytosar-U)	Neurotoxicity, ataxia, nystagmus, keratitis, nausea, vomiting, thrombocytopenia, flulike syndrome

Antimetabolite Agent (Generic Name [Brand name])	Side Effects
Floxuridine (FUDR)	Anorexia, stomatitis, cramps, ataxia, vertigo, nystagmus, seizures, nausea, vomiting, diarrhea, bleeding, leukopenia, anemia, thrombocytopenia, erythema, alopecia, hiccups, jaundice
5-Fluorouracil (Adrucil)	Ataxia, weakness, malaise, stomatitis, nausea, vomiting, diarrhea, anorexia, leukopenia, thrombocytopenia, anemia, alopecia, dermatitis, erythema, pain, burning, scaling, pruritus, confusion, disorientation
Hydroxyurea (Hydrea)	Anorexia, vomiting, diarrhea, leukopenia, thrombocytopenia, anemia, nausea, myelosuppression, skin rash, renal and neurotoxicity
Mercaptopurine (Purinethol)	Nausea, vomiting, anorexia, thrombocytopenia, anemia, jaundice, hepatic necrosis, rash, leukopenia
Methotrexate (Folex, Mexate Rheumatrex)	Pharyngitis, nausea, anemia, leukopenia, pulmonary fibrosis
Thioguanine (Lanvis)	Leukopenia, anemia, thrombocytopenia, hepatotoxicity, nausea

*Antimetabolite agents interfere with normal metabolites during DNA and RNA biosynthesis.
Source: Data from C Ciccone. Cancer Chemotherapy. Philadelphia: FA Davis, 1996; and D Moreau. Nursing '96 Drug Handbook. Springhouse, PA: Springhouse, 1996.

Table 5-A.3. Antibiotics*

Antibiotic (Generic Name [Brand name])	Side Effects
Bleomycin (Blenoxane)	Nausea, vomiting, fever, chills, anaphylaxis, alopecia, stomatitis, erythema, pulmonary toxicity (interstitial pneumonitis), general weakness and malaise, headache, leukocytosis, pulmonary fibrosis, joint swelling
Dactinomycin (Cosmegen)	Nausea, vomiting, myelosuppression, tissue necrosis, alopecia, mucositis

Table 5-A.3. *Continued*

Antibiotic (Generic Name [Brand name])	Side Effects
Daunorubicin (Cerubidine)	Nausea, vomiting, myelosuppression, tissue necrosis, stomatitis, alopecia, cardiotoxicity
Doxorubicin (Adriamycin)	Nausea, vomiting, myelosuppression, tissue necrosis, stomatitis, alopecia, cardiotoxicity
Mitomycin (Mutamycin)	Nausea, vomiting, myelosuppression, tissue necrosis, stomatitis, pulmonary and renal toxicity
Mitoxantrone (Novantrone)	Myelosuppression, cardiotoxicity (congestive heart failure, arrhythmias), nausea, vomiting, diarrhea, abdominal pain, hepatic dysfunction, seizures
Plicamycin (Mithracin)	Myelosuppression, central nervous system and renal toxicity, nausea, vomiting, coagulation abnormalities, tissue necrosis, weakness, malaise

*Antibiotics disrupt the DNA and RNA synthesis.
Source: Data from C Ciccone. Cancer Chemotherapy. Philadelphia: FA Davis, 1996; and D Moreau. Nursing '96 Drug Handbook. Springhouse, PA: Springhouse, 1996.

Table 5-A.4. Hormones*

Hormone (Generic Name [Brand Name])	Side Effects
Antiestrogens	
Tamoxifen (Nolvadex)	Nausea, vomiting, transient fall in white blood cell and platelet counts
Estrogens	
Chlorotrianisene (TACE)	Nausea, leg cramps, thromboembolism, cerebrovascular accident, pulmonary embolism, myocardial infarction
Diethylstilbestrol (DES)	Nausea, leg cramps, thromboembolism, cerebrovascular accident, pulmonary embolism, myocardial infarction
Estradiol (Oestradiol Valerate)	Thromboembolism, nausea, leg cramps

Hormone (Generic Name [Brand Name])	Side Effects
Adrenocorticosteroids	
Prednisone (Deltasone, Orasone)	Euphoria, insomnia, muscle weakness, osteoporosis, congestive heart failure, hypertension, delayed wound healing
Prednisolone (Delta-Cortef)	Euphoria, insomnia, muscle weakness, osteoporosis, congestive heart failure, hypertension, delayed wound healing
Androgens	
Fluoxymesterone (Android-F)	Edema, nausea, vomiting, thrombocytopenia
Antiandrogens	
Flutamide (Eulexin)	Drowsiness, confusion, numbness, diarrhea, nausea, vomiting, hot flashes
Gonadotropin-releasing hormone drugs	
Leuprolide (Lupron)	Hot flashes, pulmonary embolism, arrhythmia, angina, myocardial infarction
Goserelin (Zoladex)	Lethargy, pain, arrhythmia, congestive heart failure, hypertension, myocardial infarction, chronic obstructive pulmonary disease, upper respiratory tract infections
Megestrol (Megace)	Hypertension, edema, thrombophlebitis, nausea, vomiting, carpal tunnel syndrome

*Hormones are used to inhibit growth of neoplasm; they are usually combined with other chemotherapy agents.
Source: Data from C Ciccone. Cancer Chemotherapy. Philadelphia: FA Davis, 1996; and D Moreau. Nursing '96 Drug Handbook. Springhouse, PA: Springhouse, 1996.

Table 5-A.5. Plant Alkaloids*

Plant alkaloid (Generic Name [Brand Name])	Side Effects
Etoposide (VePesid)	Myelosuppression, anemia, leukopenia, thrombocytopenia, nausea, vomiting, hypotension, anaphylaxis, alopecia, headache, peripheral neuropathy, central nervous system toxicity, fever, chills

Table 5-A.5. *Continued*

Plant alkaloid (Generic Name [Brand Name])	Side Effects
Teniposide (VM 26)	Myelosuppression, tissue necrosis, fever, hypotension, anaphylaxis, alopecia
Vinblastine (Velban, Alkaban)	Myelosuppression, leukopenia, nausea, vomiting, stomatitis, alopecia, central and peripheral neuropathy, tissue necrosis
Vincristine (Oncovin, Vincasar)	Myelosuppression, nausea, vomiting, tissue necrosis, peripheral neuropathy, constipation

*Plant alkaloids disrupt the mitotic apparatus and cause death of the cancerous cell.
Source: Data from C Ciccone. Cancer Chemotherapy. Philadelphia: FA Davis, 1996; and D Moreau. Nursing '96 Drug Handbook. Springhouse, PA: Springhouse, 1996.

Table 5-A.6. Other Antineoplastic Agents

Agent (Generic Name [Brand Name])	Side Effects
Aminoglutethimide (Cytadren)	Drowsiness, dizziness, tachycardia, hypotension, myalgia
Procarbazine (Matulane)	Nausea, vomiting, myelosuppression, hallucinations, pleural effusion, central nervous system and renal toxicity
Interferons[a]	
Interferon alfa-2a	Fever, chills, malaise, dizziness, anorexia, bronchospasm, leukopenia, hepatitis
Interferon alfa-2b	Fever, chills, malaise, dizziness, anorexia, leukopenia, hepatitis
Colony-stimulating factors[b]	
Filgrastim (Neupogen)	Medullary bone pain, nausea, vomiting, skeletal pain, diarrhea
Sargramostim (Leukine, Prokine)	Fever, malaise, nausea, diarrhea, anorexia, gastrointestinal upset, edema, alopecia, rash, dyspnea

[a]Interferons provide antiviral and antineoplastic properties.
[b]Colony-stimulating factors stimulate the production of white blood cells and accelerate the recovery of bone marrow.
Source: Data from C Ciccone. Cancer Chemotherapy. Philadelphia: FA Davis, 1996; and D Moreau. Nursing '96 Drug Handbook. Springhouse, PA: Springhouse, 1996.

Appendix 5-B:
Antiemetic Agents

Antiemetic Agents (Generic Name [Brand Name])[a]	Side Effects
Phenothiazines	
Chlorpromazine (Thorazine)	Extrapyramidal reactions, sedation, tardive dyskinesia, pseudoparkinsonism, orthostatic hypotension, arrhythmias, blurred vision, ECG changes
Prochlorperazine (Compazine)	Extrapyramidal reactions, sedation, blurred vision, pseudoparkinsonism
Promethazine (Phenergan)	Sedation, drowsiness, confusion, hypotension, nausea, dry mouth, agranulocytosis
Butyrophenones	
Haloperidol (Haldol)	Severe extrapyramidal reaction, tardive dyskinesia, blurred vision, neuroleptic malignant syndrome
Droperidol (Inapsine)	Drowsiness, hypotension, extrapyramidal reaction, orthostatic hypotension
Cannabinoids	
Tetrahydrocannabinol (Marijuana)	Impaired psychomotor performance, altered sensory perception, tachycardia, paresthesia, tinnitus
Antihistamines	
Diphenhydramine (Benadryl)	Drowsiness, nausea, dry mouth, vertigo, palpitations, confusion, headache

Antiemetic Agent (Generic Name [Brand Name])[a]	Side Effects
Corticosteroids	
Dexamethasone (Decadron, Hexadrol, Dexone)	Insomnia, hypertension, edema, muscle weakness, hyperglycemia
Benzodiazepines	
Lorazepam (Ativan)	Drowsiness, lethargy, restlessness, transient hypotension, visual disturbances
Metoclopramide (Reglan)	Restlessness, anxiety, drowsiness, dizziness, extrapyramidal symptoms, tardive dyskinesia, dystonic reactions, transient hypertension
Other	
Trimethobenzamide (Tigan)	Drowsiness, hypotension, diarrhea, hepatotoxicity

[a]Antiemetics are used to control the symptoms of nausea and vomiting associated with chemotherapy, radiation treatment, or both.
Source: Data from C Ciccone. Cancer Chemotherapy. Philadelphia: FA Davis, 1996; and D Moreau. Nursing '96 Drug Handbook. Springhouse, PA: Springhouse, 1996.

6

Vascular System and Hematology

Michele Panik and Jaime C. Paz

Introduction

Alterations in the integrity of the vascular and hematologic systems can alter a patient's activity tolerance. The physical therapist must be aware of the potential impact that a change in blood composition or blood flow has on a multitude of body functions, including cardiac output, hemostasis, energy level, and healing. The objectives of this chapter are to provide the following:

1. A review of the structure and function of blood and blood vessels

2. A review of vascular and hematologic assessment, including physical examination and diagnostic and laboratory tests

3. A description of the purpose, mechanism of action, and side effects of hematologic medications

4. A description of vascular and hematologic diseases and disorders, including clinical findings, medical and surgical management, and physical therapy intervention

Structure

The network of arteries, veins, and capillaries comprises the vascular system. Living blood cells and plasma within the blood ves-

Table 6-1. Blood Vessel Layers

Layer	Description	Function
Tunica intima	Innermost layer Endothelial layer over a basement membrane	Provides a smooth surface for laminar blood flow
Tunica media	Middle layer Smooth muscle cells and elastic connective tissue with sympathetic innervation	Constricts and dilates for blood pressure regulation
Tunica adventitia	Outermost layer Composed of collagen fibers, lymph vessels, and the blood vessels that supply nutrients to the blood vessel	Protects and attaches blood vessels to nearby structures

Source: Data from The Cardiovascular System. In EN Marieb, Human Anatomy and Physiology. Redwood City, CA: Benjamin-Cummings, 1989;621.

sels are the structures that comprise the hematologic system. Another system that assists the vascular system is the lymphatic system. The lymphatic system assists the vascular system by draining unabsorbed plasma from tissue spaces and returning this fluid (lymph) to the heart via the thoracic duct, which empties into the left jugular vein. The flow of lymph is regulated by intrinsic contractions of the lymph vessels, muscular contractions, respiratory movements, and gravity [1]. Most lymphatic system disorders that physical therapists encounter are cancerous and therefore are discussed in Chapter 5.

Vascular System Structure

All arteries, capillaries, and veins are composed of three similar layers. Their wall thickness, diameter, and length vary according to location and function. Table 6-1 describes the structural characteristics of the different blood vessel layers.

Table 6-2. Blood Cell Types

Cell	Description
Erythrocyte (RBC)	Erythrocyte contains hemoglobin molecules responsible for oxygen transport to tissues Composed of four protein chains (two alpha and two beta chains) bound to four iron pigment complexes An oxygen molecule attaches to each iron atom to become oxyhemoglobin
Leukocyte (WBC)	Five types of WBCs (neutrophils, basophils, eosinophils, lymphocytes, and monocytes) are responsible for launching immune defenses and fighting infection WBCs leave the circulatory spaces to gain access to a site of infection
Thrombocyte (platelet)	Thrombocyte is the cell fragment responsible for clot formation

RBC = red blood cell; WBC = white blood cell.
Source: Data from Blood. In EN Marieb, Human Anatomy and Physiology. Redwood City, CA: Benjamin-Cummings, 1989;568.

Hematologic System Structure

Blood is composed of living cells in a nonliving plasma solution and accounts for 8% of total body weight, or 4–5 liters in females and 5–6 liters in males. Table 6-2 describes the characteristics of the different blood cells. Plasma is composed almost completely of water and contains more than 100 dissolved substances. The major solutes include albumin, fibrinogen, protein globules, nitrogenous substances, nutrients, electrolytes, and respiratory gases [2].

Function

The function of the blood vessels is to carry blood throughout the body to and from the heart. Normal alterations in the vessel diameter will occur depending on circulating blood volume and the oxygen needs of

Table 6-3. Characteristics Of Blood Vessels

Vessel	Description
Artery	Small, medium, or large in diameter Larger arteries are located closer to the heart Thick tunica media layer allows arteries to readily accommodate to pressure changes from the heart
Vein	Small, medium, or large in diameter Thin tunica media and thick tunica adventitia Valves prevent backflow of blood to maintain venous return to the heart
Capillary network	The interface of the arterial and venous systems where blood cells, fluids, and gases are exchanged Capillary beds can be open or closed depending on the circulatory requirements of the body

Source: Reprinted with permission from The Cardiovascular System: Blood Vessels. In EN Marieb, Human Anatomy and Physiology. Redwood City, CA: Benjamin-Cummings, 1989;621.

the tissues. Table 6-3 describes the unique characteristics of arteries, veins, and capillaries.

The following are the seven major functions of blood [2]:

1. The transport of oxygen and nutrients to body cells from the lungs and gastrointestinal organs, respectively

2. The transport of carbon dioxide and metabolic waste products to the lungs and kidneys, respectively

3. The transport of hormones from endocrine glands to target organs

4. The maintenance of body temperature via conduction and dispersal of heat

5. The maintenance of pH with buffers freely circulating in the blood

6. The formation of clots

7. The prevention of infection with white blood cells (WBCs), antibodies, and complement

The vascular and hematologic systems are intimately linked and the examination of these systems is often similar. For the purpose of this chapter, however, the evaluation of the vascular and hematologic systems is discussed separately.

Physical Examination

Vascular Assessment

Inspection
Observation of the following features can help delineate the location and severity of vascular disease [1]:

- Skin color (Note the presence of any discoloration of the distal extremities, which is indicative of decreased blood flow—e.g., mottled skin.)

- Hair distribution (Patchy hair loss on the lower leg may indicate arterial circulation insufficiency.)

- Venous pattern (dilation or varicosities)

- Edema or atrophy (Edema from congestive heart failure occurs bilaterally in dependent areas; edema from trauma, lymphatic, or chronic venous insufficiency is generally unilateral.)

- Presence of petechiae (small, purplish, hemorrhagic spots on the skin)

- Skin lesions (ulcers, blisters, or scars)

- Digital clubbing

Palpation
The physical therapist can assess the presence of pain and tenderness, strength and rate of peripheral pulses, respiratory rate, blood pressure, and skin temperature during the palpative portion of the examination. Changes in heart rate, blood pressure, and respiratory rate may correspond to changes in the fluid volume status of the patient. For example, a decrease in fluid volume may result in a decreased blood pressure that results in a compensatory increase in heart and respiratory rates. The decreased fluid volume and resultant increased heart rate in this

situation may then result in a decreased strength of the peripheral pulses on palpation.

The following are two methods used to grade peripheral pulses:

1. On the scale of 0–3 as [1]

   0   Absent
   +1   Weak and thready pulse
   +2   Normal
   +3   Full and bounding pulse

2. On the scale of 0–4 as [3]

   0   Absent
   1   Markedly diminished
   2   Moderately diminished
   3   Slightly diminished
   4   Normal

Peripheral pulses can be assessed in the following arteries (see Chapter 1, Figure 1-6).

- Temporal

- Carotid

- Brachial

- Ulnar

- Radial

- Femoral

- Popliteal

- Posterior tibial

- Dorsalis pedis

Clinical tip

- Peripheral pulse grades are generally denoted in the medical record by physicians in the following manner: dorsalis pedis +1.

- A small percentage of the adult population may normally have absent peripheral pulses—for example, 10–17% lack dorsalis pedis pulses [1].

Auscultation

Systemic blood pressure and the presence of bruits (whooshing sound indicative of turbulent blood flow from obstructions) are assessed through auscultation. Bruits are typically assessed by physicians and nurses (see Chapter 1 for further details on blood pressure measurement).

Diagnostic Studies

Various tests that evaluate vascular flow and integrity are described in Table 6-4.

Noninvasive Laboratory Studies

Various noninvasive procedures can examine vascular flow. The phrases *lower-extremity noninvasive studies* (LENIs) and *carotid non-invasive studies* (CNIs) are general descriptions that are inclusive of the noninvasive tests described in Table 6-5.

Invasive Vascular Studies

The most common invasive vascular study is arteriography, typically referred to as contrast angiography. This study provides anatomic and diagnostic information about the arterial system via radiopaque dye injected into the femoral, lumbar, brachial, or axillary arteries, followed by radiographic viewing (an angiogram is a picture produced by angiography). Angiography is generally performed before or during therapeutic interventions, such as percutaneous angioplasty, thrombolytic therapy, or surgical bypass grafting.

Postangiogram care includes the following:

- Bed rest for 4–8 hours

- Pressure dressings to the injection site

- Intravenous fluid administration to help with dye excretion

- Vital sign monitoring

The following are complications associated with angiography [1, 4]:

- Allergic reactions to contrast dye

Table 6-4. Vascular Tests

Test	Indication	Description	Normal Results and Values
Capillary refill time	To assess vascular perfusion and indirectly assess cardiac output	Nail beds of fingers or toes are squeezed until blanching (whitening) occurs and then they are released.	Blanching should resolve (capillary refill) in less than 3 secs.
Elevation pallor	To assess arterial perfusion	A limb is elevated 30–40 degrees and color changes are observed over 60 secs. A gray or pale (pallor) discoloration will result from arterial insufficiency or occlusion.	Grading of pallor: 0 = no pallor in 60 secs 1 = pallor in 60 secs 2 = pallor in 30–60 secs 3 = pallor in less than 30 secs 4 = pallor with limb flat (not elevated or dependent)
Trendelenburg's test	To determine which veins are involved in causing varicosities	A tourniquet is applied to the involved lower extremity, which is elevated while the patient is supine. The patient then stands and the filling of the varicosities is observed.	Greater saphenous veins are involved if the varicosities fill slowly with the tourniquet on and then suddenly dilate when the tourniquet is removed. Deep and communicating veins are involved if the varicosities fill immediately with the tourniquet still on.
Allen's test	To assess the patency of the radial and ulnar arteries	The radial and ulnar arteries are compressed at the level of the wrist while the patient clenches his or her fist. The patient then opens his or her	The pale and mottled hand that results from arterial compression and clenching should resolve in the arterial distribution of either the

		hand and either the radial or ulnar artery is released. The process is then repeated for the other artery.	radial or ulnar artery, depending on which was released.
Homans' sign	To detect presence of deep vein thrombosis	The calf muscle is gently squeezed, or the foot is quickly dorsiflexed.	Pain that is elicited with either squeezing or dorsiflexing may indicate a deep vein thrombosis.*

*A 50% false-positive rate occurs with this test. Vascular laboratory studies are more sensitive.

Source: Data from JM Black, E Matassarin-Jacobs. Luckmann and Sorensen's Medical-Surgical Nursing: A Psychophysiologic Approach (4th ed). Philadelphia: Saunders, 1993; P Lanzer, J Rosch. Vascular Diagnostics: Noninvasive and Invasive Techniques, Peri-Interventional Evaluations. Berlin: Springer-Verlag, 1994; and JW Hallet, DC Brewster, RC Darling. Handbook of Patient Care in Vascular Surgery (3rd ed). Boston: Little, Brown, 1995.

Table 6-5. Types of Noninvasive Vascular Studies

Test	Description
Doppler ultrasound	High frequency–low intensity (1–10 MHz) sound waves are applied to the skin with a Doppler probe. An acoustic gel is used as a coupling agent that detects blood flow velocity over arteries and veins with an audible signal.
Duplex scanning	Velocity patterns of blood flow along with visual images of vessel and plaque anatomy can be obtained by combining ultrasound with a pulsed Doppler detector.
Plethysmography (5 types) Pulse volume recorder (PVR) Ocular pneumoplethysmography (OPG) Impedance plethysmography (IPG) Phleborrheography (PRG) Photoplethysmography (PPG)	Plethysmography is the measurement of volume change in an organ or body region.* PVR and OPG are used to evaluate arterial flow, while IPG, PRG, and PPG are used to evaluate venous flow.
Ankle-brachial index (ABI)	Systolic blood pressures are taken in both upper extremities at the brachial arteries and both lower extremities above the ankle, with Doppler assessment of either dorsalis pedis or posterior tibialis pulses. The higher of the lower-extremity pressures is then divided by the higher of the upper-extremity pressures. (e.g., an ankle pressure of 70 mm Hg and a brachial pressure of 140 mm Hg will yield an ABI of 0.5.) Normal ABI for foot arteries is 1.0–1.2, with indexes below 1.0 indicating arterial obstruction.
Exercise testing	Exercise testing is performed to assess the nature of claudication by measuring ankle pressures and PVRs after exercise. A drop in ankle pressures is noted in arterial disease. This type of testing provides a controlled method to document onset, severity, and location of claudication.

Test	Description
	Screening for cardiorespiratory disease can also be performed as patients with peripheral vascular disease often have concurrent cardiac or pulmonary disorders (see Chapter 1).
Computed tomography (CT)	CT is used to provide visualization of the arterial wall and its structures. Indications for CT include diagnosis of abdominal aortic aneurysms and postoperative complications of graft infections, occlusions, hemorrhage, and abscess.
Magnetic resonance imaging (MRI)	MRI detects deep venous thrombosis from the pelvic iliac and lower extremity veins. It also visualizes the aorta, mesenteric, and renal arteries. It assesses cerebral edema and can stage the progression of strokes in order to determine optimal operative time for patients.

*In the case of vascular studies, *volume change* refers to blood volume changes that represent blood flow.
Source: Data from JM Black, E Matassarin-Jacobs. Luckmann and Sorensen's Medical-Surgical Nursing: A Psychophysiologic Approach (4th ed). Philadelphia: Saunders, 1993; P Lanzer, J Rosch. Vascular Diagnostics: Noninvasive and Invasive Techniques, Peri-Interventional Evaluations. Berlin: Springer-Verlag, 1994; and KL McCance, SE Huether. Pathophysiology: The Biologic Basis for Disease in Adults and Children (2nd ed). St. Louis: Mosby, 1994.

- Thrombi formation
- Vessel perforation with or without pseudoaneurysm formation
- Hematoma formation
- Hemorrhage
- Infections at the injection site
- Neurologic deficits from emboli dislodgment

Hematologic Assessment

The medical workup of the patient with a suspected hematologic abnormality emphasizes the patient history and blood tests, in addition to the patient's clinical presentation.

History

In addition to the general chart review (see Appendix I), the following information is especially relevant in the evaluation of the patient with a suspected hematologic disorder [5, 6]:

- What are the presenting symptoms?

- What was the rapidity of the onset of symptoms?

- Is the patient unable to complete daily activities secondary to fatigue?

- Is there a history of anemia or other blood disorders, cancer, hemorrhage, or systemic infection?

- Is there a history of blood transfusion?

- Is there a history of chemotherapy, radiation therapy, or other drug therapy?

- Has there been an environmental or occupational exposure to toxins?

- Have there been night sweats or fever?

- Is the patient easily bruised?

- Are menses excessive?

Other relevant data include the patient's diet (for the evaluation of vitamin- or mineral-deficiency anemia), history of weight loss (as a warning sign of cancer or altered metabolism), whether the patient abuses alcohol (a cause of anemia with chronic use), and race (some hematologic conditions have a higher incidence in certain races).

Inspection

During the hematologic assessment, the patient is observed for the following [5]:

- General appearance (e.g., lethargy)

- Degree of pallor of the skin, mucous membranes, nail beds, and palmar creases (The presence of pallor in these areas indicates low hemoglobin levels.)
- Presence of petechiae or ecchymosis (a sign of increased blood viscosity)

Palpation
Blood pressure and heart rate are measured for signs of hypovolemia (see "Palpation" in "Vascular Assessment" for a description of vital sign changes with hypovolemia).

Laboratory Studies
In addition to the history and physical examination, the clinical diagnosis of hematologic disorders is based heavily on laboratory studies.

Complete Blood Count
The standard complete blood count (CBC) consists of a red blood cell (RBC) count, WBC count, white blood cell differential, hematocrit (Hct) measurement, hemoglobin (Hgb) measurement, and platelet (Plt) count. Table 6-6 summarizes the CBC. Figure 6-1 illustrates a common method used by the physician to document portions of the CBC in daily progress notes. If a value is abnormal, it is usually circled within this "sawhorse" figure.

Erythrocyte Indices
RBC, hematocrit, and hemoglobin values are used to calculate three erythrocyte indices: (1) mean corpuscular volume (MCV), (2) mean corpuscular hemoglobin (MCH), and (3) mean corpuscular hemoglobin concentration (MCHC). At most institutions, these indices are included in the CBC. Table 6-7 summarizes these indices.

Coagulation Tests
Coagulation tests assess the blood's ability to clot. The two main tests used to determine clotting are prothrombin time (PT) and partial thromboplastin time (PTT) (Table 6-8).

Clinical tip

When confirming an order for physical therapy in the physician's orders, the therapist must be sure to differentiate between the order for physical therapy and the blood test

Table 6-6. Complete Blood Count: Values and Interpretation

Test	Description	Value	Interpretation
Red blood cell (RBC) count	Number of RBCs per μl of blood	Female: 4.2–5.4 million/μl Male: 4.6–5.9 million/μl	Used to assess blood loss or anemia Elevated RBC count may increase risk of venous stasis or thrombi formation
White blood cell (WBC)	Number of WBCs per μl of blood	4,300–10,800/μl	Used to assess the presence of infection, allergens, bone marrow integrity, or the degree of immunosuppression WBC should be monitored frequently if patient is on drugs that cause immuno-suppression
WBC differential	Proportion (percent-age) of the different types of WBCs	Neutrophils: 1,935–7,942 (45–74%) Eosinophils: 0–756 (0–7%) Basophils: 0–216 (0–2%) Lymphocytes: 688–4,860 (16–45%) Monocytes: 172–1,080 (4–10%)	Used to determine an increase or decrease in the percentages of the different types of WBCs in infectious states
Hematocrit (Hct)	Percentage of RBCs in plasma	Female: 37–48% Male: 42–52%	Used to assess blood loss and fluid balance Hct is accurate in relation to hydration sta-tus (For example, the Hct may be falsely elevated if the patient is dehydrated.) Very low Hct may cause a feeling of weak-ness, chills, or dyspnea Elevated Hct may increase the risk of thrombi formation

Hemoglobin (Hgb)	Amount of hemoglobin	Female: 12–16 g/100 ml Male: 13–18 g/100 ml	Used to assess blood loss, anemia, and bone marrow suppression Hct is approximately three times Hgb
Platelets	Amount of platelets	150,000–400,000 µl	Low platelet count increases the risk of bruising and bleeding Elevated platelet count increases the risk for thrombosis or bleeding

Source: Data from JV Corbett. Laboratory Tests & Diagnostic Procedures with Nursing Diagnoses (4th ed). Stamford, CT: Appleton & Lange, 1996.

Table 6-7. Erythrocyte Indices

Test	Description	Value	Interpretation
Mean corpuscular volume (MCV)	Mean size of an individual red blood cell (RBC) in a µl of blood	86–98 μm^3	Formula = Hct × 10/RBC count Increased MCV in some anemias, folic acid deficiency, liver disease, and recent alcohol use Decreased MCV in thalassemia, some anemias, and lead poisoning
Mean corpuscular hemoglobin (MCH)	Amount of hemoglobin (Hgb) in one RBC	28–33 pg	Formula = Hgb × 10/RBC count Used in conjunction with mean corpuscular hemoglobin concentration to assess anemia
Mean corpuscular hemoglobin concentration (MCHC)	Proportion of each RBC occupied by Hgb	32–36%	Formula = Hgb/hematocrit × 100

Source: Data from JV Corbett. Laboratory Tests & Diagnostic Procedures with Nursing Diagnoses (4th ed). Stamford, CT: Appleton & Lange, 1996.

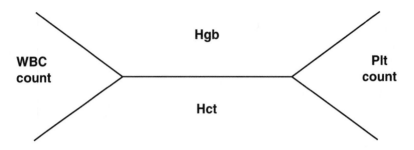

Figure 6-1. *Illustration of portions of the complete blood count in shorthand format. (WBC = white blood cell; Hgb = hemoglobin; Hct = hematocrit; Plt = platelet.)*

(i.e., the abbreviations for both physical therapy and prothrombin time are PT).

Erythrocyte Sedimentation Rate
The erythrocyte sedimentation rate, often referred to as the *sed rate*, is a measurement of how fast RBCs fall in a sample of anticoagulated blood. The normal value is 1–20 mm/hour for men and 1–13 mm/hour for women [7]. The sedimentation rate is a nonspecific screening tool used to determine the presence or stage of inflammation. It may be elevated in rheumatoid arthritis, systemic infection, or acquired immunodeficiency syndrome (AIDS). The sedimentation rate is monitored for a downward trend over time.

Peripheral Blood Smear
A blood sample may be examined microscopically so that the size and shape of the RBCs, WBCs, and platelets can be evaluated. Blood cells may form distinctive patterns or appear to stick together (Rouleaux formations).

Pathophysiology

This section is divided into a discussion of vascular and hematologic disorders.

Table 6-8. Coagulation Tests

Test	Description	Value	Interpretation
Prothrombin time (PT)	Examines clotting factors I, V, VII, X, prothrombin, and fibrinogen	11–16 secs	PT is used to assess the adequacy of warfarin (Coumadin) therapy or to screen for bleeding disorders. Elevated PT indicates risk for hemorrhage. Elevated PT should be anticipated for the patient receiving anticoagulation. Decreased PT indicates risk for thrombus formation.
Partial thromboplastin time (PTT)	Examines clotting factors VIII, IX, XI, and XII	30–45 secs	PTT is used to assess the adequacy of heparin therapy or to screen for bleeding disorders. Elevated PTT indicates risk for hemorrhage. Decreased PTT indicates risk for thrombus formation.

Source: Data from JV Corbett. Laboratory Tests & Diagnostic Procedures with Nursing Diagnoses (4th ed). Stamford, CT: Appleton & Lange, 1996.

Vascular Disorders

Vascular disorders are classified as arterial, venous, or combined arterial and venous disorders. Clinical findings differ between arterial and venous disorders, as described in Table 6-9.

Arterial Disorders

Atherosclerosis
Atherosclerosis is a diffuse and slowly progressive process characterized by areas of hemorrhage and the cellular proliferation of mono-

Table 6-9. Comparison of Clinical Findings of Arterial and Venous Disorders

Clinical Finding	Arterial Disorders	Venous Disorders
Edema	May or may not be present	Present Worse at the end of the day Improves with elevation
Muscle mass	Reduced	Unaffected
Pain	Intermittent claudication Cramping Worse with elevation	Aching pain Exercise improves pain Better with elevation Cramping at night Paresthesias, pruritus Leg heaviness, especially at end of day Commonly a positive Homans' sign
Pulses	Decreased to absent Possible systolic bruit	Usually unaffected but may be difficult to palpate if edema is present
Skin	Absence of hair Small, painful ulcers on pressure points, especially lateral malleolus Tight, shiny skin Thickened toenails	Broad, shallow, painless ulcers of the ankle and lower leg Normal toenails
Color	Pale Dependent cyanosis	Brown discoloration Dependent cyanosis
Temperature	Cool	May be warm in presence of thrombophlebitis
Sensation	Decreased Occasional itching, tingling, and numbness	Pruritus

cytes, smooth muscle, connective tissue, and lipids.* The development of atherosclerosis begins early in life with risk factors that include the following [4, 8, 9]:

- Low levels of high-density lipoproteins (HDL)

- High levels of low-density lipoproteins (LDL)

- Hyperlipidemia (12- to 14-hour fasting blood sample of cholesterol of more than 260 mg/dl or triglyceride of more than 150 mg/dl)

- Diabetes mellitus

- Sex (men are at greater risk than women)

- Smoking

- Inactivity

- Family history

Clinical manifestations of atherosclerosis result from decreased blood flow through the stenotic areas. Signs and symptoms vary according to the area, size, and location of the lesion, along with the age and physiologic status of the patient. As blood flows through a stenotic area, turbulence will occur beyond the stenosis, resulting in decreased blood perfusion past the area of atherosclerosis. Generally, a 60% blood flow reduction is necessary for patients to present with symptoms (e.g., pain). Turbulence is increased when there is an increase in blood flow to an area of the body, such as the lower extremities during exercise. A patient with no complaint of pain at rest may therefore experience leg pain (intermittent claudication) during walking or exercise as a result of decreased blood flow and the accumulation of metabolic waste (e.g., lactic acid) [4, 9].

The following are general signs and symptoms of atherosclerosis [10]:

- Slightly reduced to absent peripheral pulses

- Presence of bruits on auscultation of major arteries (i.e., carotid, abdominal aorta, iliac, and femoral)

Arteriosclerosis is a general term used to describe any wall thickening in the arteries. The term *atheroma* is applied to plaque formation with fatty material in the vessel wall.

- Coolness and pallor of skin, especially with elevation
- Presence of ulcerations, atrophic nails, and hair loss
- Increased blood pressure
- Subjective reports of continuous burning pain in toes at rest that is aggravated with elevation (ischemic pain) and relieved with walking
- Subjective reports of calf or lower-extremity pain induced by walking (intermittent claudication) and relieved by rest

---

Clinical tip

Progression of ambulation distance in the patient with intermittent claudication can be optimized if ambulation is performed in short, frequent intervals (i.e., before the onset of claudicating pain).

Symptoms similar to intermittent claudication may have a neurologic origin from lumbar canal stenosis or disk disease. These are referred to as pseudoclaudication. Table 6-10 outlines the differences between true claudication and pseudoclaudication [11].

Treatment of atherosclerotic disease is based on clinical manifestations and can range from behavioral modifications (e.g., diet, exercise, and smoking cessation) to pharmacologic therapy (e.g., anticoagulation and thrombolytics) to surgical resection and grafting.

Aneurysm
An aneurysm is a localized dilatation or outpouching of the vessel wall that results from degeneration and weakening of the supportive network of protein fibers. Aneurysms most commonly occur in the abdominal aorta [4, 12]. The exact mechanism of aneurysm formation is not fully understood but includes a combination of the following:

- Genetic abnormality in collagen (such as in Marfan's syndrome)
- Aging and natural degeneration of elastin
- Increased proteolytic enzyme activity
- Atherosclerotic damage to elastin and collagen

Table 6-10. Differentiating True Intermittent Claudication from Pseudoclaudication

Characteristic of Discomfort	Intermittent Claudication	Pseudoclaudication
Activity-induced	Yes	Yes or no
Location	Buttock, hip, thigh, calf, and foot	Same as with intermittent claudication
Nature	Cramping Tightness Tiredness	Similar to intermittent claudication or presence of tingling, weakness, and clumsiness
Occurs with standing	No	Yes
Onset	Same each time	Variable each time
Relieved by	Stopping activity	Sitting or changing body positions

Source: Reprinted with permission from JR Young, RA Graor, JW Olin, JR Bartholomew. Peripheral Vascular Diseases. St. Louis: Mosby–Year Book, 1991;183.

A true aneurysm involves the weakening of all three layers of the arterial wall and is generally fusiform and circumferential in nature. False and saccular aneurysms are the result of trauma from dissection (weakness or separation of the vascular layers) or clot formation. They primarily affect the adventitial layer [12]. Figure 6-2A and 6-2B show fusiform and saccular aneurysms, and Figure 6-2C pictures an arterial dissection.

Aneurysms will rupture if the intraluminal pressure exceeds the tensile strength of the arterial wall. The risk of rupture increases with increased aneurysm size [8].

The following are signs and symptoms of aneurysms:

- Ischemic manifestations described in "Atherosclerosis" if the aneurysm impedes blood flow

- Cerebral aneurysms, commonly found in the circle of Willis, present with increased intracranial pressure and its signs and symptoms [12]

- Low back pain (aortic aneurysms can refer pain to the low back)

- Dysphagia (difficulty swallowing) and dyspnea (breathlessness) resulting from the enlarged vessel compressing adjacent organs

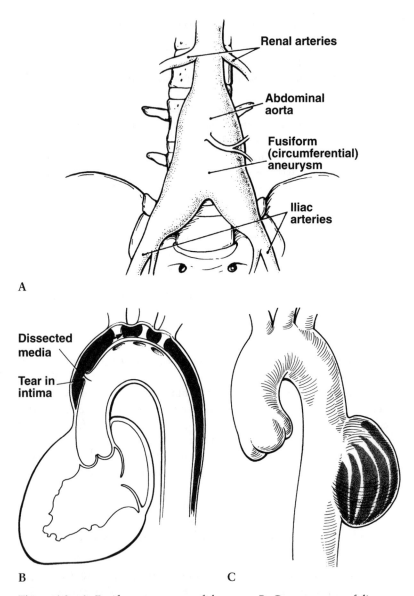

Figure 6-2. *A. Fusiform aneurysm of the aorta. B. Consequences of dissection from the ascending aorta across the arch of the aorta. C. Saccular aneurysm of the descending aorta. (Reprinted with permission from BL Bullock. Pathophysiology: Adaptations and Alterations in Function [4th ed]. Philadelphia: Lippincott–Raven, 1996;532.)*

Aneurysms that result in subarachnoid hemorrhage are discussed in Chapter 4. Surgical resection and graft replacement are generally the desired treatment for aneurysms. Nonsurgical candidates must have blood pressure and anticoagulation management [13].

Arterial Thrombosis
Arterial thrombosis occurs in areas of low or stagnant blood flow, such as atherosclerotic or aneurysmal areas. The reduced or turbulent blood flow in these areas leads to platelet adhesion and aggregation, which then activates the coagulation cycle to form a mature thrombus (clot). Blood flow may then be impeded, potentially leading to tissue ischemia [12, 13].

Arterial Emboli
Arterial emboli arise from areas of stagnant or disturbed blood flow in the heart or aorta. Conditions that predispose a person to emboli formation are (1) atrial fibrillation, (2) myocardial infarction, (3) infective endocarditis, (4) cardiac valve replacement (if not properly anticoagulated), (5) chronic congestive heart failure, and (6) aortic atherosclerosis. Areas in which arterial emboli tend to lodge and interrupt blood flow are arterial bifurcations and areas narrowed by atherosclerosis (especially in the cerebral, mesenteric, renal, and coronary arteries). Signs and symptoms of thrombi, emboli, or both depend on the size of the occlusion, the organ distal to the clot, and the collateral circulation available [12].

Treatment of thrombi, emboli, or both includes anticoagulation with or without surgical resection of the atherosclerotic area that is predisposing the formation of thrombi, emboli, or both.

Hypertension
Hypertension is an abnormally elevated arterial blood pressure, both systolic and diastolic, at rest. Table 6-11 outlines normal and hypertensive blood pressures for a given age group. Signs and symptoms that can result from hypertension and its effects on target organs are described in Table 6-12. Two general forms of hypertension exist: essential and secondary.

Essential, or idiopathic, hypertension is an elevation in blood pressure that results without a specific medical cause but is related to the following risk factors:

- Smoking
- Sedentary lifestyle
- Type A personality

Table 6-11. Hypertension As It Relates to Different Age Groups

Age	Normal Blood Pressure (Systolic/Diastolic)	Hypertensive Blood Pressure (Systolic/Diastolic)
Infants	80/40	90/60
Children	100/60	120/80
Teenagers (12–17 yrs)	115/70	130/80
Adults		
20–45 yrs	120–125/75–80	135/90
45–65 yrs	135–140/85	140–160/90–95
Older than 65 yrs	150/85	160/90

Source: Reprinted with permission from B Bullock. Pathophysiology: Adaptations and Alterations in Function (4th ed). Philadelphia: Lippincott, 1996;517.

- Family history
- Obesity
- Diabetes
- Diet high in fat, cholesterol, and sodium
- Atherosclerosis

Secondary hypertension results from a known medical cause, such as renal disease and others listed in Table 6-13. If the causative factors are treated sufficiently, systolic blood pressure may return to normal limits [12].

Management of hypertension consists of behavioral (e.g., diet, smoking cessation, activity modification) and pharmacologic intervention to maintain blood pressure within acceptable parameters. The primary medications used are diuretics, beta-blockers, calcium channel blockers, angiotensin-converting enzyme inhibitors, and vasodilators. A summary of these medications, their actions, and their side effects can be found in Chapter Appendix 1-C [12, 14].

Table 6-12. Hypertensive Effects on Target Organs

Organ	Hypertensive Effect	Clinical Manifestation
Brain	Cerebrovascular accident	Severe occipital headache Paralysis Speech disturbances Coma
	Encephalopathy	Rapid development of confusion, agitation, convulsions, and death
Eyes	Blurred or impaired vision	Nicking arteries and veins Hemorrhages and exudates on visual exam
	Encephalopathy	Papilledema
Heart	Myocardial infarction	Electrocardiographic changes Enzyme elevations
	Congestive failure	Decreased cardiac output Auscultation of S3 or gallop Cardiomegaly on radiograph
	Myocardial hypertrophy	Increased angina frequency ST- and T-wave changes
	Dysrhythmias	Ventricular or conduction defects
Kidneys	Renal insufficiency	Nocturia Proteinuria Elevated blood urea nitrogen and creatinine levels
	Renal failure	Fluid overload Accumulation of metabolites Metabolic acidosis

Source: Reprinted from B Bullock. Pathophysiology: Adaptations and Alterations in Function (4th ed). Philadelphia: Lippincott, 1996;522.

Systemic Vasculitis

Systemic vasculitis is a general term referring to the inflammation of arteries and veins that progresses to necrosis that leads to narrowing of the vessels. The precise etiology is unknown; however, an autoimmune mechanism is being investigated. The secondary manifestations of vasculitis are numerous and may include thrombosis, aneurysm formation, hemorrhage, and arterial occlusion. The recognized forms of vasculitis are discussed below [8, 9].

Table 6-13. Causes of Secondary Hypertension

Origin	Description
Coarctation of the aorta	Congenital constriction of the aorta at the level of the ductus arteriosus, which results in increased pressure above the constriction and decreased pressure below
Cushing's disease or syndrome	See "Pituitary Gland" in Chapter 11
Oral contraceptives	May be related to an increased secretion of glucocorticoids from adrenal or pituitary dysfunction
Pheochromocytoma	Tumor of the adrenal medulla causing increased catecholamine secretion
Primary aldosteronism	Increased aldosterone secretion primarily as a result of an adrenal tumor
Renin-secreting tumors	See "Adrenal Gland" in Chapter 11
Renovascular disease	Parenchymal disease, such as acute and chronic glomerulonephritis Narrowing stenosis of renal artery as a result of atherosclerosis or congenital fibroplasia

Source: Adapted from B Bullock. Pathophysiology: Adaptations and Alterations in Function (4th ed). Philadelphia: Lippincott, 1996;517.

Polyarteritis Nodosa. Polyarteritis nodosa (PAN) is a disseminated disease with focal transmural arterial inflammation resulting in necrosis of small- and medium-sized arteries. The most frequently involved organs are the kidney, heart, liver, and gastrointestinal tract, with symptoms representative of the dysfunction of the involved organ. Aneurysm formation with destruction of the medial layer is the hallmark characteristic of PAN. Pulmonary involvement can occur; however, most cases of vasculitis in the respiratory tract are associated with Wegener's granulomatosis.

Current management of PAN includes steroid therapy along with cyclophosphamide use. Elective surgical correction of PAN is not feasible given its diffuse nature. Patients diagnosed with PAN have a poor survival rate [8].

Wegener's Granulomatosis. Wegener's granulomatosis is a granulomatous inflammatory disease that affects small- and medium-sized blood vessels throughout the body, with primary manifestations in the pulmonary and renal systems. The etiology is unknown; diagnosis and treatment are still in development. Onset of symptoms generally occurs after 40 years of age and is slightly more common in males. Pulmonary signs and symptoms mimic those of pneumonia (i.e., fever, productive cough at times with negative sputum cultures and chest pain). Treatment of Wegener's disease may consist of a combination of immunosuppressive agents, corticosteroids, and plasmapheresis [14].

Thromboangiitis Obliterans. Thromboangiitis obliterans (Buerger's disease) is a clinical syndrome that is found mainly in young men ages 20–45 who have a smoking history. The disease is characterized by segmental thrombotic occlusions of the small- and medium-sized arteries in the lower and upper extremities. The thrombotic occlusions consist of microabscesses that are inflammatory in nature, suggesting a collagen or autoimmune origin, although the exact etiology is still unknown.

Treatment of Buerger's disease can include smoking cessation, corticosteroids, prostaglandin E_1 infusion, vasodilators, hemorheologic agents, antiplatelet agents, and anticoagulants [8, 12].

Giant Cell Arteritis. Giant cell arteritis (GCA) is another granulomatous inflammatory disorder of an unknown etiology. It predominantly affects the large arteries and is characterized by destruction of the internal elastic lamina. Two clinical presentations of GCA have been recognized: temporal arteritis and Takayasu's arteritis [12].

Temporal arteritis is a more common and mild presentation of GCA that occurs after 50 years of age. The primary signs and symptoms are persistent headache (temporal areas), transient visual disturbances (amaurosis fugax and graying or blurring of vision), and jaw claudication. Polymyalgia rheumatica, a clinical syndrome characterized by pain on active motion and acute onset of proximal muscular stiffness, is frequently associated with temporal arteritis. The primary treatment of temporal arteritis is prednisone [11].

Takayasu's arteritis generally affects young Asian females but has been known to occur in both sexes of blacks and Hispanics as well. It is a form of generalized GCA that primarily involves claudication of the upper extremities and the aorta and its major branches. Lower-extremity involvement is less common. Management of Takayasu's arteritis may consist of prednisone and cyclophosphamide, along with surgical intervention if the disease progresses to aneurysm, gangrene, or both [11].

Raynaud's Disease

Raynaud's disease is a form of intermittent arteriolar vasoconstriction that occurs in patients who have concurrent immunologic disease. The exact etiology is unknown but may be linked to defects in the sympathetic nervous system. Evidence exists both for and against the theory of sympathetic overactivity, which is said to lead to Raynaud's disease. Women ages 16–40 are most commonly affected, especially in cold climates or during the winter season. Other than cold hypersensitivity, emotional factors can also trigger the sudden vasoconstriction. Areas generally affected are the fingertips, toes, or the tip of the nose.

Raynaud's Phenomenon. *Raynaud's phenomenon* may result from Raynaud's disease and is the term used to describe the localized and intermittent episodes of vasoconstriction that cause unilateral color and temperature changes in the areas mentioned above. The color changes of the affected skin progress from white to blue to red (reflecting the vasoconstriction, cyanosis, and vasodilation process, respectively). Numbness, tingling, and burning pain may also accompany the color changes. Raynaud's phenomenon can also be associated with diseases such as systemic lupus erythematosus, rheumatoid arthritis, and obstructive arterial disease and trauma [11, 14].

Management of Raynaud's disease and phenomenon may consist of any of the following: conservative measures to ensure warmth of the body and extremities; pharmacologic intervention, including calcium channel blockers and sympatholytics; plasmapheresis; conditioning and biofeedback; and sympathectomy [11].

Reflex Sympathetic Dystrophy

Reflex sympathetic dystrophy is constant, extreme pain that occurs after the healing phase of minor or major trauma, fractures, surgery, or any combination of these. Injured sensory nerve fibers may transmit constant signals to the spinal cord that result in increased sympathetic activity to the limbs. Affected areas initially present as dry, swollen, and warm but then progress to being cold, swollen, and pale or cyanotic. Raynaud's phenomenon can occur later on. Management may consist of physical therapy, pharmacologic sympathetic blocks, surgical sympathectomy, or any combination of these [11].

Compartment Syndrome

Compartment syndrome is the swelling in the muscle compartments (myotendon, neural, and vascular structures contained within a fascial compartment of an extremity) that can occur after traumatic injury to the arteries (fractures are common causes of compartment syndrome) or after revascularization procedures. External factors, such as casts and circular dressings that are too constrictive, may also lead to compartment syndrome. A common symptom of compartment syndrome is leg or forearm pain associated with tense, tender muscle groups. Numbness or paralysis may also be accompanied by a gradual diminution of peripheral pulses. Pallor, which indicates tissue ischemia, can progress to tissue necrosis if fasciotomy (incisional release of the fascia) is not performed [4, 11].

Venous Disorders

Varicose Veins

Varicose veins are chronic dilations of the veins that result from downward reflux of blood from improper closure of the saphenous vein valve cusps and ultimate weakening of the vessel walls. A genetic predisposition, as well as the occurrence of venous thrombosis, can promote varicose vein formation. Patients generally complain of tired, heavy-feeling legs after prolonged standing.

Management of varicose veins may consist of any of the following: behavioral modifications (e.g., avoiding prolonged sitting or standing and constrictive clothing), weight loss (if obesity is an issue), elevating the feet for 10–15 minutes three or four times a day, gradual exercise, applying well-fitting support stockings in the morning, showering or bathing in the evening, sclerotherapy (to close dilated veins), and surgical ligation and stripping of incompetent veins [4].

Venous Thrombosis

Venous thrombosis can occur in the superficial or deep veins (deep venous thrombosis [DVT]) and can result from a combination of venous stasis, injury to the endothelial layer of the vein, and hypercoagulability. The primary complication of venous thrombosis is pulmonary embolism [4].

The following are risk factors associated with venous thrombosis formation [11]:

- Surgery and nonsurgical trauma
- Increasing age
- Malignancy

- Immobilization
- Heart failure or myocardial infarction
- Previous DVT
- Obesity
- Pregnancy
- Use of oral contraceptives
- Limb paresis or paralysis

Signs and symptoms of venous thrombosis can include the following:

- Pain and swelling distal to the site of thrombus
- Redness and warmth in the area around the thrombus
- Dilated veins
- Low-grade fever

Clinical tip

Homans' sign (pain in upper calf with forced ankle dorsi-flexion) has been used as a screening tool for venous thrombosis, but it is an insensitive and nonspecific test that has a 50% false-positive rate [1]. A positive Homans' sign accompanied by swelling, redness, and warmth may be more clinically indicative of a DVT than a positive Homan's sign alone. Ultimately, examination by vascular noninvasive tests and laboratory testing of clotting times (prothrombin time and partial thromboplastin time) are better methods to evaluate the presence of DVT. Physical therapy intervention should be withheld until cleared by a physician.

Management and prevention of venous thrombosis may consist of any of the following: avoidance of immobilization; lower-extremity elevation, application of compression stockings (elastic or pneumatic), or both if bed rest is required; anticoagulation medications (intravenous heparin or oral warfarin [Coumadin]); thrombolytic therapy (streptokinase and urokinase); and surgical thrombectomy (limited uses) [4].

Pulmonary Embolism

Pulmonary embolism (PE) is the primary complication of venous thrombosis, with emboli commonly originating in the lower extremities. Other sources are the upper extremities and pelvic venous plexus. Mechanical blockage of a pulmonary artery or capillary, depending on clot size, results in an acute ventilation-perfusion mismatch that leads to a decrease in partial pressure of oxygen and oxyhemoglobin saturation, which ultimately manifests as tissue hypoxia. Chronic physiologic sequelae from PE include pulmonary hypertension, chronic hypoxemia, and right congestive heart failure. See Chapter 2 for more details on ventilation-perfusion mismatches, as well as the respiratory sequelae from PE. Early detection of PE, along with thorough anticoagulation therapy, the placement of an inferior vena cava filter, or both, is the preferred management course, with full resolution of cardiopulmonary function generally occurring [4].

Chronic Venous Insufficiency and Postphlebitic Syndrome

Chronic venous insufficiency and postphlebitic syndrome are similar disorders that result from venous outflow obstruction, valvular dysfunction from thrombotic destruction of veins, or both. Valvular dysfunction is generally the most significant cause of either disorder. Within 5 years of sustaining a DVT, approximately 50% of patients will develop signs of these disorders. The hallmark characteristics of both are the following:

- Chronic swollen limbs
- Thick, coarse, brownish skin (induration) around the ankles
- Venous stasis ulceration

Management of these disorders may consist of any of the following: leg elevation above the level of the heart 2–4 times daily for 10–15 minutes; application of proper elastic supports (knee-length preferable); skin hygiene; avoidance of crossing legs, poorly fitting chairs, garters, and sources of pressure above the legs (e.g., tight girdles); pneumatic compression stockings (if the patient needs to remain in bed); exercise to aid muscular pumping of venous blood; and surgical ligation of veins [1, 4].

Combined Arterial and Venous Disorders

Arteriovenous Malformations

Arteriovenous malformations (AVMs) involve shunting of blood directly from the artery to the vein, bypassing the capillary bed. The

presence of an arteriovenous fistula in the AVM is usually the cause of the shunt. The majority of AVMs occur in the trunk and extremities, with a certain number of cases also presenting in the cerebrovascular region [8].
Signs of AVMs may include the following [8]:

- Skin color changes (erythema or cyanosis)
- Venous varices
- Edema
- Limb deformity
- Skin ulceration
- Pulse deficit
- Bleeding
- Ischemic manifestations in involved organ systems

Congenital Vascular Malformations
Congenital vascular malformations (CVMs) are rare developmental abnormalities that may involve all components of the peripheral circulation (i.e., arteries, veins, capillaries, and lymphatics). Signs and symptoms of CVMs are similar to those of AVMs, with tissue hypoxia being the most significant clinical finding. Although CVMs can be self-limiting or incurable, management of certain cases may consist of arteriogram with embolization, elastic supports, and limb elevation [8].

Hematologic Disorders

Erythrocytic Disorders
Disorders of RBCs are generally categorized as either a decrease or an increase in the number of RBCs in the circulating blood.

Anemia
Anemia is a decrease in the number of RBCs. Anemia can be described according to etiology as (1) a decrease in RBC production, (2) abnormal RBC maturation, or (3) an increase in RBC destruction [5]. Anemia can also be described according to morphology based on RBC size or color [15]. RBCs that are of normal size are *normocytic*; RBCs that

are smaller than normal are *microcytic;* and RBCs that are larger than normal are *macrocytic.* RBCs of normal color are *normochromic;* RBCs of decreased color are *microchromic.* Some of the most common anemias are described in this section.

Aplastic Anemia. Aplastic anemia is characterized by a decreased RBC production secondary to bone marrow damage. The bone marrow damage either causes irreversible changes to the stem cell population, rendering these cells unable to produce RBCs, or alters the stem cell environment, which inhibits RBC production. The exact mechanism of stem cell damage is unknown; however, present theories include exposure to radiation and chemotherapy, the use of drugs (i.e., diuretics, antiarrhythmics, antihypertensives, anti-inflammatory agents, or antidepressants), or the presence of infection or malignancy. Signs and symptoms of aplastic anemia may include the following:

- Fatigue and dyspnea
- Fever
- Anorexia
- Sore throat
- Hematuria, painful urination, fecal blood
- Bleeding gums
- Petechiae

Management of aplastic anemia may include any of the following: investigation of and removal of causative agent, blood transfusion, bone marrow transplantation, corticosteroids, and antibiotics [6, 15, 16].

Folic Acid Anemia. Decreased folic acid causes the production of macrocytic, normochromic RBCs. Folic acid deficiency is associated with alcoholism, pregnancy, impaired intestinal absorption of folic acid, or the use of anticonvulsant medications. Folic acid anemia is diagnosed by clinical presentation, blood smear, and lactate dehydrogenase (LDH) and MCV values [17]. Management of folic acid anemia consists of folic acid supplementation [6, 15, 16].

Hemolytic Anemia. The two types of hemolytic anemia are extravascular and intravascular hemolytic anemia. Extravascular hemolytic anemia involves the destruction of RBCs outside of the circulation, usually in the spleen. This condition is usually the result of an inherited defect of the RBC membrane or structure, but it can be an autoimmune process in which antibodies in the blood cause RBC destruction through mononuclear phagocytosis.

Intravascular hemolytic anemia is the destruction of RBC membrane within the circulation. It results in the deposition of hemoglobin in plasma. This may occur because of a genetic enzyme deficit, the attack of oxidants on RBCs, or infection. It may also occur traumatically when RBCs are torn apart at sites of blood flow turbulence, near a tumor, through prosthetic valves, or with aortic stenosis.

Signs and symptoms of hemolytic anemia may include the following:

- Fatigue and weakness

- Nausea and vomiting

- Fever and chills

- Decreased urine output

- Jaundice

- Abdominal or back pain and splenomegaly (intravascular only)

Management of hemolytic anemia may include any of the following: investigation and removal of the causative factor, fluid replacement, blood transfusion, corticosteroids, or splenectomy [6, 15, 16].

Iron-Deficiency Anemia. Iron-deficiency anemia occurs when decreased iron storage in the bone marrow causes the production of microcytic, normochromic RBCs. Iron deficiency can be caused by a diet low in iron, the malabsorption of iron, rapid body development, frequent blood donation, excessive menses, pregnancy, acute or chronic blood loss, inflammation, or hookworm. Iron deficiency is diagnosed by clinical presentation and serum ferritin laboratory values. Signs and symptoms of iron-deficiency anemia include the following:

- Fatigue and dyspnea on exertion

- Tachycardia

- Headache

- Irritability

- Mouth soreness, difficulty swallowing, and gastritis

- Softening of nails or pale ear lobes, palms, and conjunctivae

Management of iron-deficiency anemia may consist of a medical workup to identify a possible blood loss site, iron supplementation, or nutritional counseling [6, 15, 16].

Posthemorrhagic Anemia. Posthemorrhagic anemia can occur with rapid blood loss from traumatic artery severance, aneurysm rupture, or arterial erosion from malignant or ulcerative lesions. Blood loss results in a normocytic, normochromic anemia. Signs and symptoms of posthemorrhagic anemia may include the following:

- Tachycardia, tachypnea, hypotension, and palpitations

- Dizziness

- Fatigue

- Stupor

- Decreased urine output, thirst

- Pallor, diaphoresis

Management of posthemorrhagic anemia may consist of any of the following: control of bleeding at the source, blood and blood product transfusion, intravenous and oral fluid administration, and supplemental oxygen [6, 15, 16].

Sickle Cell Anemia. Sickle cell anemia is an autosomal recessive trait characterized by RBCs that become sickle (crescent)-shaped when deoxygenated. Over time, these normal cells become rigid and occlude blood vessels, thus increasing the risk of cerebrovascular accident and the infarction of muscles or other organs. Symptoms and physical findings of sickle cell anemia may include the following:

- Headache

- Neck, chest, abdominal, bone, and joint pain

- Blindness, nystagmus

- Cranial nerve palsy

- Paresthesias

- Nocturia, hematuria, pyelonephritis, renal failure, splenohepatomegaly

Management of sickle cell anemia may include the prevention or supportive treatment of symptoms and the use of corticosteroids [6, 15, 16].

Vitamin B$_{12}$ Anemia. Decreased levels of vitamin B$_{12}$ cause the production of macrocytic, normochromic RBCs. Vitamin B$_{12}$ deficiency can be caused by a diet low in vitamin B$_{12}$, poor absorption of vitamin B$_{12}$, or abnormal use of Vitamin B$_{12}$. There may be numbness or tingling of the extremities, with progression to ataxia and degeneration of the lateral and posterior spinal columns. Vitamin B$_{12}$ deficiency is diagnosed by clinical presentation, blood smear, measurement of LDH and MCV values, and urine sampling. Management of vitamin B$_{12}$ anemia consists of vitamin B$_{12}$ supplementation and nutritional counseling (note: the term *pernicious anemia* refers to a type of vitamin B$_{12}$ anemia in which there is atrophy of gastric cells, causing decreased vitamin B$_{12}$ absorption) [6, 15, 16].

Polycythemia
The three types of polycythemia are primary polycythemia (polycythemia vera), secondary polycythemia, and relative polycythemia. They involve the abnormal increase in the number of RBCs and result in increased blood viscosity.

1. *Primary polycythemia*, or *polycythemia vera*, is an increase in the number of RBCs, WBCs, and platelets [18]. The origin of this disease is unknown; however, it often progresses to leukemia.

2. *Secondary polycythemia* is the overproduction of RBCs due to a high level of erythropoietin. The increased erythropoietin level is a result of either altered stem cells, which automatically produce erythropoietin, or chronic low oxygenation of tissues, in which the body attempts to compensate for hypoxia. It is common in individuals with chronic obstructive pulmonary disease, patients with cardiopulmonary disease, or patients with exposure to high altitudes.

3. *Relative polycythemia* is the temporary increase in RBCs secondary to decreased fluid volume, as with excessive vomiting, diarrhea, diuretic use, or after a burn injury.

Signs and symptoms of polycythemia may include the following:

- Fatigue

- Decreased mental acuity

- Irritability

- Headache

- Dizziness

- Fainting

- Blurred vision

- Altered sensation in the hands and feet

- Onset of gout

- Ruddy cyanosis

- Clubbing or bruising

- Hypertension

- Splenomegaly (polycythemia vera only)

Management of polycythemia may include any of the following: antineoplastic agents, radioactive phosphorus, and venesection (for primary polycythemia); smoking cessation and phlebotomy (for secondary polycythemia); and fluid resuscitation (for relative polycythemia).

Thrombocytic Disorders

Disseminated Intravascular Coagulation

Disseminated intravascular coagulation (DIC) involves the introduction of thromboplastic substances into the circulation that initiate a massive clotting cascade accompanied by fibrin, plasmin, and platelet activation. DIC can be acute or chronic.

The onset of acute DIC usually occurs in the presence of illness. This condition is associated with infection, trauma, burn injury, shock, tissue acidosis, antigen-antibody complexes, or the entrance of amniotic fluid or placenta into the maternal circulation.

Chronic DIC is associated with hemangioma and other cancers (particularly pancreatic or prostate cancer), systemic lupus erythematosus, or missed abortion.

Signs and symptoms of DIC may include the following:

- Abrupt (in acute DIC) or slow (in chronic DIC) blood loss from an injury site, nose, gums, or gastrointestinal or urinary tracts

- Thrombosis (for chronic DIC)
- Tachypnea, tachycardia, hypotension, and dysrhythmia
- Altered consciousness, anxiety, fear, or restlessness
- Ecchymosis, petechiae, and purpura
- Weakness
- Decreased urine output
- Acute renal failure (for acute DIC)

Management of DIC may include any of the following: treatment of the causative condition; blood and blood product transfusion; fluid, hemodynamic, and shock management; antibiotics; antineoplastics; and heparin therapy (this is controversial) [19].

Hemophilia
Hemophilia is a disease characterized by excessive spontaneous hemorrhaging at mucous membranes, into joint spaces and muscles, or intracranially. It is the result of a genetic deficiency of a clotting factor. There are four basic types:

1. Hemophilia A is characterized by the lack of factor VIII and is inherited as an X-linked recessive trait.

2. Hemophilia B is characterized by the lack of factor IX and is inherited as an X-linked recessive trait.

3. Hemophilia C is characterized by the lack of factor XI and is inherited as an autosomal recessive trait.

4. von Willebrand's disease is characterized by the lack of factor VIII and is inherited as an autosomal dominant trait.

Symptoms and physical findings of hemophilia may include the following:

- Petechiae, purpura, and ecchymosis
- Tachycardia, tachypnea, and hypotension
- Disorientation
- Convulsions

- Decreased reflexes

Management of hemophilia may include any of the following: methods to stop active bleeding (e.g., direct pressure), factor replacement therapy, immunosuppressive drugs, and antifibrinolytics [19].

Thalassemia
Thalassemia is an autosomal recessive disease characterized by abnormal formation of hemoglobin chains in RBCs, resulting in RBC membrane damage and abnormal erythropoiesis and hemolysis.
Hemoglobin is composed of two alpha and two beta chains. Alpha-thalassemia is a defect in alpha chain synthesis in which one (alpha trait), two (alpha-thalassemia minor), three (hemoglobin H disease), or four (alpha-thalassemia major) genes are altered. Each type of alpha-thalassemia varies in presentation from a lack of symptoms (alpha trait) to minor or severe hemolytic anemia. Beta-thalassemia is a defect in beta chain synthesis in one of two beta chains (beta-thalassemia minor) or a severe reduction or absence in beta chain production (Cooley's anemia) [19].

Thrombocytopenia
Thrombocytopenia is an acute or chronic decrease in the number of platelets (less than 100,000/µl) in the circulation. It can result from decreased platelet production (caused by infection, drug or immune responses, or blood vessel damage), increased platelet destruction (caused by malignancy or the use of myelosuppressive drugs), or altered platelet distribution (caused by cardiac surgery–induced hypothermia, portal hypertension, or splenomegaly).
Signs and symptoms of thrombocytopenia may include the following:

- Bleeding of nose, gums, or puncture sites or blood in emesis, urine, or stool

- Ecchymosis and petechiae

- Tachycardia and tachypnea

- Signs of increased intracranial pressure if a cranial bleed is present

- Renal failure

- Splenomegaly

Management of thrombocytopenia may include any of the following: plasma transfusion or plasmapheresis, corticosteroids, or splenectomy [19].

Thrombotic Thrombocytopenic Purpura
Thrombotic thrombocytopenic purpura (TTP) is the rapid accumulation of thrombi in small blood vessels. The etiology of TTP is unknown; however, it is associated with bacterial or viral infections and autoimmune disorders such as AIDS.

Signs and symptoms of TTP may include the following:

- Fatigue and weakness
- Thrombocytopenia
- Hemolytic anemia
- Fever
- Seizure
- Coma
- Abdominal pain
- Acute renal failure

Management of TTP may include any of the following: plasma exchange, antiplatelet agents, corticosteroids, immunosuppressive agents, or splenectomy [19].

Management

The management of vascular disorders includes pharmacologic therapy and vascular surgical procedures. Hematologic disorders may be managed with pharmacologic therapy as well as with nutritional therapy and blood transfusions.

Pharmacologic Therapy

Chapter Appendix 6-A describes the various pharmacologic agents used in managing vascular and hematologic disorders.

Table 6-14. Blood Type Characteristics

Type	Agglutinogen	Agglutinin	May Transfuse
A	A	B	A, O
B	B	A	B, O
AB	A, B	—	A, B, AB, O
O	—	A, B	O

Nutritional Therapy

Nutritional therapy is the treatment of choice for anemia caused by vitamin and mineral deficiency. Chapter Appendix 6-A describes the use and general side effects of the agents used to manage vitamin B_{12}, folic acid, and iron-deficiency anemias.

Blood Transfusion

Blood and blood products are transfused to replete blood volume, maintain oxygen delivery to tissues, or maintain proper coagulation [20]. Chapter Appendix 6-B lists the most common transfusion products and the rationale for their use. Before transfusing blood or blood products, the substance to be given must be typed and crossed. This process ensures that the correct type of blood is given to a patient to avoid hemolytic reactions. Blood is typed according to agglutinogen or the type of antigen present on the RBC. Agglutinin, or the antibody opposite the agglutinogen, is present in plasma. Table 6-14 lists blood type characteristics. There are a variety of transfusion reactions that can occur with the administration of blood products. Table 6-15 lists the signs and symptoms of various types of adverse transfusion reactions. In addition to these reactions, complications of blood transfusion include circulation overload (from a rapid increase in volume) or air embolism (if the blood is pumped into the patient).

Clinical tip

If the patient is receiving blood products, the physical therapist should observe the patient, speak to the nurse, or both

Table 6-15. Adverse Blood Reactions

Reaction	Cause	Signs and Symptoms
Allergic reaction	Patient's blood is sensitive to transfused plasma protein	(Mild) Bronchial wheezing Flushed and itchy skin
	Patient's blood and transfused blood create an antibody-antigen reaction	(Severe) Dyspnea Chest pain Cardiac arrest
Febrile reaction	Patient's blood is sensitive to transfused plasma protein, platelets, or white blood cells	Fever Headache Chills Flushed skin Muscle pain
Hemolytic reaction	Patient's blood and transfused blood are not compatible	Tachycardia Hypotension Dyspnea Cyanosis Chest pain Fever Chills Headache or backache
Septic reaction	Transfused blood is contaminated	Hypotension Fever Chills Emesis Diarrhea

Source: Adapted from B Kozier, G Erb, K Blais, JM Wilkinson. Fundamentals of Nursing: Concepts, Process and Practice (5th ed). Redwood City, CA: Benjamin-Cummings, 1995;110.

before physical therapy intervention. If possible, the therapist may defer out-of-bed or vigorous activities until the transfusion is complete.

Vascular Surgical Procedures

Surgical management of vascular disorders such as angioplasty, arthrectomy, and stent placement are described in Chapter 1 under "Cardiac

Surgical Procedures." This section therefore concentrates on embolization therapy, endarterectomy, bypass grafting, and aneurysm repair and replacement with synthetic grafts.

Embolization Therapy

Embolization therapy is the process of purposely occluding a vessel with Gel-foam, coils, balloons, polyvinyl alcohol, and various glue-like agents, which are injected as liquids and solidify in the vessel.* Embolization therapy is performed with a specialized intravascular catheter after angiographic evaluation has outlined the area to be treated.

Indications for embolization therapy include disorders characterized by inappropriate blood flow, such as arteriovenous malformations or less commonly for persistent hemoptysis.

Complications of embolization therapy include tissue necrosis, inadvertent embolization of normal tissues, and passage of embolic materials through arteriovenous communications [13].

Peripheral Vascular Bypass Grafting

To reperfuse an area that has been ischemic from peripheral vascular disease, two general bypass grafting procedures (with many specific variations of each type) can be performed. The area of vascular occlusion can be bypassed with either an inverted portion of the saphenous vein or with a synthetic material such as Gore-Tex or Lycra. (The synthetic graft is referred to as a prosthetic graft.) Vascular surgeons generally describe and illustrate in the medical record what type of procedure was performed on the particular vascular anatomy. The terminology used to describe each bypass graft procedure indicates which vessels were involved. (For example, a *fem-pop bypass graft [FPBPG]* involves bypassing an occlusion of the femoral artery with another conduit to the popliteal artery distal to the area of occlusion.) After a bypass procedure, patients, depending on premorbid physiologic status and extent of surgery, require approximately 24–48 hours to become hemodynamically stable and are usually monitored in an intensive care unit setting.

Complications that can occur after bypass grafting include the following [4]:

---

*The term *embolization* is general and can either refer to a pathologic occlusion of a vessel by a dislodged portion of a thrombus, fat, air, or to the therapeutic procedure described in this section. The context in which *embolization* is discussed must be considered in order to avoid confusion.

- Hemorrhage (at graft site or in gastrointestinal tract)
- Thrombosis
- Infection
- Colon ischemia
- Pseudoaneurysm formation at the anastomosis
- Sexual dysfunction
- Spinal cord ischemia
- Renal failure

Endarterectomy

Endarterectomy is a process in which the stenotic area of an artery wall is excised and the noninvolved ends of the artery are reanastomosed. It can be used to correct localized occlusive vascular disease, eliminating the need for bypassing the area [13].

Aneurysm Repair and Reconstruction

Aneurysm repair and reconstruction involves isolating the aneurysm by clamping off the vessel proximal and distal to the aneurysm, excising the aneurysm, and replacing the aneurysmal area with a synthetic graft. Performing the procedure before the aneurysm ruptures (elective surgery) is preferable to repairing a ruptured aneurysm (emergency surgery) because a ruptured aneurysm requires an extremely challenging and difficult operative course due to the hemodynamic instability from hemorrhage. The cross-clamp time of the vessels is also crucial because organs distal to the site of repair can become ischemic if the clamp time is prolonged. Complications that may occur after aneurysm repair are similar to those discussed in "Peripheral Vascular Bypass Grafting" [4].

Clinical tip

- It is important to examine incision sites for mobility and range-of-motion treatments. Incisions should be inspected before and after mobility to assess the patency of the incision, as drainage or weeping may occur during activity. If drainage or weeping occurs, notify the nurse promptly and document it accordingly in the medical record. Abdominal incisions or other incisional pain can limit a patient's cough effectiveness and lead to pulmonary infection. Diligent attention to position changes, deep breathing, assisted coughing, and manual techniques (e.g., percussion and vibration techniques as needed) can help prevent pulmonary infections. Grafts that cross the hip joint, such as aortobifem grafts, require clarification by the surgeon regarding the amount of flexion allowed at the hip.

• After a patient is cleared to be out of bed, specific orders from the physician should be obtained regarding weight bearing on the involved extremities, particularly those with recent bypass grafts.

• Patients may have systolic blood pressure limitations postoperatively to maintain adequate perfusion of the limb or to ensure the patency of the graft area. Blood pressures that are below the specified limit may decrease perfusion, whereas pressures above the limit may lead to graft damage. Thorough vital sign monitoring before, during, and after activity is essential [5].

Physical Therapy Interventions for Patients with Vascular and Hematologic Disorders

The primary physical therapy goals for patients with vascular and hematologic disorders are optimizing functional mobility and optimizing activity tolerance. In addition to these goals, patients with vascular disorders require patient education to prevent skin breakdown, to manage edema, and to prevent joint contractures and muscle shortening.

Guidelines for the physical therapist working with the patient who has either vascular or hematologic dysfunction include the following:

• Patients with peripheral vascular disease commonly have concurrent coronary artery disease; therefore, monitoring vital signs during therapy sessions is essential.

• Patients with peripheral vascular disease may also have concurrent chronic obstructive pulmonary disease; therefore, activity tolerance may have pulmonary limitations as well.

- Patients with peripheral vascular disease may have impaired sensation from arterial insufficiency, comorbid diagnosis of diabetes mellitus, or peripheral edema; therefore, sensation testing is an important component of the physical therapy evaluation.

- Assessing laboratory values of patients with hematologic disorders on a daily basis is important because of the high risk for bruising or bleeding and because exercise parameters should be adjusted in accordance with fluctuations in components of the CBC.

- Progression of activity tolerance in patients with hematologic disorders does not occur at the same rate as in patients with normal blood composition; therefore, the time frame for goal achievement should be modified.

References

1. Black JM, Matassarin-Jacobs E. Luckmann and Sorensen's Medical-Surgical Nursing: A Psychophysiologic Approach (4th ed). Philadelphia: Saunders, 1993;1286.
2. Marieb EN. Blood. In EN Marieb (ed), Human Anatomy and Physiology. Redwood City, CA: Benjamin-Cummings, 1989;568.
3. Lanzer P, Rosch J. Vascular Diagnostics: Noninvasive and Invasive Techniques, Peri-Interventional Evaluations. Berlin: Springer-Verlag, 1994.
4. Hallet JW, Brewster DC, Darling RC. Handbook of Patient Care in Vascular Surgery (3rd ed). Boston: Little, Brown, 1995.
5. Hillman RS, Ault KA. Hematology in Clinical Practice: A Guide to Diagnosis and Management. New York: McGraw-Hill, 1995;17.
6. Goodman CC, Snyder TK. Overview of Hematology: Signs and Symptoms. In CC Goodman, TK Snyder (eds), Differential Diagnosis in Physical Therapy: Musculoskeletal and Systemic Conditions. Philadelphia: Saunders, 1990;114.
7. Corbett JV. Laboratory Tests & Diagnostic Procedures with Nursing Diagnoses (4th ed). Stamford, CT: Appleton & Lange, 1996;25.
8. Moore WS. Vascular Surgery: A Comprehensive Review (4th ed). Philadelphia: Saunders, 1993;90.
9. McCance KL, Huether SE. Pathophysiology: The Biologic Basis for Disease in Adults and Children (2nd ed). St. Louis: Mosby, 1994;1001.
10. Thompson JM, McFarland GK, Hirsch JE, et al. Clinical Nursing. St. Louis: Mosby, 1986;85.
11. Young JR, Graor RA, Olin JW, Bartholomew JR. Peripheral Vascular Diseases. St. Louis: Mosby, 1991.
12. Bullock BL. Pathophysiology: Adaptations and Alterations in Function (4th ed). Philadelphia: Lippincott, 1996;524.

13. Strandness DE, Breda AV. Vascular Diseases: Surgical & Interventional Therapy (Vols. 1 and 2). New York: Churchill Livingstone, 1994.
14. Smeltzer SC, Bare BG. Brunner and Suddarth's Textbook of Medical-Surgical Nursing (8th ed). Philadelphia: Lippincott, 1995;722.
15. Purtillo DT, Purtillo RP. A Survey of Human Diseases (2nd ed). Boston: Little, Brown, 1989;287.
16. Erythrocyte Disease. In AE Belcher, Blood Disorders. St. Louis: Mosby–Year Book, 1993;51.
17. Roper D, Stein S, Payne M, Coleman M. Anemias Caused by Impaired Production of Erythrocytes. In BF Rodak (ed), Diagnostic Hematology. Philadelphia: Saunders, 1995;181.
18. Babior BM, Stossel TP. Hematology: A Pathophysiological Approach (3rd ed). New York: Churchill Livingstone, 1994;359.
19. Thrombolytic Disorders. In AE Belcher, Blood Disorders. St. Louis: Mosby–Year Book, 1993;112.
20. Harkness GA, Dincher JR. Medical-Surgical Nursing: Total Patient Care (9th ed). St. Louis: Mosby–Year Book, 1996;656.

Appendix 6-A:
Anticoagulation, Thrombolytic, and Nutritional Therapy Agents

Table 6-A.1. Pharmacologic Management for Excessive Clotting

Medication	Indication	Action	Side Effects
Anticoagulant agents Heparin (Calciparine, Hep-Lock, Lipo-Hepin, Liquaemin Sodium) Warfarin (Coumadin) Anisindione Phenprocoumon	Prevent DVT formation to treat preexisting DVT, PE, or both	Delays clotting time of blood by inhibiting synthesis and function of clotting factors Cannot dissolve preexisting thrombus	Hemorrhage exhibited by hematuria, bruises, nose-bleeds, and bleeding gums Thrombocytopenia Allergic reactions Osteoporosis (prolonged use)
Antithrombotic agents Aspirin Dipyridamole (Persantine, Pyramode) Sulfinpyrazone (Antazone, Anturan, Anturane, Apo-Sulfinpyrazone, Apra-zone, Noropyrazone, Salazopyrin, Zynol)	Prevent formation of arterial thrombus	Platelet aggregation and clotting inhibition	Gastrointestinal bleeding Syncope Weakness Headache, nausea, vomiting
Thrombolytic agents* Urokinase (Abbokinase, Open-Cath) Streptokinase (Kabikinase, Streptase) Tissue plasminogen activator	Treatment of preexisting thrombus or embolus	Dissolves preexisting clots by enhancing the fibrinolytic system	Side effects are similar to those of anticoagulants

DVT = deep venous thrombosis; PE = pulmonary embolism.
*Contraindications for thrombolytic agents include active bleeding, recent stroke, surgery or organ biopsy within the previous 10 days, and coagulopathy.
Source: Data from JW Hallet, DC Brewster, RC Darling. Handbook of Patient Care in Vascular Surgery (3rd ed). Boston: Little, Brown, 1995; KL McCance, SE Huether. Pathophysiology: The Biologic Basis for Disease in Adults and Children (2nd ed). St. Louis: Mosby, 1994; JB Clark, SF Queenir, VB Karb. Pharmacologic Basis of Nursing Practice (4th ed). St. Louis: Mosby-Year Book, 1993; and CD Ciccone. Treatment of Coagulation Disorders. Pharmacology in Rehabilitation. Philadelphia: FA Davis, 1990.

Table 6-A.2. Summary of Nutritional Therapy Agents for Vitamin- and Mineral-Deficiency Anemias

Agent	Use	General Side Effects
Iron therapy agents	Iron-deficiency	Gastric discomfort
Ferrous fumarate (Femiron,	anemia	Constipation
Feostat, Fersamal. Fumasorb,		Dark stools
Fumerin, Hemocyte,		Hypotension
Ircon-FA, Palmiron)		
Ferrous gluconate (Fergon,		
Ferralet, Fertinic, Noro-		
ferrogloc, Simron)		
Ferrous sulfate (Feosol, Fer-In-		
Sol, Fero-Gradumet, Fero-		
space, Ferralynx, Ferra-TD,		
Fesofor, Hematinic,		
Mol-Iron, Slow-Fe)		
Iron dextran (Imfed, Imferon)		Headache
		Dizziness
		Syncope
		Arrhythmia
		Hypotension
		Nausea
		Vomiting
		Abdominal pain
Vitamin B$_{12}$ therapy	Vitamin B$_{12}$	Itchy skin or rash
Hydroxocobalamin (Alpham-	anemia	Congestive heart
iné, AlphaPedisol, Hydro-	Pernicious	failure
bexan, Hydro-12, LA-12)	anemia	Pulmonary edema
Cyanocobalamin (Betalin 12,		Diarrhea
Cobex, Crystamine,		Hypokalemia
Crysti-12, Cyanabin,		Thrombosis
Cyanoject, Kayborite,		
Redisol, Robesol,		
Rubramin PC)		
Folic acid therapy	Folic acid	None known
Folic acid (Folacin, Folvite)	anemia	
Leucovorin calcium (calcium		
folinate, citrovorum factor,		
folinic acid, Wellcovorin)		

Source: Data from MT Shannon, BA Wilson, CL Stang. Govoni and Hayes Drugs and Nursing Implications (8th ed). East Norwalk, CT: Appleton & Lange, 1995.

Appendix 6-B:
Blood Products

Table 6-B.1. Common Blood Products and Their Uses

Product	Description	Use
Albumin	Contains albumin cells	To increase albumin level or to replete circulating intravascular volume, as in shock management or acute liver failure
Plasma (fresh frozen)	Contains all plasma components, namely blood factors and protein	To increase clotting factor levels
Platelets	Contains concentrated platelets only	To restore clotting function after blood loss
Red blood cells (packed cells)	Contains red blood cells only	After blood loss or decreased hematocrit Treatment for anemia
Whole blood	Contains all blood cells with an anticoagulation preservative	After major blood loss when RBC and plasma need replacement (rarely used)

Source: Adapted from GA Harkness, JR Dincher. Medical-Surgical Nursing: Total Patient Care (9th ed). St. Louis: Mosby–Year Book, 1996;659; and B Kozier, G Erb, K Blais, JM Wilkinson. Fundamentals of Nursing: Concepts, Process and Practice (5th ed). Redwood City, CA: Benjamin Cummings, 1995;1111.

7

Burns and Wounds

Michele Panik and Marie Jarrell-Gracious

Introduction

Treating a patient with a major burn injury or other skin wound is often a specialized area of physical therapy.* Physical therapists should, however, have a basic understanding of normal and abnormal skin integrity, including the etiology of skin breakdown and the factors that influence wound healing. The main objectives of this chapter are therefore to provide a fundamental review of the following:

1. The structure and function of the skin or integument

2. The etiology of different types of wounds and the process of wound healing

3. The evaluation and physiologic sequelae of burn injury including medical-surgical management and physical therapy intervention

4. The evaluation and management of wounds, including physical therapy intervention

*For the purpose of this chapter, an alteration in skin integrity secondary to a burn injury is referred to as a "burn." Alteration in skin integrity from any other etiology is referred to as a "wound."

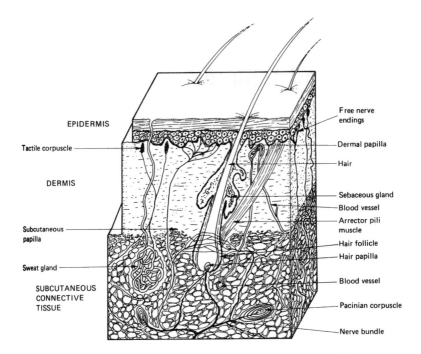

EPIDERMIS

Tactile corpuscle

DERMIS

Subcutaneous
papilla

Sweat gland

SUBCUTANEOUS
CONNECTIVE
TISSUE

Free nerve
endings

Dermal papilla

Hair

Sebaceous gland

Blood vessel

Arrector pili
muscle

Hair follicle

Hair papilla

Blood vessel

Pacinian corpuscle

Nerve bundle

Figure 7-1. *Three-dimensional representation of the skin and subcutaneous connective tissue layer showing the arrangement of hair, glands, and blood vessels. (Reprinted with permission from N Palastanga, D Field, R Soames, et al. Anatomy and Human Movement [2nd ed]. Oxford: Butterworth–Heinemann, 1989;49.)*

Structure and Function: The Normal Integument

Structure

The integumentary system consists of the skin and its appendages (hair and hair shafts, nails, and sebaceous and sweat glands), which are located throughout the skin, as pictured in Figure 7-1. Skin is 0.5–4.0 mm thick and is composed of two major layers: the epidermis and the dermis. These layers are supported by subcutaneous tissue and fat that connect the skin to muscle and bone. The thin, avascular epidermis is composed mainly of cells containing keratin. The epidermal cells are in different stages of growth and degeneration. The thick, highly vascularized dermis is composed mainly of connective tissue. Table 7-1 lists the major contents of each skin layer.

The skin has a number of clinically significant variations: (1) males have thicker skin than females; (2) the young and elderly have thinner skin than adults [1]; and (3) the skin on various parts of the body varies in thickness, number of appendages, and blood flow [2]. These variations affect the severity of a burn injury or skin breakdown and the process of tissue healing.

Function

The integument has seven major functions [3]:

1.   Temperature regulation. Body temperature is regulated by increasing or decreasing sweat production, superficial blood flow, or both.

2.   Protection. The skin acts as a barrier to protect the body from microorganism invasion, ultraviolet (UV) radiation, abrasion, chemicals, and dehydration.

3.   Sensation. Multiple sensory cells within the skin detect pain, temperature, and touch.

4.   Excretion. Heat, sweat, and water can be excreted from the skin.

5.   Immunity. Normal periodic loss of epidermal cells removes microorganisms from the body surface, and immune cells in the skin transport antigens from outside the body to the antibody cells of the immune system.

6.   Blood reservoir. Large volumes of blood can be shunted from the skin to central organs or muscles as needed.

7.   Vitamin D synthesis. Modified cholesterol molecules are converted to vitamin D when exposed to UV radiation.

Pathophysiology of Burns

Skin and body tissue destruction occurs from the absorption of heat energy and results in tissue coagulation. This coagulation is depicted in zones (Figure 7-2). The zone of coagulation, located in the center of the burn, is the area of greatest damage and contains nonviable tissue

Table 7-1. Normal Skin Layers: Structure and Function

Layer	Composition	Function
Epidermis		
Stratum corneum	Dead keratinocytes	Tough outer layer that protects deeper layers of epidermis
Pigment layer	Melanocytes	Produces melanin to prevent ultraviolet absorption
Stratum granulosum	Mature keratinocytes	Produces keratin to make the skin waterproof
	Langerhans' cells	Interacts with immune cells
Stratum spinosum	Keratinocytes	Undergoes mitosis to continue skin cell development but to a lesser degree than basale
Stratum basale	New keratinocytes	The origin of skin cells, which undergoes mitosis, then moves superficially
	Merkel's cells	Detects touch
Dermis		
Papillary layer	Areolar connective tissue	Binds epidermis and dermis together
	Meissner's corpuscles	Detects light touch
	Blood and lymph vessels	Provides circulation and drainage
	Free nerve endings	Detects heat and pain
Reticular layer	Collagen, elastin, and reticular fibers	Provides strength and resilience
Hypodermis	Subcutaneous fat	Provides insulation and shock absorption
	Pacinian cells	Detects pressure
	Free nerve endings	Detects cold

Source: Data from GA Thibodeau, KT Patton. Structure and Function of the Body (9th ed). St. Louis: Mosby–Year Book, 1992.

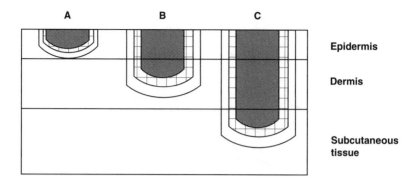

Figure 7-2. *The zones of coagulation. A. Superficial burn. B. Partial-thickness burn. C. Full-thickness burn. (Modified from WG Williams, LG Phillips. Pathophysiology of the Burn Wound. In DN Herndon [ed], Total Burn Care. London: Saunders, 1996;65.)*

referred to as *eschar.* Although eschar covers the surface and may appear to take the place of skin, it does not have any of the characteristics or functions of normal skin. Instead, eschar is constrictive, attracts microorganisms, and houses burn toxins that may circulate throughout the body [1]. The zone of stasis, which surrounds the zone of coagulation, contains marginally viable tissue. The zone of hyperemia, the outermost area, is the least damaged and heals rapidly.

Physiologic Sequelae of Burn Injury

A series of physiologic events occurs after a burn (Figure 7-3). The physical therapist must appreciate the multisystem effects of a burn injury, namely, that the metabolic demands of the body increase dramatically. Tissue damage or organ dysfunction can be immediate or delayed, minor or severe, and local or systemic. A summary of the most common complications of burns is listed in Table 7-2 [4].

Types of Burns

Thermal Burns
Thermal burns can be the result of conduction or convection, as in contact with a hot object, hot liquid, or flame (conduction) or steam (con-

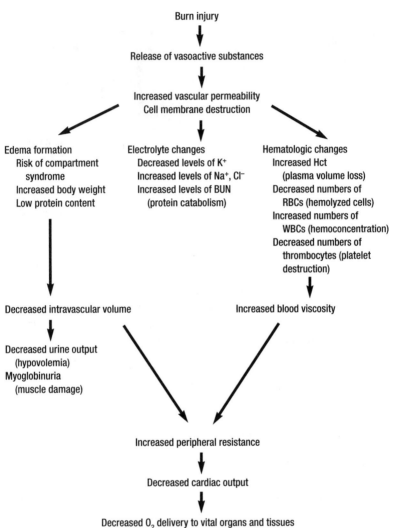

Figure 7-3. *The physiologic sequelae of major burn injury. (K⁺ = potassium; Na⁺ = sodium; Cl⁻ = chlorine; BUN = blood urea nitrogen; Hct = hematocrit; RBC = red blood cell; WBC = white blood cell; O₂ = oxygen.) (Modified from J Marvin. Thermal Injuries. In VD Cardona, PD Hurn, PJ Bastnagel Mason, et al. [eds], Trauma Nursing: From Resuscitation Through Rehabilitation [2nd ed]. Philadelphia: Saunders, 1994;740; and RH Demling, C Lalonde. Burn Trauma. New York: Thieme, 1989;99.)*

Table 7-2. Systemic Complications of Burns Injury

Body System	Complications
Respiratory	Inhalation injury, restrictive respiratory pattern (which may occur with a burn on the trunk), atelectasis, pneumonia, microthrombi, and acute respiratory distress syndrome
Cardiovascular	Hypovolemia, hypertension, subendocardial ischemia, myocardial necrosis (from electrical burns), anemia, and disseminated intravascular coagulopathy (see Chapter 6, "Thrombotic Disorders")
Gastrointestinal	Stress ulceration, hemorrhage, gastroduodenitis, ischemic colitis, cholestasis, and liver failure
Renal	Edema, hemorrhage, and tubular necrosis

Source: Data from HA Linares. The Burn Problem: A Pathologist's Perspective. In DN Herndon (ed), Total Burn Care. London: Saunders, 1996.

vection). The severity of burn depends on the location of the burn, the temperature of the burn source, and the duration of contact [4].

Electrical Burns

The severity of an electrical burn depends on the voltage of the source, the type and pathway of current, duration of contact with the source, and the amperage and resistance through the body tissues [5]. Electrical burns are characterized by deep *entrance* and *exit wounds*. The entrance wound is usually an obvious necrotic and depressed area, whereas the exit wound varies in presentation. The exit wound can be a single wound or multiple wounds located where the patient was grounded during injury [5]. Tissue damage is superficial and deep, occurring along the path of the electrical current.

Complications specific to electrical injury include the following [5]:

- Cardiovascular. Cardiac arrest or arrhythmia secondary to alterations in electrical conductivity of the heart

- Neurologic. Coma, seizures, or both and peripheral nerve injury, resulting from ischemia or spinal cord paralysis from demyelination during the burn injury

- Orthopedic. Dislocations or fractures secondary to sustained muscular contraction

- Other. Corneal damage and tympanic membrane rupture

Lightning

Lightning, considered a form of electrical current, causes injury via four mechanisms [6]:

1. Direct strike, in which the person is the grounding site
2. Flash discharge, in which an object deviates the course of the lightning current before striking the person
3. Ground current, in which lightning strikes the ground and a person within the grounding area creates a pathway for the current
4. Shock wave, in which lightning travels outside the person and static electricity vaporizes moisture in the skin

Chemical Burns

Chemical burns can be the result of reduction, oxidation, corrosion, or desecration of body tissue with or without an associated thermal injury [7]. The severity of burn depends on the type of chemical and its concentration, duration of contact, and mechanism of action. Unlike thermal burns, chemical burns significantly alter systemic tissue pH and metabolism. These changes can cause serious pulmonary complications (e.g., airway obstruction from bronchospasm, edema, or epithelial sloughing) and metabolic complications (e.g., liver necrosis or renal dysfunction from prolonged chemical exposure).

Ultraviolet and Ionizing Radiation Burns

A sunburn is a superficial partial-thickness burn from the overexposure of the skin to UV radiation. Ionizing radiation burns with or without thermal burn occur when electromagnetic or particulate radiation energy is transferred to body tissues, resulting in the formation of chemical free radicals [8]. Ionizing radiation burns usually occur in laboratory or industrial settings. The severity of the ionizing radiation burn depends on the dose, dose rate, and the tissue sensitivity of exposed cells. Often referred to as acute radiation syndrome, complications of ionizing radiation burns include the following [8]:

- Gastrointestinal. Cramps, nausea, vomiting, diarrhea, and bowel ischemia

- Hematologic. Pancytopenia (decreased number of red blood cells, white blood cells, and platelets), granulocytopenia (decreased number of granular leukocytes), thrombocytopenia (decreased number of platelets), and hemorrhage

- Vascular. Endothelium destruction

Burn Assessment and Acute Care Management of Burn Injury

Classification of a Burn

The extent and depth of the burn determines its severity and dictates acute care treatment.

Assessing the Extent of a Burn

The assessment of the extent of a burn is necessary to calculate fluid volume therapy and is a predictor of morbidity [9]. The extent of a burn injury is referred to as total body surface area (TBSA) and can be calculated by the Rule of Nines or the Lund and Browder formula.

Rule of Nines

The Rule of Nines divides the body into sections, seven of which are assigned 9% of TBSA. The genitalia is assigned 1%, and the anterior and posterior trunk are each assigned 18% (Figure 7-4). This formula is quick and easy to use, especially when a rapid initial estimation of TBSA is needed in the field or the emergency room. To use the Rule of Nines, the area of burn is filled in on the diagram, and the percentages are added for a TBSA. Modifications can be made if an entire body section is not burned. For example, if only the posterior left arm is burned, the TBSA is 4.5%.

Lund and Browder Formula

Table 7-3 describes the Lund and Browder formula. The body is divided into 19 sections, and each is assigned a different percentage of TBSA. These percentages vary with age from infant to adult to accommodate for relative changes in TBSA with normal growth. The Lund and Browder formula is a more accurate predictor of TBSA than the Rule of Nines because of the inclusion of a greater number of body divisions along with the adjustments for age and normal growth.

Estimating the Extent of Irregularly Shaped Burns

It is important to note that using the Rule of Nines or the Lund and Browder formula may not be accurate for irregularly shaped burns. To

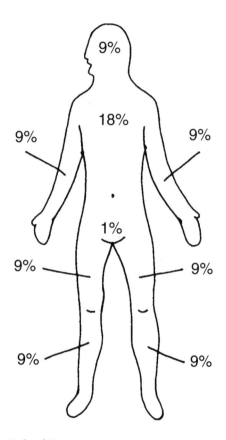

Figure 7-4. *The Rule of Nines.*

estimate TBSA with irregularly shaped burns, the patient's palm is used to measure the shape of the burn. The palm represents 1% TBSA [9].

Assessing the Depth of a Burn

The depth of a burn can be described as superficial, moderate, deep partial thickness, or full thickness. Each type has its own appearance, healing time, and level of pain (Table 7-4). The assessment of burn depth allows an estimation of the proper type of burn care or surgery and the expected functional outcome and cosmesis [10]. Burn depth may also be assessed by detection of pinprick (if the patient can sense a pinprick, the burn is superficial; if the patient cannot detect a pinprick [because of the destruction of nerve endings], the burn is deeper).

Table 7-3. Lund and Browder Method of Assessing the Extent of Burns*

	Birth	1–4 yrs	5–9 yrs	10–14 yrs	15 yrs	Adult
Head and trunk						
Head	19	17	13	11	9	7
Neck	2	2	2	2	2	2
Anterior trunk	13	13	13	13	13	13
Posterior trunk	13	13	13	13	13	13
Left buttock	2.5	2.5	2.5	2.5	2.5	2.5
Right buttock	2.5	2.5	2.5	2.5	2.5	2.5
Genitalia	1	1	1	1	1	1
Upper extremity						
Left upper arm	4	4	4	4	4	4
Right upper arm	4	4	4	4	4	4
Left forearm	3	3	3	3	3	3
Right forearm	3	3	3	3	3	3
Left hand	2.5	2.5	2.5	2.5	2.5	2.5
Right hand	2.5	2.5	2.5	2.5	2.5	2.5
Lower extremity						
Left thigh	5.5	6.5	8	8.5	9	9.5
Right thigh	5.5	6.5	8	8.5	9	9.5
Left lower leg	5	5	5.5	6	6.5	7
Right lower leg	5	5	5.5	6	6.5	7
Left foot	3.5	3.5	3.5	3.5	3.5	3.5
Right foot	3.5	3.5	3.5	3.5	3.5	3.5

*Values represent percentage of total body surface area.
Source: Adapted from WF McManus, BA Pruitt. Thermal Injuries. In DV Feliciano, EE Moore, KL Mattox (eds), Trauma. Stamford, CT: Appleton & Lange, 1996;941; and CC Lund, NC Browder. The estimation of areas of burns. Surg Gynecol Obstet 1944;79:355.

Acute Care Management of Burn Injury

This section discusses the admission guidelines and resuscitative and reparative phases of burn care.

Table 7-4. Burn Depth Characteristics

Depth	Appearance	Healing	Pain
Superficial partial thickness (first-degree) Epidermis injured	Pink to red With or without edema Dry appearance No blisters Blanches Skin intact when rubbed	3–5 days	Tenderness to touch or painful
Moderate partial thickness (second-degree) Superficial dermis injured	Pink to mottled red or red with edema Moist appearance Blisters present May blanch Skin disrupted when rubbed	5 days to 3 weeks	Very painful
Deep partial thickness (second-degree) Deep dermis injured	Pink to pale ivory Dry appearance Blisters present Does not blanch Hair readily removed	3 weeks to months	Very painful
Full thickness (third-degree) Fat, muscle, and bone injured	Black, brown, red, or white Dry appearance May be blistered Does not blanch Thrombosed blood vessels Depressed wound	Not able to regenerate	No pain, perhaps an ache

Admission Guidelines

In addition to the burn's extent and depth, the presence of associated pulmonary, orthopedic, or visual injuries determines what level of care is optimal for the patient. The American Burn Association recommends medical care at a burn center if the patient suffers from any of the following [9]:

- Second- and third-degree burns that are greater than or equal to 10% of TBSA in patients younger than 10 years of age or older than 50 years of age

- Burns of any type that are greater than 20% of TBSA in patients between 10 and 50 years of age

- Full-thickness burns that are greater than or equal to 5% of TBSA

- Burns of the eyes, ears, face, hands, feet, or perineum

- High-voltage electric or lightning injury

- Inhalation injury or other trauma

- A significant chemical burn

- Preexisting disease in which the burn could increase mortality

The American Burn Association recommends medical care at a general emergency room or hospital if a patient suffers from any of the following [9]:

- Second- and third-degree burns of less than 10% of TBSA in patients younger than 10 years of age or older than 50 years of age

- Burns of any type that are less than 20% of TBSA in patients between 10 and 50 years of age

- No other associated injury or preexisting disease

Resuscitative Phase
The objectives of emergency room management of the patient who has a major burn injury include simultaneous general systemic stabilization and burn care [11]. The prioritization of care and precautions during this initial time period have a great impact on survival and illustrate some key concepts of burn care.

General Systemic Stabilization

General systemic stabilization involves (1) the assessment of inhalation injury and carbon monoxide poisoning and the maintenance of the airway and ventilation with supplemental oxygen or mechanical ventilation (see Appendix III); (2) vital sign monitoring and electrolyte and laboratory analysis; (3) the placement of lines, including venous and Foley catheters and a nasogastric tube (see Appendix IV); (4) fluid resuscitation; and (5) the use of analgesia (see Appendix VI).

Inhalation Injury and Carbon Monoxide Poisoning. The inhalation of smoke, gases, or poisons, which may be related to burn injuries, can cause asphyxia, direct cellular injury, or both. Inhalation injury varies depending on the inhalant. There is no strict definition of inhalation injury. Inhalation injury is suspected if the patient was exposed to noxious inhalants, especially in an enclosed space, or if the patient has one or more of the following: (1) altered mental status; (2) burns on the face, neck, or upper chest; (3) laryngeal edema; (4) arterial blood gas levels consistent with hypoxia; (5) abnormal breath sounds; (6) the presence of soot in sputum; or (7) positive blood test results for chemicals.

The pathophysiology of inhalation injury generally occurs in three stages: (1) inhalation injury (0–36 hours after injury), (2) pulmonary edema (6–72 hours after injury), and (3) bronchopneumonia (3–10 days after injury). The oropharynx and tracheobronchial tree are usually damaged by thermal injury, whereas the lung parenchyma is damaged by the chemical effects of the inhalant. There are edema formation throughout the airways and de-epithelialization, exudate formation, and fibrin production in the distal airways. There is an elaborate activity of histamine, serotonin, leukocytes, and other cells, which are recruited to the lung. This mechanism is not yet fully understood. Decreased lung compliance and hypoxia are the primary effects of inhalation injury. The degree of these effects depends on the location and severity of the injury. Supplemental oxygen, elective intubation, bronchoscopy, bronchodilators, and fluid resuscitation are initiated to maximize gas exchange and reverse hypoxia [12–14].

The inhalation of carbon monoxide (CO), which is a colorless, odorless, tasteless, combustible, nonirritating gas produced by the incomplete combustion of organic material, results in asphyxia. CO molecules displace oxygen molecules from hemoglobin and shift the oxyhemoglobin curve to the left, thereby decreasing the release of oxygen. Additionally, CO molecules increase pulmonary secretions and decrease the effectiveness of the mucociliary elevator [15].

Burn Care in the Resuscitative Phase
During the first 72 hours after a burn injury, medical management consists of fluid resuscitation, infection control, body temperature maintenance, and pain and anxiety management. Further care of the burn involves the following:

- Burn source neutralization, including removal of clothing and jewelry and lavage (for a chemical burn)

- Determination of the extent and depth of the burn, including the presence of secondary injuries

- Infection control, including aseptic conditions, topical antibiotics, dressings for burn coverage, and tetanus prophylaxis

- Hypothermia prevention

Initial Burn Care. Initially a burn is debrided, cleaned, and dressed with the hospital's or burn unit's antimicrobial agent of choice. Topical antimicrobial agents attempt to prevent or minimize bacterial growth in a burn and expedite eschar separation. There are a variety of antimicrobial agents, each with its own application, advantages, and disadvantages. Chapter Appendix 7-A lists the most common antimicrobial agents available. The physician determines whether to cover the burn or leave it open and estimates the time frame for burn repair, the need for surgical intervention, or both.

Fluid Resuscitation. After a burn, fluid shifts from vascular to interstitial and intracellular spaces. In burns of more than 20% TBSA, this fluid shift becomes massive and requires immediate fluid repletion [10]. This fluid shift, referred to as *burn shock*, is a life-threatening condition. Plasma, sodium-rich solutions, and other fluids are infused over a 48-hour period according to a standard formula derived from individual TBSA and body weight. The formula used varies according to hospital preference.

After fluid administration, the patient is monitored closely for adequacy of fluid resuscitation. Heart rate, blood pressure, urine output, urine glucose level, and bowel sounds provide valuable information about the effectiveness of fluid resuscitation.

Infection Control. Prevention of infection at the burn site(s) is crucial in both the resuscitative and reparative phases of burn care. The patient with a major burn is considered immunocompromised because of the loss of skin and the inability to keep microorganisms from entering the body. Infection control is achieved by the following [10]:

- Observation of the patient for signs and symptoms of sepsis (see Chapter 10, "Pathophysiology")

- Minimization of the presence of microorganisms in the patient's internal and external environment

- Use of aseptic techniques in all interactions with the patient

- Use of topical antimicrobial agents or antibiotics as needed

Body Temperature Maintenance. The patient with a major burn injury is at risk for hypothermia from skin loss and the inability to thermoregulate. Body heat is lost through conduction to the surrounding atmosphere and to the surface of the bed. Initially, dry dressings may be placed on the patient to minimize heat loss. Once stabilized, the patient should be placed in a warm atmosphere to maintain body temperature.

Pain Management. A patient with a burn injury can experience pain as a result of any of the following:

- Free nerve ending exposure to air currents, potassium, substance P, and prostanoids

- Edema

- Exudate accumulation [15]

- Burn debridement and dressing changes

- Mobility

Patients may also experience fear from the injury and burn treatment, which can exacerbate pain. Analgesia, given intravenously, is therefore started as soon as possible (see Appendix VI).

Reparative Phase

The reparative phase consists of further burn healing, surgical and non-surgical burn management, pain control, skilled mobilization with physical and occupational therapies, and nutritional and psychosocial support. It is beyond the scope of this chapter to discuss the nutritional and psychosocial management of patients with burn injuries. It must be emphasized that each hospital or burn team can have a unique method or professional approach to burn care.

Burn Management in the Reparative Phase

Tissue healing at burn sites occurs according to the depth of the burn and is described in "The Process of Wound Healing." After the healing process, a scar forms (see "Factors That Can Delay Wound Healing" for a discussion of factors that can slow the process of burn healing). A burn scar may be *normotrophic,* with a normal appearance from the dermal collagen fibers that are arranged in an organized parallel formation, or *hypertrophic,* with an abnormal appearance as a result of the disorganized formation of dermal collagen fibers [16]. A full-thickness burn is unable to initiate repair secondary to dermal destruction before grafting [10]. Burn management can be divided into two major categories: the surgical management of burns and burn cleansing and debridement. It is beyond the scope of this chapter to discuss in detail the indications, advantages, and disadvantages of specific surgical interventions that facilitate burn closure. Instead, surgical procedures related to burn care are defined below.

Surgical Procedures. The cornerstone of present surgical burn management is early burn excision and grafting. *Excision* is the surgical removal of eschar and exposure of viable tissue to minimize infection and promote burn closure. Early burn closure minimizes infection, the incidence of multisystem organ failure, and morbidity. Table 7-5 describes the different types of excision and grafting.

Surgical excision and grafting are completed at any site if patient survival will improve. They are otherwise performed to maximize functional outcome and cosmesis, with the hands, arms, face, feet, and joint surfaces grafted before other areas of the body [17].

Grafts, which typically adhere in 2–5 days, may not adhere or "take" in the presence of any of the following [17]:

- An incomplete eschar excision
- Movement of the graft on the recipient site
- A septic recipient site
- A hematoma at the graft site

Clinical tip

To promote grafting success, restrictions to movement of a specific joint or entire limb may be present postoperatively.

Table 7-5. Types of Excision and Grafting

Procedure	Description
Tangential excision	Removal of eschar in successive layers down to the dermis
Full-thickness excision	Removal of eschar as a single layer down to the subcutaneous tissue
Autograft	Surgical harvesting of a patient's own skin from another part of the body (donor site) and placing it permanently on the burn (recipient site)
Split-thickness skin graft	Autograft consisting of epidermis and a portion of dermis
Full-thickness skin graft	Autograft consisting of epidermis and the entire dermis
Mesh graft	Autograft placed through a mesher (a machine that expands the size of the graft usually 3–4 times) before being placed on the recipient site
Sheet graft	Autograft placed on the recipient site as a single piece without meshing
Cultured epidermal autograft	Autograft of unburned epidermal cells cultured in the laboratory
Composite skin graft	Autograft of unburned epidermal and dermal cells cultured in the laboratory
Allogenic graft	Autograft of unburned epidermal cells and cadaver skin cultured in the laboratory
Homograft	Temporary graft from cadaver skin
Heterograft (xenograft)	Temporary graft from another animal species, typically of porcine skin
Amnion graft	Temporary graft from placental membrane

Source: Data from SF Miller, MJ Staley, RL Richard. Surgical Management of the Burn Patient. In RL Richard, MJ Staley (eds), Burn Care and Rehabilitation: Principles and Practice. Philadelphia: FA Davis, 1994.

The therapist should become familiar with the surgeon's procedures and protocols and alter range of motion (ROM), therapeutic exercise, and functional mobility accordingly. The therapist should check with the physician to determine if the graft crosses a joint, to determine how close the graft borders the joint, or to observe the graft during dressing changes.

Nonsurgical Procedures

Burn cleansing and debridement may be performed many times a day to minimize infection and promote tissue healing. These procedures may be performed by a physician, nurse, or physical therapist depending on the hospital's or burn unit's protocol. See "Wound Cleansing and Debridement" and "Dressings and Topical Agents" for a discussion of these aspects of burn care.

Physical Therapy Intervention in Burn Care

History

In addition to the general chart review (see Appendix I), the following questions are especially relevant in the evaluation, treatment planning, and understanding of the psychological status of a patient with a burn.

- How, when, where, and why did the burn occur?

- Did the patient get thrown (as in an explosion) or fall during the burn incident?

- Is there an inhalation injury or carbon monoxide poisoning?

- What are the secondary injuries?

- What is the extent and depth of the burn?

- Does the patient have a condition(s) that might impair tissue healing?

- Was the burn self-inflicted? If so, is there a history of self-injury or suicide?

- Were friends or family members also injured?

Inspection

To assist with treatment planning, pertinent data that can be gathered from the observation of a patient include the following:

- Level of consciousness

- The presence of agitation, pain, and stress

- Location of the burn, including the proximity of the burn to a joint
- Presence and location of dressings
- Presence and location of edema
- Posture
- Position of head, trunk, and extremities
- Respiratory rate and pattern

Clinical tip

To minimize the risk of infection, the physical therapist must use a sterile technique according to the burn unit procedures when entering a patient's room or approaching the patient's bedside. The physical therapist should take the time to familiarize himself or herself with the institution's policies regarding the use and disposal of protective barriers such as gloves, gowns, and masks.

Pain Assessment

Good pain control increases patient participation and activity tolerance; therefore, pain assessment occurs daily. For the conscious patient, the physical therapist should note the presence, quality, and grade of (1) resting pain; (2) pain with passive, active assisted, or active ROM; (3) pain at the burn site versus the donor site; and (4) pain before, during, and after physical therapy intervention.

Clinical tip

- The physical therapist should become familiar with the patient's pain medication schedule and arrange for physical therapy treatment when pain medication is most effective and the patient is as comfortable as possible.

- Restlessness and vital sign monitoring (i.e., heart rate, blood pressure, and respiratory rate increases) may be the best indicator of pain in sedated or unconscious patients who cannot verbally report pain.

Range of Motion

ROM of the involved joints typically requires goniometric measurements. Exact goniometric values can be difficult to measure when the patient has bulky dressings; therefore, some estimation of ROM may be necessary. The uninvolved joints or extremities can be grossly addressed either actively or passively, depending on the patient's level of alertness or level of participation.

Clinical tip

• The physical therapist should be aware of the presence of tendon damage before ROM assessment. ROM should not be performed on joints with exposed tendons.

• The physical therapist should always have a good view of the extremity during ROM exercise to observe for banding or areas of tissue that appear white when stretched.

• The physical therapist should pay attention to the position of adjacent joints when measuring ROM to account for any length-tension deficits of healing skin or muscle.

• The physical therapist should appreciate the fact that a major burn injury is usually characterized by burns of different depths and types. The physical therapist must be aware of the various qualities of combination burns when performing ROM or functional activities.

Strength

Strength on the uninvolved side is usually assessed grossly by function. More formal strength testing, such as resisted isometrics or manual muscle testing, is indicated on either the involved or uninvolved side if there is severe edema, electrical injury, or suspected secondary injury [18].

Girth

Circumferential girth may be measured in the involved extremity to monitor edema formation. Edema may be severe enough (and in conjunction with constrictive eschar) to cause compartment syndrome. Distal pulses can become decreased. If that happens, an escharotomy or fasciotomy is performed to avoid loss of the limb. An *escharotomy* is the surgical incision through eschar on the trunk or extremities (while at the bedside or in the operating room) that allows deeper tissues to expand and improve tissue perfusion distal to the eschar. A *fasciotomy* is an incision through fascia of an extremity that allows all tissues within the fascia to decompress.

Functional Mobility

Functional mobility is the ability to perform bed mobility, transfers, ambulation, and activities of daily living. Functional mobility may be limited depending on state of illness, medication, need for warm or sterile environment, and pain. The physical therapist should evaluate functional mobility, as much as possible, according to medical stability and precautions.

Goals

The primary goal of physical therapy intervention for patients with burn injuries is to maximize function with ROM exercise, stretching, positioning, and functional activity. The specific methods of accomplishing this goal have not been discussed because the emphasis of this chapter is to enhance understanding of medical-surgical aspects of burn care.

Pathophysiology of Wounds

The different types of wounds, their etiologies, and the factors that contribute to or delay wound healing are discussed in the following sections.

Types of Wounds

Trauma Wounds

A trauma wound is an injury caused by an external force, such as a laceration from broken glass or a knife or penetration from a bullet.

Surgical Wounds

A surgical wound is the residual skin defect after a surgical incision. For individuals who do not have problems healing, these wounds are sutured or stapled, and they heal without special intervention. When complications such as infection, arterial insufficiency, diabetes, or venous insufficiency are present, however, surgical wound healing can be delayed and require additional care.

Arterial Insufficiency Wounds

A wound resulting from arterial insufficiency is secondary to ischemia of the tissue, which causes irreversible damage. This type of ulceration is frequently caused by atherosclerosis, which obstructs blood supply to the tissue. These wounds, described in Table 7-6, are most commonly seen in the lower leg because of a lack of collateral circulation to this area. Clinically, arterial ulcers are frequently seen in the pretibial areas and the dorsum of the toes and feet [19, 20].

Venous Insufficiency Wounds

Although a wound resulting from venous insufficiency is caused by the improper functioning of the venous system, which causes poor nutrition to the tissues, the exact mechanism by which this occurs has not been established. These wounds, described in Table 7-6, are frequently present on the medial malleolus [19–21].

Pressure Wounds

A pressure ulcer is caused by ischemia that develops as a result of pressure on the tissue. The pressure usually originates from weight bearing on a bony prominence, causing internal ischemia at the point of pressure that continues to necrotize externally until a wound is created at the skin surface. By this time, there is significant internal tissue damage. All bed- or chair-bound individuals or any individuals who have an impaired ability to reposition themselves and weight shift are at risk of developing pressure ulcers.

There are three elements to be considered when discussing pressure wounds: (1) the amount of force, (2) the duration of force, and (3) the direction of the force. A minimal amount of force for a long period of time can cause damage equal to a large amount of force for a short period of time [19, 20, 22, 23].

Neuropathic Ulcers

A neuropathic ulcer is the secondary result of peripheral neuropathy that may result in decreased sensation or structural changes due to muscular atrophies. Individuals who have decreased sensation may not be aware of trauma, shearing forces, excessive pressure, or warm temperatures, which can cause ulcers. Structural changes in the foot such as "hammer toes" or excessive pronation or supination can also create pressure points that lead to ischemia and a subsequent ulcer [24, 25].

Table 7-6. Clinical Indicators of Insufficiency Wounds and Diabetic Ulcers

Type of Insufficiency Wound	Clinical Indicator
Arterial insufficiency	Intermittent claudication
	Extreme pain
	Decreased pain with rest
	Frequently in pretibial areas or dorsum of toes or feet
	Decreased or absent pedal pulses
	Decreased temperature
	Distinct, well-defined wound edges
	Increased pain with elevation
	Cyanosis
	Deep wound bed
Venous insufficiency	Localized limb pain
	Pain with deep pressure or palpation
	Pain increased with standing, relieved with elevation
	Increased temperature around the wound or ulcer
	Edema around the wound or ulcer
	Frequently located over medial malleolus
	Indistinct, irregular wound edges
	Substantial drainage
	Shallow wound bed
	Pedal pulses present
Diabetic neuropathic ulcer	Occurs in high-pressure areas (heels, metatarsal heads)
	Shiny skin on distal extremity
	Ulcer painless, but lower-extremity pain present
	Deep wound bed
	Decreased temperature in distal extremity
	Pedal pulses absent

The Process of Wound Healing

Epidermal wounds heal by re-epithelialization. Within 24–48 hours after an injury, new epithelial cells proliferate and mature. Deeper wounds, which involve the dermal tissues and even muscle, go through a rather complex and lengthy sequence of (1) inflammatory response, (2) fibroplastic phase, and (3) remodeling phase [19, 20].

In the inflammatory phase, platelets aggregate and clots form. Leukocytes, followed by macrophages, migrate to the area, and phagocytosis begins. Macrophages also provide amino acids and sugars, which are needed for wound repair. In preparing the wound for healing, they stimulate the fibroplastic phase. During the fibroplastic phase, granulation begins. Granulation is indicative of capillary buds growing into the wound bed. Concurrently, fibrocytes and other undifferentiated cells multiply and migrate to the area. These cells network to transform into fibroblasts, which begin to secrete strands of collagen, forming immature pink scar tissue. In the remodeling phase, scar tissue matures. New scar tissue is characterized by its pink color, as it is composed of white collagen fibers and a large number of capillaries. The amount of time the entire healing process takes depends on the size and type of wound. It may take from 3 days to several months for complete closure to occur.

Factors That Can Delay Wound Healing

With deep or large wounds or a critically ill state, wound healing can be delayed by age, lifestyle, nutrition, cognitive and self-care ability, vascular status, medical complications, and medications [10, 19, 21, 24].

Age
The patient's risk of delayed healing increases with age, especially when complicating factors exist, such as diabetes, peripheral neuropathies, and related vascular problems. Diabetic amputations as a result of nonhealing wounds and diabetic ulcers are reported to increase with advancing age, indicating that difficulty with healing increases with age.

Lifestyle
The patient's occupation and hobbies can indicate how many hours are spent on his or her feet and what kind of elements he or she is exposed to. Smoking delays wound healing because nicotine constricts blood vessels, and in a patient with an already compromised vascular system, continued use of tobacco can exponentially increase further health risk and significantly impede healing.

Nutrition
Generally poor nutrition decreases the body's ability to heal. Inadequate diet control in diabetic patients exacerbates all symptoms of diabetes, including impaired circulation and sensation and delayed healing.

Cognition and Self-Care Ability

If an individual or caregiver does not have the cognitive ability to properly care for wounds, there is an increased risk of infection and other complications. The home situation has a great influence on discharge planning, including determining the level of care and type of dressing.

Vascular Status

In addition to arterial and venous insufficiency and pressure as causes of ischemia and wound development, edema can also result in decreased circulation. These alterations in vascular status also delay healing of an existing wound.

Medical Complications

Compromised health generally causes a decrease in the body's ability to progress through the healing process. A history of cancer, chemotherapy, radiation, or acquired immunodeficiency syndrome or other immunodeficiency disorders causes an increased risk of infection. Cardiac problems such as congestive heart failure, hypertension, renal problems, and preexisting infection also slow wound healing.

Medications

Steroids, antihistamines, nonsteroidal anti-inflammatory drugs, and oral contraceptives may delay wound healing, as can chemotherapy and radiation. Anticoagulants indicate a need for the patient and health care providers to diligently monitor bleeding during dressing removal and debridement.

Wound Assessment and Acute Care Management of Wounds

The assessment of a patient with a skin wound includes history and wound evaluation, as well as a general functional mobility, ROM, and strength assessment.

History

In addition to the general chart review (see Appendix I), the following questions are especially relevant for determining wound etiology and risk factors, a treatment plan, and outcome [19, 21, 24]:

- How and when did the wound occur?

- What has been done for the wound thus far?

- Is there a history of previous wounds? If so, what was the etiology, intervention, and time frame of healing?

- Does the patient have risk factors for delayed healing?

- Does the patient have a medical condition that increases his or her risk of infection or immunodeficiency?

- Does the patient have a medical condition that causes altered sensation?

- Does the patient take medications that can delay wound healing?

- Does the patient take an anticoagulant?

- What is the patient's occupation or hobby?

A review of vascular tests, radiographic studies, and tissue biopsy results lends valuable information about the integrity of the vascular and orthopedic systems and the presence of underlying disease.

Wound Inspection and Evaluation

Wound observation and measurements objectively record a baseline status of the wound and determine the best intervention to facilitate wound healing.

Clinical tip

The location of the wound should be documented in relation to anatomic landmarks. Multiple wounds can be documented relative to each other if the wounds are numbered—for example, Wound #1: Left lower extremity, 3 cm proximal to the medial malleolus. Wound #2: 2 cm proximal to Wound #1.

Size, Depth, and Orientation

Wound length, width, and depth, as well as the presence of undermining (tunneling), are essential measurements in wound assessment. Length typically refers to the distance from the top to the bottom of the wound, whereas width usually refers to the distance across the wound. The orientation of the wound must be determined to ensure consistent length and width measurements, particularly for a wound with an abstract shape or odd location. One method of determining wound orientation is to consider the wound in terms of a clock, with the patient's head being 12 o'clock. When documenting length, the measurement is the distance of the wound (measured in the direction of the patient's head to toe), and the width is the lateral measurement. There are many means of measuring wounds. A calibrated grid on an acetate sheet on which the wound can be traced is optimal, especially for irregularly shaped wounds.

Depth can be measured by placing a sterile cotton tip applicator perpendicular to the wound bed. The applicator is then grasped or marked at the point of the wound edge and measured. If the wound has varying depths, this measurement is repeated.

Undermining or *tunneling* describes a continuation of the wound underneath intact skin and is assessed by taking a sterile cotton tip applicator and placing it underneath the skin parallel to the wound bed and grasping or marking the applicator at the point of the wound edge. Assessment of undermining should be done all around the wound. It can be documented using the clock orientation (e.g., undermining: 2 cm at 12 o'clock, 5 cm at 4 o'clock).

Clinical tip

To ensure consistency and accuracy in wound assessments, a consistent unit of measure should be used among all individuals measuring the wound. Centimeters are more universally used in the literature than inches.

Color

The color of the wound should be documented because it is an indicator of the general condition and vascularity of the wound. Different colors have different meanings, as listed in Table 7-4. Pink indicates recently epithelized tissue. Red indicates healing, possibly granulating tissue. Yellow indicates infection, necrotic material being sloughed off from the wound, or both. Black indicates eschar, frequently thick and resilient. It is important to document the percentage of each color in the wound bed—an increase in the amount of pink and red tissue, a decrease in the amount of yellow and black tissue, or both are indicative of progress. An increase in the amount of black (necrotic) tissue is indicative of regression.

Drainage

Wound drainage is described by type, amount, and odor. Drainage can be (1) serous (clear, thin; this drainage may be present in a healthy, healing wound), (2) serosanguineous (containing blood; this drainage may also be present in a healthy, healing wound), (3) purulent (thick, white, pus-like; this drainage may be indicative of infection and should be cultured), or (4) green (usually indicative of *Pseudomonas* infection and should also be cultured). The amount of drainage is also important because a large amount of drainage can indicate infection. Conversely, a reduction in the amount of drainage can indicate that an infection is resolving. The amount of drainage can be documented as absent, minimal, moderate, or large. The presence and degree of odor can be documented as absent, mild, or foul.

Despite a lack of better objective measurements of drainage, it is still important to document drainage because an increase in the amount of wound drainage could indicate a new infection, or a change in drainage from thick and white to clear can indicate improvement.

Wound Culture

A culture is a sampling of microorganisms from the wound bed that is subsequently grown in a nutrient medium and assessed as to the type and number of organisms present. By determining the type of organisms present, the appropriate antibiotic can be prescribed. A wound culture is indicated if there are clinical signs of infection such as purulent drainage, large amounts of drainage, increased local or systemic temperature, inflammation, or foul odor. All wounds are contaminated, which does not necessarily mean they are infected. Cultures may be performed by a physical therapist, nurse, or physician, depending on the protocol of the institution. The results of aerobic and nonaerobic cultures determine the type of microorganism in the wound and the antibiotic needed [26].

Clinical tip

Cultures should be taken after debridement of thick eschar and necrotic material and cleansing of the wound; otherwise, the culture will reflect the growth of the microorganisms of the external wound environment rather than the internal environment.

Assessing Surrounding Areas

The area surrounding the wound should also be assessed. Statements should be made about skin color, which can indicate the vascularity of the area. Other indications of the status of the skin, such as the absence of hair, shiny or flaky skin, the presence of reddened or darkened areas, the presence of edema, or changes in the nails, can all indicate vascular abnormalities. Increased localized temperature can indicate local infection; decreased temperature can indicate decreased blood supply.

Wound Stage and Classification

Superficial wounds involve only the epidermis. Partial-thickness wounds further involve the superficial layers of the dermis; full-thickness wounds may continue through to muscle and bone. Pressure ulcers have a unique classification system because of their unique characteristic of developing from "inside out." Pressure ulcers are traditionally described by a four-stage system [22]:

Stage I is characterized by a reddened area on the skin on which the epidermis is still intact.

Stage II is a wound similar to a blister or abrasion on which the dermis is exposed.

Stage III is characterized by a wound that exposes subcutaneous tissue down to, but not through, underlying fascia.

Stage IV is characterized by a wound that exposes muscle, bone, or other supporting structures, such as a tendon or joint capsule.

Physical Therapy Intervention in Wound Care

The responsibility and autonomy of the physical therapist in the treatment of wounds varies greatly among facilities. The physical therapist can and should play a key role in the patient's clinical course and the initiation of wound healing. Unless the wound is superficial and caused by trauma, wound closure does not occur during the acute care phase. The ultimate long-term goal of complete wound closure, which may occur over many months, occurs at a different level of care, usually outpatient or home care.

The following are the primary goals of physical therapy for wound treatment in the acute care setting:

- The promotion of wound healing through wound and dressing assessment and cleansing and debridement
- Patient and family education for wound care and prevention of further breakdown and future wounds
- Recommendations and referrals for follow-up care

To fulfill these responsibilities, the therapist must consider all information gathered during the evaluation process to set appropriate goals and time frames. The etiology of the wound, risk factors, and other data guide the therapist toward the proper method of treatment. Objective, measurable, and functional goals are as important in wound care as in any other aspect of physical therapy.

Wound Cleansing and Debridement
It is beyond the scope of this chapter to discuss in detail the method of wound cleansing and debridement. Instead, general descriptions and indications of each are provided.

Wound Cleansing
Wound cleansing is not synonymous with wound debridement or wound decontamination. The purpose of cleansing a wound is to remove loosely attached cellular debris and bacteria from the wound bed. Use of sterile saline, with pressure such as that created with a spray bottle or pulsed lavage if needed, is sufficient for cleansing [20]. Many cleansing agents currently used are actually cytotoxic to living tissues— they destroy cells and actually delay healing. The goal of cleansing should always be kept in mind and aggressive agents used only if necessary. Cleansing should be discontinued when the majority of a wound bed is granulating or when re-epithelialization is occurring. Hydrotherapy, although commonly and perhaps even habitually used, is not always indicated for wound cleansing. Actually, the use of whirlpool jets is mechanical debridement and therefore should be used only if mechanical debridement is indicated. In terms of whirlpool additives for cleansing, again, creating a normal saline solution is the most neutral and least damaging to viable tissue. In infected wounds that have foul odors, copious amounts of drainage, and a great deal of exudate and necrotic tissue, more aggressive additives such as bleach or chlorazene may be used.

Wound Debridement

Debridement has three primary purposes. The first is to remove necrotic tissue or foreign matter from the wound bed. The presence of this tissue prevents re-epithelialization and can split the wound open, which prevents contraction and closure. The second purpose is to prevent infection. The necrotic tissue itself can be the source of the pathogenic organisms. Additionally, debridement of the slough and eschar increases the effectiveness of topical agents. The third purpose is to correct abnormal wound repair.

There are two types of debridement: selective and nonselective. Selective debridement removes nonviable tissue only (such as with sharp or autolytic debridement). Nonselective debridement removes both viable and nonviable tissues (such as mechanical or enzymatic debridement) [20].

Selective Debridement

Sharp Debridement. Sharp debridement involves the use of scalpels, scissors, and forceps to remove necrotic tissue. It is a highly skilled technique best done under the direct supervision of or by an experienced clinician. Sharp debridement is especially expedient in the removal of large amounts of thick, leathery eschar or in the patient with immunocompromise, as the underside of eschar can provide a medium for bacterial growth. Because the true selectivity of sharp debridement depends on the skill of the clinician, sharp debridement can result in damage to healthy tissues that can cause bleeding and a risk of infection. Sharp debridement can be painful; it is therefore recommended that pain medications or topical analgesics be administered before treatment. When debriding, the clinician should spare as much tissue as possible and be careful to have the technique remain selective by not removing viable tissue. Because of the potential for excessive bleeding, extra care should be taken with patients who are taking anticoagulants.

Autolytic Debridement. Autolytic debridement is the natural form of debridement. The body uses its own enzymes to lyse necrotic tissue. It is painless and does not harm healthy tissues. Moist dressings facilitate autolytic debridement, as do films, hydrocolloids, and calcium alginates. Autolytic debridement is the most selective form of debridement. It is a normal process and may be used for any wound; however, because it will take some time for the necrotic material to be removed, sharp debridement of eschar first is recommended. Because of the risk of infection, autolytic debridement is contraindicated as the primary method of debridement in patients who are immunosuppressed or otherwise require quick elimination of necrotic material.

Nonselective Debridement
Nonselective debridement is indicated in severely necrotic wounds with minimal to no healthy tissue. It is contraindicated in clean wounds that have granulating and epithelializing tissues.

Mechanical Debridement. Mechanical debridement involves agitating the necrotic tissue of the wound. Gauze dressings, scrubbing, whirlpool, and irrigation are all examples of mechanical debridement.

Enzymatic Debridement. Enzymatic debridement is achieved through the topical application of enzymes that lyse collagen, fibrin, and elastin. Different enzymatic debriding agents are effective with each of these tissues. Wounds with heavy black eschar are best debrided by proteinases and fibrolytic enzymes (e.g., Elase). Collagenases are used when necrotic collagen, which generally appears yellowish, is present. Santyl is an example of a collagenase. All of these agents are indicated on stage III and IV wounds with yellow and black necrotic material. The use of these agents should be discontinued as soon as the wound is clean, as they can also be damaging to viable tissue. Because it takes a long time for these agents to work, if sharp debridement can be used first to remove tissue, followed by the use of agents for the removal of residual necrotic tissue, it is recommended.

Dressings and Topical Agents

When applying dressings, the therapist should always follow universal precautions and use a clean technique to prevent cross contamination. When choosing a dressing for a wound, four factors related to the wound itself should be considered: (1) the color of the wound, (2) the amount of drainage, (3) the wound depth, and (4) the surrounding skin. Other significant factors include the patient's cognitive and physical ability to apply the dressing and the accessibility of physical therapy or nursing services to the patient. Cost is also frequently a consideration. Table 7-7 is a summary of the advantages and disadvantages of different dressings [19, 20, 25, 27].

A large number of wound care products are available, and it is virtually impossible to be aware of application instructions and purpose of every available dressing. It is the responsibility of the therapist to read manufacturer's instructions for application, to know the purpose of the dressing, and to make educated decisions when choosing the appropriate dressing for a given wound at each stage of the healing process. Clin-

Table 7-7. Advantages and Disadvantages of Wound Dressings

Dressing	Advantages	Disadvantages
Wet-to-wet gauze	Allows for moist wound healing Causes less tissue disruption Mechanical debridement	Can cause skin maceration Frequent changes required Can cause some tissue disruption
Wet-to-dry gauze	Allows for moist wound healing Mechanical debridement	Can cause skin maceration Can cause tissue disruption
Dry gauze	Mechanical debridement	Can cause tissue disruption No moist environment
Vaseline gauze	Causes less tissue disruption Nontoxic Nonirritating	Can cause some tissue disruption
Transparent and occlusive dressings	Protective Autolytic debridement Allow for moist wound healing Require less frequent changes	Can adhere to wound Nonporous, which may facilitate bacterial growth
Hydrogels	Absorbent Mechanical debridement	Difficult to retain in place Expensive Can cause skin maceration
Hydrocolloids	Autolytic debridement Moist environment Cost effective	Can cause increased odor May be difficult to remove Unable to see wound
Calcium alginates	Absorbent Can be used in sinuses	Frequent dressing changes necessary
Foams	Thermal insulation	Expensive

icians should not rely on manufacturer's claims of efficacy to justify a dressing's effectiveness. Although it is not possible to identify every dressing, it is possible to catalog most dressings into some basic categories.

Gauze

Gauze is usually readily available and cost effective. Gauze may be applied dry, wet-to-dry, or wet-to-wet (i.e., the absorbent layer is also wet). Gauze can be used for mechanical debridement, but it should be remembered that viable tissue may be damaged in gauze removal. Gauze removal can be painful. As a highly permeable dressing, gauze is also permeable to bacteria. Frequent dressing changes are usually necessary, because the absorbency level of gauze is limited.

Nonadherent Dressings

Nonadherent dressings may be nonimpregnated or impregnated. Nonadherent dressings may be used when surrounding skin is fragile, as they are less likely to adhere to the wound. A nonimpregnated, nonadherent dressing contains inert materials that conform to the wound surface and have a low to medium absorption rate. They may be used as a contact layer for minor lacerations and abrasions or as a secondary dressing for deep full-thickness wounds. An example of a nonimpregnated dressing is Telfa pads. An impregnated dressing has a nonadhering substance such as Vaseline integrated into the dressing. These nonadherent dressings are indicated for partial- to full-thickness wounds.

Hydrocolloids

Hydrocolloids are wafers that contain absorptive particles that interact with moisture, such as wound exudate, to form a gelatinous mass. They are impermeable to water, oxygen, and bacteria and absorb minimal to moderate amounts of drainage. They adhere with body heat and are easy to apply in difficult areas because they mold well. Because they are impermeable, they can prevent secondary wound infection. They are especially indicated for ischial wounds and other wounds at risk to exposure to urine and stool. They promote autolysis and provide a moist wound environment. Hydrocolloids can be used for acute and chronic wounds, both partial and full thickness. They are indicated with granular or partially necrotic wounds. Because hydrocolloid dressings absorb moisture, they are not indicated for wounds with dry eschar because it takes longer to create the fluid environment needed for leukocyte migration. They can be used for moderately draining wounds when combined with absorptive granules, powders, or pastes. They are not, however, indicated for heavily exudating wounds. Because these dressings are impermeable to oxygen, they are not recommended in the presence of anaerobic infections in the wound.

These dressings are changed every 3–7 days or as needed due to leakage or wrinkling. Because these dressings need to be changed infrequently, they may be indicated for patients with the appropriate types of wounds who also have difficulty changing dressings. They may also be indicated for outpatients who may have several days between visits.

Clinical tip

When applying hydrocolloids, it is important for the therapist to dry the skin surrounding the wound and to remember that the dressing should be approximately 1.5–2.0 in. larger than the wound to allow for adherence to the skin.

Semipermeable Films

Semipermeable films are constructed from transparent polyurethane and coated on one side with a water-resistant adhesive. They are highly conforming and allow for visual wound monitoring. The films are semipermeable to water and oxygen but are impermeable to bacteria and are minimally absorbent. They trap exudate and provide a moist wound environment, which facilitates autolytic debridement. Semipermeable films are not indicated for moderate or greater exudating wounds. They can be difficult to apply because they are thin and highly adhesive. The therapist must take care with application to fragile skin, as removal can cause skin tears. They are applied in a manner similar to that of hydrocolloids.

Hydrogels

Hydrogels are composed of 96% water or glycerin. They are transparent and highly conformable and maintain a clean, moist wound surface. If properly applied, hydrogels require no adhesion. These dressings also facilitate autolysis and are indicated for light to moderate absorption. The amount of absorption varies with the nature of the absorptive fluid. Most of these dressings are permeable to oxygen. Hydrogels are indicated for partial-thickness wounds and are especially good for patients with skin breakdown and very fragile skin. They can also be used on full-thickness wounds and to keep the wound surface moist and clean in conjunction with other dressings. Application depends on the individual product. Individual product application instructions should be followed by the therapist.

Foams

Foams are composed of polyurethane. They are hydrophilic on the wound surface and hydrophobic on the outer surface; thus, they repel water, urine, stool, and other environmental contaminants. They are permeable to oxygen, which reduces the risk of anaerobic infection. If used properly, foam dressings are nonadherent and highly conformable. They are capable of filling wound cavities. Foams are indicated for partial- and full-thickness wounds with small to moderate amounts of exudate. They are not indicated for wounds with dry eschar.

To apply foams, the ulcer should be cleaned and the surrounding skin should be patted dry. Skin sealant, which can be applied to intact skin around the wound, is recommended. The foam should be cut with at least a 1-in. border and then secured with an elastic bandage, tape, or a transparent adhesive dressing.

Calcium Alginates

Calcium alginates include powders, pastes, and beads that absorb several times their weight. They are therefore indicated for highly draining wounds. Calcium alginates can be used in combination with other dressings. They convert into a viscous hydrophilic gel after contact with exudate. The dressings are highly conformable and can fill deep, uneven wounds. They provide a moist wound environment and facilitate autolysis. These dressings can be used with both partial- and full-thickness wounds.

References

1. Williams WG, Phillips LG. Pathophysiology of the Burn Wound. In DN Herndon (ed), Total Burn Care. London: Saunders, 1996;63.
2. Falkel JE. Anatomy and Physiology of the Skin. In RI Richard, MJ Staley (eds), Burn Care Rehabilitation Principles and Practice. Philadelphia: FA Davis, 1994;10.
3. Totora GJ, Grabowski SR. Principles of Anatomy and Physiology (7th ed). New York: Harper-Collins College, 1989;126.
4. Johnson C. Pathologic Manifestations of Burn Injury. In RI Richard, MJ Staley (eds), Burn Care and Rehabilitation Principles and Practice. Philadelphia: FA Davis, 1994;29.
5. High-Tension Electrical Burns. In RH Demling, C LaLonde, Burn Trauma. New York: Thieme, 1989;223.
6. Lightning. In RH Demling, C LaLonde, Burn Trauma. New York: Thieme, 1989;242.
7. Milner SM, Rylah LTA, Nguyen TT, et al. Chemical Injury. In DN Herndon (ed), Total Burn Care. London: Saunders, 1996;424.

8. Milner SM, Nguyen TT, Herndon DN, Rylah LTA. Radiation Injuries and Mass Casualties. In DN Herndon (ed), Total Burn Care. London: Saunders, 1996;425.

9. McManus WF, Pruitt BA. Thermal Injuries. In DV Feliciano, EE Moore, KL Mattox (eds), Trauma. Stamford, CT: Appleton & Lange, 1996;937.

10. Marvin J. Thermal Injuries. In VD Cardona, PD Hurn, PJ Bastnagel Mason, et al. (eds), Trauma Nursing: From Resuscitation Through Rehabilitation (2nd ed). Philadelphia: Saunders, 1994;736.

11. Wardrope J, Smith JA. The Management of Wounds and Burns. New York: Oxford University Press, 1992;202.

12. Desai MH, Herndon DN. Burns. In DD Trunkey, FR Lewis, BC Decker (eds), Current Therapy of Trauma (3rd ed). Philadelphia: Mosby–Year Book, 1991;315.

13. Abraham E. Toxic Gas and Inhalation Injury. In BE Brenner (ed), Comprehensive Management of Respiratory Emergencies. Rockville, MD: Aspen Publications, 1995;241.

14. Traber DL, Herndon DN. Pathophysiology of Smoke Inhalation. In EF Haponik, AM Munster (eds), Respiratory Injury: Smoke Inhalation and Burns. New York: McGraw-Hill, 1990;61.

15. Crapo RO. Causes of Respiratory Injury. In EF Haponik, AM Munster (eds), Respiratory Injury: Smoke Inhalation and Burns. New York: McGraw-Hill, 1990;47.

16. Linares HA. Pathophysiology of Burn Scar. In DN Herndon (ed), Total Burn Care. London: Saunders, 1996;383.

17. Miller SF, Staley MJ, Richard RL. Surgical Management of the Burn Patient. In RL Richard, MJ Staley (eds), Burn Care and Rehabilitation Principles and Practice. Philadelphia: FA Davis, 1994;177.

18. Richard RL, Staley MJ. Burn Patient Evaluation and Treatment Planning. In RL Richard, MJ Staley (eds), Burn Care and Rehabilitation Principles and Practice. Philadelphia: FA Davis, 1994;201.

19. Gogia PP. Clinical Wound Management. Thorofare, NJ: Slack, 1995.

20. Kloth LC. Miller KH. Wound Healing: Alternatives in Management. Philadelphia: FA Davis, 1990.

21. Burton CS. Venous ulcers. Am J Surg 1994;1:37.

22. The National Pressure Ulcer Advisory Panel's Summary of the AHCPR Clinical Practice Guideline: Pressure Ulcers in Adults: Prediction and Prevention (AHCPR Publication No. 92-0047). Rockville, MD. May 1992.

23. Leigh, IH. Pressure ulcers: prevalence, etiology, and treatment modalities, a review. Am J Surg 1994;1:25.

24. Laing P. Diabetic foot ulcers. Am J Surg 1994,1:31.

25. Levin ML, O'Neal LW, Bowker JH. The Diabetic Foot (5th ed). St. Louis: Mosby, 1993.

26. Thompson PD, Smith DJ. What is infection? Am J Surg 1994,1:7.

27. Lawrence JC. Dressings and wound infection. Am J Surg 1994,1:21.

Appendix 7-A:
Topical Agents for Burn
and Wound Care

Agent[a,b]	Uses	Advantages	Disadvantages	Comments[c]
Creams				
Silver sulfadiazine (Silvadene, SSD, Thermazene) 1% cream	Partial- and full-thickness burns Infected burns Donor sites	Wide antibacterial spectrum, including *Pseudomonas* Comfortable and easy to apply Deeply penetrating Moderate absorbency Softens eschar	Sulfa allergy (transient) Leukopenia seen, especially in patients with major burns Regular cleansing and debridement essential	Introduced in 1968 as an antipseudomonal agent, it is the most widely used topical agent in America and is probably the agent of choice for treating most large and deep burns.
Mafenide acetate (Sulfamylon) 0.5% cream	Deep or infected injuries As an alternative to sulfadiazine	Very wide antibacterial spectrum, including *Pseudomonas* and yeast Penetrates deeply into eschar	Sulfa allergy Carbonic anhydrase inhibitor causes hyperventilation Painful following application Mafenide acetate also available as solution for wet dressings	It is a powerful and effective alternative to sulfadiazine. Its use on large areas should be monitored.
Nitrofurazone (Furacin cream and impregnated gauze) 0.2% compound	Routine treatment of partial- and full-thickness burns Can be used as	Wide antibacterial spectrum, but less effective against *Pseudomonas* Comfortable	Hypersensitivity Dermatitis Superinfection and development of resistant organisms	It is a widely used product for routine burn care. It is less effective for complicated (very deep or infected) wounds.

	dry dressing for grafts and donor sites	Soothing	Less effective against yeast	
Nystatin (Mycostatin, Nilstat) 100,000 units/g	Burn wounds, grafts, or donor sites colonized with yeast Can be combined with other topicals for mixed infections	Activity restricted to yeast, especially *Candida* Also available as ointment	Infrequent hypersensitivity	It is a good product for yeast infections. It is also available as an ointment or powder for soaks.
Ointments				
Gentamicin (Garamycin) 0.1% Ointment	Smaller partial- and full-thickness burns General ointment for donor sites and skin grafts	Effective against gram-negatives, some *Pseudomonas*, most staphylococci, and streptococci	Hypersensitivity Nephrotoxic in large volumes Resistance common with prolonged use Ineffective against yeast	Its use is probably best restricted to small and superficial burns. Routine use can promote the emergence of resistant strains.
Bacitracin ointment, 50 U/g (plus neomycin, 0.5% and polymyxin B, 5,000 U/g)	Partial- and full-thickness burns Outpatient burns Healing wounds Donor sites	Effective against gram-positive organisms Soothing and comfortable	Hypersensitivity, rashes Not a powerful antibiotic Superinfection with yeast Ineffective for gram-negative bacteria	It is a good general burn ointment. Prolonged use, especially on healed skin, can lead to rash or skin breakdown. It is available as a solution for soaks.

Agent[a,b]	Uses	Advantages	Disadvantages	Comments[c]
				A variety of formulations are available.
Povidone iodine ointment (Betadine)	Partial- and full-thickness burns Some skin grafts	Wide-spectrum antiseptic	Dermatitis Tends to harden eschar Metabolic acidosis reported Retards healing	Contraindicated for large injuries because of systemic toxicity.
Enzymes (Santyl, Elase)	Enzymatic debridement of deep partial- and full-thickness burns	Speeds eschar removal Prepares wound for grafting without excision (in theory)	Liquefies eschar, producing a film that must be cleansed and debrided Possible problematic bleeding Infections hard to detect Painful on application	It is a controversial substance with a unique action. Advocates claim that the "chemical excision" is quick and preserves tissue. Critics claim that normal tissue may be damaged. Graft adherence is poor, and infections are frequent.
Solutions				
Silver nitrate 0.5% solution	Wet dressings for partial- and full-thickness burns Applied as soaks	Wide spectrum of antibiotic activity Less effective against *Pseudomonas* or yeast	Painful on application Stains wounds, dressings, and bedding dark brown Hypotonic solution that	It is an "old-fashioned" burn dressing, which has been largely replaced by more powerful creams (e.g., sulfadiazine,

	Use	Activity/Advantages	Disadvantages	Comments
	to gauze dressings at 2- to 3-hr intervals. Poor penetration limits use in large burns		"leaches" sodium and chloride	mafenide). Electrolyte problems result from prolonged use, especially on large burns. It is not available commercially and must be made by a pharmacy.
Acetic acid 0.5% solution	Fresh grafts or infected wounds	Excellent activity against *Pseudomonas*		It is an effective antipseudomonal. It is probably best restricted to small wounds.
Sodium hypochlorite (Dakins solution)	Dilute chlorine bleach for soaking fresh grafts. Infected wounds	General bactericidal. Cleans and dries infected wounds	Acidosis results from prolonged use on large wounds. Not effective against all organisms	It is probably best used on small wounds.
Mafenide acetate 0.5% solution	See Creams, above, for a general description		Painful following application. Can cause bleeding. Acidosis. Must be made in hospital	Mafenide soaks are very effective in treating infected burns, contaminated grafts, and for "wet-to-moist" dressings for untidy wounds. Mafenide solution is not available commercially

Agent[a,b]	Uses	Advantages	Disadvantages	Comments[c]
				and must be made by the hospital pharmacy from powder.
				It can be combined with Nystatin powder for use in mixed fungal infections.
Bacitracin/ neomycin/ polymyxin	See Ointments, above, for a general description			It is formulated as a triple antibiotic solution.
				This is excellent as a soak for fresh grafts and in wet-to-moist dressings for infected wounds.
				It must be prepared by the hospital pharmacy.
				It can be combined with Nystatin powder in mixed fungal infections.

[a]This table is restricted to antibiotic agents that are used commonly in burn treatment (agents used primarily for moisturizing are not included). Liquid formulations (mafenide acetate, silver nitrate, acetic acid) are not available commercially.

[b]Agents are listed by their proper name, the commonly used brand name, and their usual formulation.

[c]Comments reflect the opinions of the authors, particularly with regard to the relative usefulness of various agents.

Source: Reprinted with permission from RI Richard, MJ Staley. Burn Care and Rehabilitation: Principles and Practice. Philadelphia: FA Davis, 1994;172.

8

Gastrointestinal System

Jaime C. Paz

Introduction

Disorders of the gastrointestinal (GI) system account for the majority of hospitalizations in the United States [1]. GI system disorders may affect nutrition and activity tolerance, which in turn may influence physical therapy interventions. In addition, physical therapists must be aware of pain referral patterns from the GI system that may mimic musculoskeletal symptoms (Table 8-1). The objectives of this chapter are to provide the following:

1. A basic understanding of the structure and function of the GI system

2. Information on the clinical assessment of the GI system, including physical examination and diagnostic studies

3. A basic understanding of the various diseases and disorders of the GI system

4. Information on the management of GI disorders, including pharmacologic therapy and surgical procedures

5. Guidelines for physical therapy intervention in patients with GI diseases and disorders

Table 8-1. Gastrointestinal System Pain Referral Patterns

Structures	Segmental Innervation	Areas of Pain Referral
Esophagus	T4–6	Substernal region Upper abdomen
Stomach	T6–10	Upper abdomen Middle and lower thoracic spine
Small intestine	T7–10	Middle thoracic spine
Pancreas	T6–10	Upper abdomen Lower thoracic spine Upper thoracic spine
Gallbladder	T7–9	Right upper abdomen Right, middle, and lower thoracic spine
Liver	T7–9	Right middle and lower thoracic spine Right cervical spine
Common bile duct	T6–10	Upper abdomen Middle thoracic spine
Large intestine	T11–L1	Lower abdomen Middle lumbar spine
Sigmoid colon	T11–12	Upper sacral region Suprapubic region Left lower quadrant of abdomen

Source: Reprinted with permission from WG Boissonnault, C Bass. Pathological origins of trunk and neck pain: part I. Pelvic and abdominal visceral disorders. J Orthop Sports Phys Ther 1990;12:194.

Structure and Function

The basic structure of the GI system is shown in Figure 8-1, with the primary and accessory organs of digestion and their respective functions described in Tables 8-2 and 8-3.

Clinical Assessment

Assessment of the GI system involves combining information gathered through physical examination and diagnostic studies.

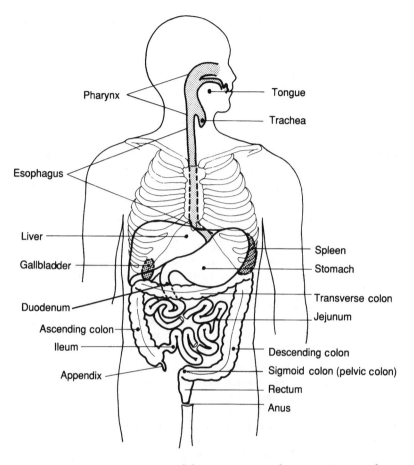

Figure 8-1. *Anatomic overview of the gastrointestinal system. (Reprinted with permission from MB Koopmeiners. Screening for Gastrointestinal System Disease. In WG Boissonnault [ed], Examination in Physical Therapy Practice. New York: Churchill Livingstone, 1991;106.)*

Physical Examination

Physical examination of the abdomen consists of inspection, auscultation, percussion, and palpation. Physicians and nurses usually perform this examination on a daily basis in the acute care setting; however, physical therapists can also perform this examination to help delineate between systemic and musculoskeletal pain. Before performing the

Table 8-2. The Structure and Function of the Primary Organs of Digestion

Structure	Function
Oral cavity (mouth, buccal cavity)	The oral cavity is the entrance to the gastrointestinal system, where mechanical and chemical digestion begins.
Pharynx	The pharynx is involved in swallowing and mechanical movement of food.
Esophagus	The esophagus connects the mouth to the stomach and transports and disperses food. The lower esophageal sphincter prevents the backflow of food.
Stomach (fundus, body, pylorus)	Mechanical functions of the stomach include storage, mixing and grinding of food, and regulation of outflow to small intestine. Exocrine functions of the stomach include secretion of acid, intrinsic factor, pepsin, mucus, and bicarbonate necessary for digestion. Endocrine functions of the stomach include secretion of hormones that trigger the release of digestive enzymes from the pancreas, liver, and gallbladder into the duodenum.
Small intestine (duodenum, jejunum, ileum)	The duodenum neutralizes acid in food transported from the stomach and mixes pancreatic and biliary secretions with food. The jejunum absorbs nutrients, water, and electrolytes. The ileum absorbs bile acids and intrinsic factors to be recycled in the body (which is necessary to prevent vitamin B_{12} deficiency).
Large intestine (cecum; appendix; ascending, transverse, descending, and sigmoid colon; rectum; anus)	The large intestine absorbs water and electrolytes. It also stores and eliminates indigestible material as feces.

Source: Data from JC Scanlon, T Sanders. Essentials of Anatomy and Physiology (2nd ed). Philadelphia: FA Davis, 1993;362.

Table 8-3. Structure and Function of the Accessory Organs of Digestion

Structure	Function
Teeth	The teeth break down food to combine with saliva.
Tongue	The tongue provides sensory innervation by CN VII (taste) and motor innervation by CN XII. It also keeps food between teeth to maintain efficient chewing action for food to mix with saliva.
Salivary glands (parotid, submandibular, sublingual)	Salivary glands produce saliva, which dissolves food for tasting and moistens food for swallowing.
Liver	The liver regulates serum levels of fats, proteins, and carbohydrates. Bile is produced in the liver and is necessary for the absorption of lipids and lipid-soluble substances. The liver also assists with drug metabolism and red blood cell and vitamin K production.
Gallbladder	The gallbladder is located beneath the liver. It stores and releases bile into the duodenum via the hepatic duct when food enters the stomach.
Pancreas	Exocrine portion secretes bicarbonate and digestive enzymes into duodenum. Endocrine portion secretes insulin, glucagon, and numerous other hormones, all of which are essential in regulating blood glucose levels.
Spleen*	The spleen filters out foreign substances and degenerated blood cells from the bloodstream.

CN = cranial nerve.
*The spleen is not part of gastrointestinal system but is located near other gastrointestinal components in the abdominal cavity.
Source: Data from JC Scanlon, T Sanders. Essentials of Anatomy and Physiology (2nd ed). Philadelphia: FA Davis, 1993.

examination, the presence or absence of items related to GI pathology are ascertained through patient interview, questionnaire completion, or chart review. For a list of these items, see Table 8-4. Appendix I also describes the general medical record review.

Table 8-4. Items Associated with Gastrointestinal Pathology

Signs and symptoms
  Nausea
  Vomiting
  Hemoptysis
  Constipation
  Diarrhea
  Jaundice

Urine and stool characteristics
  Change in urine color
  Change in stool color
  Hematochezia (bright red blood in stool)
  Melena (black tarry stools)

Associated disorders
  History of hepatitis
  History of hernia
  Drug and alcohol abuse
  Fatty food intolerance

Source: Adapted from MB Koopmeiners. Screening for Gastrointestinal System Disease. In WG Boissonnault (ed), Examination in Physical Therapy Practice. New York: Churchill Livingstone, 1991;113.

Inspection

Figure 8-2 demonstrates the abdominal regions associated with organ location. During inspection the physical therapist should note asymmetries in size and shape in each quadrant, umbilicus appearance, and the presence of abdominal scars indicative of previous abdominal procedures or trauma. The presence of incisions, tubes, and drains should also be noted during inspection because these may require particular handling or placement during mobility exercises [2].

Clinical tip

Changes in abdominal girth, especially enlargement, should be documented by the physical therapist. In addition, the nurses and physicians should be notified. Abdominal enlargement may hinder the patient's respiratory and mobility status.

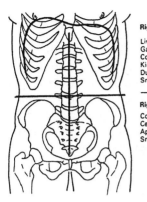

Right upper	Left upper
Liver	Stomach
Gallbladder	Spleen
Colon (hepatic flexure and transverse)	Pancreas
Kidney and adrenal gland	Kidney and adrenal gland
Duodenum with head of pancreas	Colon (splenic flexure and transverse)
Small intestine	Small intestine (jejunum)
Right lower	**Left lower**
Colon (ascending)	Colon (descending)
Cecum	Sigmoid colon
Appendix	
Small intestine	Small intestine

Figure 8-2. *The four abdominal quadrants showing the viscera found in each. (Reprinted with permission from N Palastanga, D Field, R Soames. Anatomy and Human Movement: Structure and Function [2nd ed]. Oxford: Butterworth–Heinemann, 1989;783.)*

Auscultation

The abdomen is auscultated for the presence or absence of bowel sounds and bruits (murmurs) to help evaluate gastric motility and vascular flow, respectively. Bowel sounds can be altered postoperatively, as well as in cases of diarrhea, intestinal obstruction, paralytic ileus, and peritonitis. The presence of bruits may be indicative of renal artery stenosis [2].

Percussion

Mediate percussion is used to evaluate liver and spleen size and borders as well as to identify ascitic fluid, solid, or fluid-filled masses and air in the stomach and bowel [2]. The technique for mediate percussion is described in the physical examination section of Chapter 2.

Palpation

Light palpation and deep palpation are used to identify abdominal tenderness, muscular resistance, and superficial organs and masses. The presence of rebound tenderness (i.e., abdominal pain worsened by a quick release of palpatory pressure) is an indication of peritoneal irritation from possible abdominal hemorrhage and requires immediate medical attention. Muscle guarding during palpation may also indicate a protective mechanism for underlying visceral pathology [2].

Diagnostic Studies

Evaluation of the GI system by laboratory studies can be subdivided into (1) direct evaluation of contents of the GI system, (2) contrast radiography, (3) computed tomography scan, and (4) ultrasonography (Tables 8-5 through 8-8). Other diagnostic procedures used to evaluate the GI system are radionuclide imaging, laparoscopy, magnetic resonance imaging, positron emission tomography (PET) scans, and liver function tests (LFTs). These methods are described below.

Radionuclide Imaging

Radionuclide imaging involves injecting a radionuclide into the circulation and performing a series of imaging scans to evaluate areas of increased or decreased uptake. Imaging of the liver or spleen is performed to screen patients for the presence of hepatic metastases, cirrhosis, and hepatitis. Lesions, such as tumors, cysts, abscesses, splenic

Table 8-5. Direct Evaluation of Gastrointestinal System

Test	Description
Esophageal acidity test (pH monitoring)	Esophageal acidity test evaluates competency of lower esophageal sphincter by measuring intraesophageal pH. It also indicates gastric reflux. Normal esophageal pH is 6.0 or more.
Esophageal acid perfusion test (Bernstein test)	The acid perfusion test evaluates esophageal mucosa, esophagitis, and gastric reflux by dripping acidic and neutral solutions into a nasogastric tube. Test differentiates between esophageal and cardiac chest pain.
Esophageal manometry	Esophageal manometry measures upper and lower esophageal sphincter pressure for presence of achalasia, diffuse esophageal spasm, and esophageal scleroderma. Normal baseline pressure is 20 mm Hg. Normal relaxation pressure is 18 mm Hg.
Basal gastric secretion test (gastric analysis)	Basal gastric secretion test measures basal secretions under fasting conditions by aspirating stomach contents through a nasogastric tube. It is indicated for anorexia, weight loss, and epigastric pain.

Test	Description
	Normal values are 0.2–3.8 mEq/hr for women, and 1–5 mEq/hr for men.
Gastric acid stimulation test	The gastric acid stimulation test follows the basal gastric secretion test.
	Pentagastrin is given to stimulate gastric acid output and is used to help diagnose duodenal ulcers, Zollinger-Ellison syndrome, gastric carcinoma, and pernicious anemia.
	Normal values are 11–21 mEq/hr for women and 18–28 mEq/hr for men.
Peritoneal fluid analysis	Peritoneal fluid is sampled through paracentesis to determine composition of ascitic fluid to help diagnose abdominal trauma.
Fecal occult blood test	Three separate stool specimens are collected to detect gastrointestinal bleeding and to screen for colorectal cancer.
Fecal fat	Stool specimens are collected and examined for excessive presence of lipids indicative of malabsorption syndromes.
Fecal urobilinogen	Stool specimens are collected and examined for bilirubin and urobilinogen levels in order to help detect hepatobiliary and hemolytic disorders.
Esophagogastroduodenoscopy	Direct visual examination of the esophagus, stomach, and upper duodenum is performed to help diagnose inflammatory disease, ulcers, tumors, structural abnormality, and Mallory-Weiss tears.
Colonoscopy	Colon and rectum are examined to diagnose inflammatory bowel diseases, including ulcerative colitis and granulomatous colitis. Sources of gastrointestinal bleeding, biopsies, and polyp removal may also be performed.
Proctosigmoidoscopy	Proctosigmoidoscopy is the examination of the sigmoid colon, rectum, and anal canal to visualize mucosa and perform biopsies.

Source: Adapted from DC Broadwell. Gastrointestinal System. In JM Thompson, JE Hirsch, GK MacFarland, et al. (eds), Clinical Nursing Practice. St. Louis: Mosby, 1986;1141.

Table 8-6. Contrast Radiographic Evaluation of the Gastrointestinal System

Test	Description
Barium swallow	Barium swallow is a fluoroscopic examination of esophagus and pharynx after ingestion of barium sulfate. It is indicated to diagnose or detect hiatal hernia, achalasia, diverticulum, varices, strictures, ulcers, tumors, motility disorders, polyps, and surgical site integrity.
Upper and lower gastrointestinal series	Fluoroscopic examination of the esophagus, stomach, and small intestine is performed after ingestion of barium sulfate. Upper and lower gastrointestinal series are indicated for detecting or diagnosing hiatal hernias, diverticulum, varices, ulcers, strictures, tumors, regional enteritis, and motility disorders.
Barium enema	Barium sulfate or barium sulfate and air are instilled into the large intestine through the anus as a method to diagnose colorectal cancer and inflammatory bowel disease. Polyps, diverticula, and other colorectal changes may also be detected.
Oral cholecystography	A contrast medium is administered orally the evening before the test, which is followed by radiographic examination of the gallbladder.
Intravenous cholangiography	Radiographic and tomographic studies are performed after intravenous infusion of a contrast medium to provide better visualization of biliary ducts. It is indicated for patients with right upper quadrant pain after cholecystectomy and to evaluate congenital abnormalities of the biliary system in children.
Celiac and mesenteric arteriography	A contrast medium is injected into the celiac, superior mesenteric, or inferior mesenteric artery for radiographic visualization of the vasculature. Sites of gastrointestinal bleeds can be located and treated. Evaluation of cirrhosis, portal hypertension, vascular damage, intestinal ischemia, and tumors can also be performed.

Source: Adapted from DC Broadwell. Gastrointestinal System. In JM Thompson, JE Hirsch, GK MacFarland, et al. (eds), Clinical Nursing Practice. St. Louis: Mosby, 1986;1144.

Table 8-7. Computed Tomography of the Gastrointestinal System

Test	Description
Computed tomography (CT) scan of biliary tract and liver	Multiple uses include (1) identification of focal points found on nuclear scans as solid, cystic, inflammatory, or vascular hematomas after trauma; (2) determination of obstructive or nonobstructive jaundice etiology; (3) defining the relationships of organs; and (4) identifying the presence of tumors.
CT scan of the pancreas	Pancreatic carcinoma and pancreatitis can be diagnosed. It can also distinguish between pancreatic disorders and disorders of the retroperitoneum.

Source: Adapted from DC Broadwell. Gastrointestinal System. In JM Thompson, JE Hirsch, GK MacFarland, et al. (eds), Clinical Nursing Practice. St. Louis: Mosby, 1986;1149.

Table 8-8. Ultrasonographic Evaluation of the Gastrointestinal System

Test	Description
Ultrasonography of the gallbladder and biliary system	Purposes include (1) confirming cholelithiasis, (2) diagnosing acute cholecystitis, and (3) distinguishing between obstructive and nonobstructive jaundice
Ultrasonography of the liver	Purposes include (1) to distinguish between obstructive and nonobstructive jaundice, (2) to screen or diagnose hepatocellular disease and hepatic metastases, and (3) to detect hematoma after abdominal trauma
Ultrasonography of the spleen	Evaluates changes in splenic size and splenic condition after abdominal trauma
Ultrasonography of the pancreas	Detects alterations in size, contour, and parenchymal texture of the pancreas that are found in abnormalities such as pseudocysts or carcinoma

Source: Adapted from DC Broadwell. Gastrointestinal System. In JM Thompson, JE Hirsch, GK MacFarland, et al. (eds), Clinical Nursing Practice. St. Louis: Mosby, 1986;1149.

Table 8-9. Summary of the Uses for Laparoscopy

Indications
    Liver biopsy
    Determination of the etiology of ascites (free fluid in the peritoneal cavity)
    Staging of Hodgkin's disease and non-Hodgkin's lymphoma
    Evaluation of patients with fever of unknown origin
    Evaluation of patients with chronic or intermittent abdominal pain

Contraindications
    Perforated viscus
    Abdominal wall infections
    Diffuse peritonitis
    Clinically significant coagulopathy

Interventions
    Aspiration of cysts and abscesses
    Lysis of adhesions
    Ligation of fallopian tubes
    Ablation of endometriosis or cancer by laser

Surgical procedures
    Cholecystectomy (gallbladder removal)
    Appendectomy
    Inguinal herniorrhaphy (hernia repair)
    Gastrectomy
    Colectomy
    Vagotomy

Source: Data from GL Eastwood, C Avunduk. Manual of Gastroenterology (2nd ed). Boston: Little, Brown, 1994;27.

infarcts can be identified, as well as hepatomegaly and splenomegaly, which indicate organ dysfunction. Liver or spleen imaging scans can also be performed after abdominal trauma [1].

Laparoscopy

Laparoscopy is the insertion of a laparoscope (a fiberoptic tube) into the abdominal cavity through a small incision to the left of and above the umbilicus. To perform this procedure, a local anesthetic is given and gas (i.e., nitric oxide or carbon dioxide) is infused into the abdominal cavity to allow better visualization and manipulation of the scope. Table 8-9 describes the evaluations and treatments that may be performed with a laparoscope [3].

Table 8-10. Liver Function Tests for Specific Diseases

Disease	Clinical Evidence
Primary biliary cirrhosis	The presence of mitochondrial antibody
Autoimmune chronic hepatitis	The presence of smooth muscle antibody
Wilson's disease	Low levels of ceruloplasmin
α_1-Antitrypsin deficiency	Low levels of α_1-antitrypsin
Hemochromatosis	Increased levels of iron, ferritin, and transferrin
Hepatocellular carcinoma	Increased levels of α-fetoprotein
Metastatic liver cancer (primary site of colon or pancreas)	The presence of carcinoembryonic antigen
Biliary obstructions	Reduced or absent urine urobilinogen

Source: Data from B Kapelman. Approach to the Patient with Liver Disease. In DS Sachar, JD Waye, BS Lewis (eds), Pocket Guide to Gastroenterology. Baltimore: Williams & Wilkins, 1991;90.

Magnetic Resonance Imaging

The use of magnetic resonance imaging of the GI system is primarily limited to imaging of the liver for hepatic tumors, iron overload, and hepatic and portal venous occlusion. Computed tomography scans are preferred for the visualization of other abdominal organs [4].

Positron Emission Tomography

PET is the use of positively charged ions to create color images of organs and their functions. Clinical uses of PET for the GI system include evaluation of liver disease, pancreatic function, and GI cancer [4].

Liver Function Tests

Liver function tests is a broad term that refers to a battery of measures that evaluate liver function. Briefly, LFTs include tests for hepatocellular injury and dysfunction, the presence of cholestasis and other related liver diseases, and hepatobiliary pathology. Tests for hepatocellular injury and dysfunction and the presence of cholestasis are described below [5]. Tests for the presence of related liver diseases and hepatobiliary pathology are described in Tables 8-10 and 8-11, respectively.

Hepatocellular injury results in cellular damage in the liver, which causes increased levels of the following enzymes: aspartate amino-

Table 8-11. Liver Function Tests of Hepatobiliary Pathology

Hepatobiliary Pathology	Clinical Evidence
Hepatocyte damage	Reduced levels of serum albumin (produced in liver)
Common bile duct obstruction or pancreatic dysfunction	Increased levels of amylase
Acute hepatic dysfunction	Reduced levels of cholesterol
Prolonged cholestasis	Increased levels of cholesterol
Hemolysis (blood cell damage)	Increased levels of bilirubin
Hepatic encephalopathy	Increased levels of ammonia
Portal hypertension	Low levels of platelets
Macrocytosis	Presence of large blood cells

Source: Data from B Kapelman. Approach to the Patient with Liver Disease. In DS Sachar, JD Waye, BS Lewis (eds), Pocket Guide to Gastroenterology. Baltimore: Williams & Wilkins, 1991;90.

transferase (AST) (previously called serum glutamic-oxaloacetic transaminase [SGOT]), alanine aminotransferase (ALT) (previously called serum glutamate pyruvate transaminase [SGPT]), and lactate dehydrogenase (LDH) [5].

Hepatocellular dysfunction can be identified when bilirubin levels are elevated or when clotting times are increased (denoted by an increased prothrombin time [PT]). The liver produces all coagulation factors except factor VIII, and therefore an increased PT implicates impaired production of coagulation factors.

Cholestasis is the impairment of bile flow from the liver to the duodenum that results in elevations of the following serum enzymes: alkaline phosphatase (AP), aspartate transaminase (previously known as γ-glutamine-oxaloacetic transaminase (GOT), or γ-glutamyl transpeptidase (GGTP), and 5'-nucleotidase [5].

Pathophysiology

GI disorders can be classified regionally by the structure involved and may consist of the following:

- Motility disorders

- Inflammation or hemorrhage

- Enzymatic dysfunction

- Neoplasms

Esophageal Disorders

Dysphagia

Dysphagia, or difficulty swallowing, can be classified as proximal (cervical), distal, multifactorial, or dysphagia lusoria (which is rare). Dysphagia should be characterized by (1) whether it occurs with ingestion of solids, liquids, or both; (2) whether it is accompanied by chest pain or heartburn; and (3) whether it is intermittent, constant, or progressive. The location at which the food becomes stuck should also be noted [6].

Proximal Dysphagia
Proximal dysphagia is difficulty swallowing in the upper, or proximal, region of the esophagus. Proximal dysphagia may result from the following reasons:

- Neurologic or neuromuscular etiology (e.g., stroke, myasthenia gravis, or polymyositis)

- Cricopharyngeal dysfunction

- Cervical osteophytes

- Diffuse idiopathic skeletal hyperostosis

- Thyrotoxicosis

- Transfer dysphagia (difficulty transferring food from the mouth and pharynx to esophagus)

Distal Dysphagia
Distal dysphagia is difficulty swallowing in the lower, or distal, portion of the esophagus. Distal dysphagia is usually the result of mechanical obstruction to flow from peptic strictures, mucosal rings, or neoplasms.

Multifactorial Dysphagia
Multifactorial dysphagia is characterized by fibrosis of smooth muscle in the distal two-thirds of the esophagus that reduces normal peri-

stalsis. Scleroderma, or progressive systemic sclerosis, is generally the cause of this type of dysphagia, which can possibly lead to gastroesophageal (GE) reflux and stricture formation.

Dysphagia Lusoria

Dysphagia lusoria is a congenital condition caused by external compromise of the esophagus by vascular structures, such as an aberrant right subclavian artery. Symptoms may be latent until adulthood.

Motility Disorders and Angina-Like Chest Pain

Poor esophageal motility from spasms or abnormal contraction patterns can present as anterior chest pain and mimic anginal symptoms. Systematic cardiac and GI workup should establish the differential diagnosis. The following are common esophageal motility disorders [7]:

Achalasia is a neuromuscular disorder of esophageal motility characterized by esophageal dilation and hypertrophy, along with failure of the lower esophageal sphincter to relax. A definitive etiology is currently unknown. Suspected causes include autoimmune dysfunction and genetic predisposition [8].

Nutcracker esophagus is characterized by high-amplitude distal esophageal contractions that accompany normal peristalsis [7].

Diffuse esophageal spasm is characterized by the intermittent occurrence of normal peristalsis that is disrupted by nonperistaltic, simultaneous contractions of the esophagus that occur in 10% of all wet swallows [7].

Hypertensive lower esophageal sphincter is characterized by the occurrence of normal peristalsis of the esophagus that is accompanied by increased sphincter pressures on closure and relaxation that is normal [7].

Gastroesophageal Reflux Disease

GE reflux (e.g., heartburn, esophagitis) is characterized by gastric acid backflow into the esophagus as a result of improper lower esophageal sphincter relaxation. Although the exact etiology of GE reflux is unknown, smoking along with the consumption of fats, alcohol, or chocolate have been associated with this inappropriate relaxation. Esophageal and gastric motility disorders may also contribute to GE reflux. Depending on the severity, treatment can range from antacids to surgery [9].

Barrett's Esophagus

Barrett's esophagus is a disorder in which columnar epithelium replaces the normal stratified squamous mucosa of the distal esophagus and is associated with chronic GE reflux. Associated signs and symptoms include dysphagia, esophagitis, ulceration, perforations, strictures, bleeding, or adenocarcinoma. Treatment for Barrett's esophagus ranges from dietary modifications to antacids to surgery [10].

Esophageal Cancer

A description of esophageal cancers with respect to diagnosis and treatments can be found in Chapter 5, "Cancers of the Body Systems."

Esophageal Diverticula, Rings, and Webs

Esophageal diverticula, rings, and webs are anatomic abnormalities that disrupt the normal cylindrical shape of the esophagus and result in an interruption of esophageal motility, leading to dysphagia. Webs and diverticula tend to occur proximally, whereas rings generally occur distally at the GE junction [11].

Infectious Esophagitis

Infection by *Candida* or herpes viruses (herpes simplex, cytomegalovirus) can cause inflammation of the esophagus in chronically debilitated or immunocompromised patients. Infectious esophagitis may be asymptomatic or may present with difficult swallowing (dysphagia), painful swallowing (odynophagia), or both. Treatment is generally aimed at the infectious agent [12].

Esophageal Varices

Varices are dilated blood vessels in the esophagus caused by portal hypertension and may result in hemorrhage that necessitates immediate medical and usually surgical management. Alcohol abuse is an associated risk factor [13].

Stomach Disorders

Upper Gastrointestinal Bleed

GI hemorrhage can result from one or more of the following: (1) duodenal ulcers, (2) gastric erosion, (3) gastric ulcers, and (4) esophageal varices. Eighty percent of GI bleeds are small and require no intervention; 20%

are massive and constitute medical emergencies because of hemodynamic instability, which leads to shock. Dark brown ("coffee ground") emesis or black tarry stools from acid degradation of hemoglobin are the primary clinical manifestations and indications of GI bleeds. Patients are stabilized hemodynamically before the cause of bleeding is searched for. Nasogastric tubes (Appendix IV-B) are mandatory in GI bleeds. Endoscopy is performed to evaluate or treat the source of hemorrhage [14].

Gastritis

Diffuse inflammatory lesions in the mucosal layer of the stomach are classified as acute, chronic erosive, or chronic nonerosive. Etiology of acute gastritis includes associations with aspirin, anti-inflammatory agents, alcohol, and corticosteroid use, along with physiologic stress, intense emotional reactions, and bacterial infections. Treatment includes removal of the irritant(s), fluid replacement, antibiotics, and surgery (if perforations occur). Chronic gastritis is subdivided into erosive and nonerosive. Chronic nonerosive gastritis can further be subdivided into type A (primarily involving the body of the stomach) and type B (involves the antrum of the stomach). Chronic gastritis is managed with antacids, vitamins C and B_{12}, and routine endoscopies to assess formation of gastric polyps, carcinomas, or both [15].

Gastric Ulcer

A well-defined perforation in the gastric mucosa that extends into the muscularis mucosa characterizes ulceration in the stomach. Symptoms may include abdominal pain during or after a meal or at night, nausea with or without vomiting, or both. A strong correlation exists between gastric ulcers and alcohol and aspirin abuse. Management of gastric ulcers may consist of any or all of the following: diet modification, elimination of irritants, anti-inflammatory agents, antacids, and surgery (partial gastrectomy or vagotomy) [16].

Duodenal Ulcer

Duodenal ulcers are more common than gastric ulcers and are defined as a chronic circumscribed break in the mucosa that extends through the muscularis mucosa layer and leaves a residual scar with healing. Duodenal ulcers are linked with gastric acid hypersecretion and genetic predisposition. Consequences are thrombosis, endarteritis, inflammatory changes resulting in avascular scarring, upper GI bleeding, gastric outlet obstruction, perforation, and intractable pain. Management is similar to that of gastric ulcers [17].

Gastric Emptying Disorders

Abnormal gastric emptying is described as either decreased or increased emptying. Decreased gastric emptying is also referred to as *gastric retention* and may result from or be associated with (1) pyloric stenosis as a consequence of duodenal ulcers, (2) hyperglycemia, (3) diabetic ketoacidosis, (4) electrolyte imbalance, (5) autonomic neuropathy, (6) postoperative stasis, and (7) pernicious anemia. Pharmacologic intervention to promote gastric motility is indicated for patients with gastric emptying disorders.

Enhanced gastric emptying is associated with an interruption of normal digestive sequencing that results from vagotomy, gastrectomy or gastric or duodenal ulcers. Gastric peristalsis, mixing, and grinding are disturbed, resulting in rapid emptying of liquids, slow or increased emptying of solids, and prolonged retention of indigestible solids. With enhanced gastric emptying, blood glucose levels are subsequently low and can result in signs and symptoms of anxiety, sweating, intense hunger, dizziness, weakness, and palpitations. Nutritional and pharmacologic management are the usual treatment choices [18].

Zollinger-Ellison Syndrome

Zollinger-Ellison is a clinical triad that includes gastric acid hypersecretion, recurrent peptic ulcerations, and a non-beta islet-cell tumor in the pancreas. Symptoms mimic peptic ulcer disease, but consequences are more severe if left untreated. Management is directed at the gastric acid hypersecretion and tumor with antacids and resection, respectively [19].

Gastric Cancer

The most common malignant neoplasms found in the stomach are adenocarcinomas, which arise from normal or mucosal cells. Benign tumors are rarely found but do include leiomyomas and polyps. For a more detailed discussion of gastric oncology see Chapter 5, "Cancers of the Body Systems."

Intestinal Disorders

Appendicitis

Inflammation of the appendix of the large intestine can be classified as simple, gangrenous, or perforated. Simple appendicitis involves an inflamed but intact appendix. Gangrenous appendicitis is the presence of focal or extensive necrosis accompanied by microscopic perforations. Perforated appendicitis is a gross disruption of the appendix wall [1].

Signs and symptoms of appendicitis include the following:

- Right lower quadrant, epigastric, or periumbilical abdominal pain that fluctuates in intensity
- Vomiting with presence of anorexia
- Constipation and failure to pass flatus
- Low-grade fever (no greater than 102°F or 39°C)
- Shallow and rapid respirations (possibly)

Management of appendicitis involves the use of anti-infective agents or surgical appendectomy [1].

Diverticular Disease

Diverticulosis is an out-pocketing, or herniation, of the mucosa of the large colon through the muscle layers. Diverticulitis is the result of an inflammatory process and localized peritonitis that occurs after the perforation of a single diverticulum [1].

Signs and symptoms of diverticular disease include the following:

- Achy, left lower quadrant pain and tenderness (pain intensifies with acute diverticulitis)
- Pain referred to low back region
- Urinary frequency
- Distended and tympanic abdomen
- Elevated white blood cell count (acute diverticulitis)
- Constipation, bloody stools, or both
- Nausea, vomiting, anorexia

Management of diverticular disease includes any of the following:

- Surgical repair of herniation, resection, or both (possible colostomy)
- Dietary modifications (e.g., increased fiber)

- Insertion of nasogastric tube in cases of severe nausea, vomiting, abdominal distention, or any combination of these

- Laxatives

- Intravenous (IV) fluids

- Pain medications

- Anti-infective agents

Herniation

Muscle weakening from abdominal distention that occurs in obesity, surgery, or ascites can lead to an abnormal protrusion of bowel through the muscle wall, or herniation. Herniation may also develop congenitally [1].

Signs and symptoms of herniation include the following:

- Abdominal distention, nausea, and vomiting

- Observable bulge with position changes, coughing, or laughing

- Pain of increasing severity with fever, tachycardia, and abdominal rigidity (if the herniated bowel is strangulated)

Management of herniation includes any of the following:

- Wearing a binder or corset

- Herniorrhaphy (surgical repair)

- Hernioplasty (surgical reinforcement of weakened area with mesh, wire, or fascia)

- Temporary colostomy in cases of intestinal obstruction

Intestinal Obstructions

Failure of intestinal contents to propel forward can occur by mechanical or functional obstructions. Blockage of the bowel by adhesion, herniation, volvulus (twisting of bowel on itself), tumor, inflammation, impacted feces, or invagination of an adjacent bowel segment constitute mechanical obstructions. Loss of the propulsive activity of the intestines leads to functional obstructions (ileus). Obstructions may result from abdominal surgery, intestinal distention, hypokalemia, peritonitis, severe trauma, spinal fractures, ureteral distention, or use of narcotics [1].

Signs and symptoms of intestinal obstructions include the following:

- Sudden onset of "crampy" abdominal pain that may be intermittent in nature as peristalsis occurs

- Localized tenderness

- Vomiting

- Constipation

- High-pitched or absent bowel sounds (depending on extent of obstruction)

- Tachycardia and hypotension in presence of dehydration or peritonitis

- Bloody stools

Management of intestinal obstructions includes any of the following:

- Insertion of a nasogastric tube

- Supportive management of functional etiologies (as able)

- Surgical resection of mechanical obstructions from adhesions, necrosis, tumor, or unresolved inflammatory lesions

- Colostomy placement and eventual colostomy closure. (Colostomy closure is also referred to as "colostomy takedown.")

Intestinal Ischemia

Intestinal ischemia results from thrombosis or emboli to the superior mesenteric artery, strangulation obstructions, chronic vascular insufficiency, anoxia, or hypotension. All of these factors can lead to an insufficient mesenteric blood supply that may be acute or chronic [1].

Signs and symptoms of intestinal ischemia include the following:

- Abdominal pain varying in severity according to acuity

- Nausea and vomiting

- Diarrhea or rectal bleeding

- Rebound tenderness, abdominal distention, and rigidity (with necrosis)

- Tachycardia, hypotension, and fever (with necrosis)

Management of intestinal ischemia includes any of the following:

- Revascularization procedures, including balloon angioplasty, bypass grafting, embolectomy, and endarterectomy
- Resection of necrotic segments with temporary colostomy or ileostomy placement and subsequent reanastomosis of functional segments as indicated
- Anti-infective agents
- Vasodilators or vasopressors (blood perfusion enhancement)
- Anticoagulation therapy
- IV fluid replacement
- Insertion of nasogastric tube
- Dietary modifications

Irritable Bowel Syndrome
Irritable bowel syndrome is characterized by inconsistent motility of the large bowel (i.e., constipation or diarrhea). Motility of the large bowel can be affected by emotions, food, neurohumoral agents, GI hormones, toxins, prostaglandins, and colon distention. Organic pathologic manifestations are usually nondetectable [1].

Signs and symptoms of irritable bowel syndrome include the following:

- Diffuse abdominal pain
- Constipation or diarrhea
- Correlation of GI symptoms with high emotional states or stress
- No weight loss
- Tender sigmoid colon on palpation

Management of irritable bowel syndrome includes any of the following:

- Laxatives or antidiarrheal agents
- Antispasmodic agents

- Dietary modifications
- Counseling or psychotherapy
- Surgery (in rare cases)

Malabsorption Syndromes

Malabsorption syndromes is a general term for disorders that are characterized by the intestines' failure to absorb or digest carbohydrates, proteins, fats, vitamins, and electrolytes. Malabsorption syndromes can result from any of the following [1]:

- Chronic pancreatitis
- Pancreatic carcinoma
- Crohn's disease (see "Crohn's Disease")
- Celiac sprue (small intestine mucosal damage from glutens [wheat, barley, rye, and oats])
- Amyloidosis (disorder of protein metabolism)
- Lactase deficiency
- Zollinger-Ellison syndrome (see "Zollinger-Ellison Syndrome")
- Postgastrectomy disorders

Signs and symptoms of malabsorption syndromes include the following:

- Diarrhea
- Anorexia and weight loss
- Abdominal bloating
- Bone pain
- Steatorrhea (excessive fat excretion)

Management of malabsorption syndromes includes any of the following:

- Dietary modifications and nutritional support
- Fluid, electrolyte, vitamin, and mineral support

Peritonitis

Peritonitis is general or localized inflammation in the peritoneal cavity as a result of bacterial or chemical contamination. Etiologies can include bacterial infection, ascites, perforation of the GI tract, gangrene of the bowel, trauma, and surgical irritants [1].

Signs and symptoms of peritonitis include the following:

- Abdominal guarding with diffuse tenderness and rigidity
- Abdominal distention
- Diminished or absent bowel sounds
- Nausea, vomiting, or both
- Pain with deep inspirations (therefore shallow and rapid respirations)
- Tachycardia
- Hypotension
- Fever
- Decreased urinary output

Management of peritonitis includes any of the following:

- Surgical correction of primary etiology
- Fluid management with electrolytes and colloids
- Pain management
- Antibiotics
- Nasogastric suctioning
- Invasive monitoring of central hemodynamic pressures

Polyps

GI polyps are usually adenomas that arise from the epithelium above the mucosal surface of the intestine. Polyps are benign in and of themselves but may proliferate to carcinoma of the colon.

Signs and symptoms of polyps include the following [1]:

- Rectal bleeding (occult or overt)

- Constipation or diarrhea

- Lower abdominal crampy pain

Management of polyps includes the following:

- Colonoscopy or proctosigmoidoscopy

- Surgical resection with or without ileostomy

Crohn's Disease

Crohn's disease is a chronic, idiopathic, inflammatory disorder occurring in any part of the GI system. The small intestine, particularly the ileum, is most commonly involved, whereas the esophagus and stomach are rarely affected. Suspected causes of Crohn's disease include genetic predetermination, altered immunologic mechanisms, infectious agents, psychological factors, dietary factors, and environmental factors [1].

Signs and symptoms of Crohn's disease include the following:

- Constant crampy abdominal pain, often in right lower quadrant, not relieved by bowel movement

- Right lower quadrant abdominal mass

- Diarrhea

- Low-grade fever

- Fistula formation

Management of Crohn's disease includes any of the following:

- Surgical resection of involved area, with or without need for ileostomy

- Antibiotics

- Anti-inflammatory medications

- IV fluids and dietary modification and support (possible total parenteral nutrition use)

- Nasogastric suctioning

- Activity limitations (in acute phases)

Complications of Crohn's disease can include the following:

- Arthritis, ankylosing spondylitis
- Inflammation of eyes, skin, and mucous membranes
- Hepatitis, bile duct carcinoma
- Gallstones
- Amyloidosis
- Vitamin B_{12} deficiency
- Obstructive hydronephrosis

Ulcerative Colitis

Ulcerative colitis is a chronic inflammation of the intestine limited to the mucosal layer of the colon and rectum. The definitive etiology of ulcerative colitis is unknown, but suspected causes are similar to those of Crohn's disease. Inflammation can be mild, moderate, or severe [1].

Signs and symptoms of ulcerative colitis include the following:

- Crampy lower abdominal pain that is relieved by a bowel movement
- Small, frequent stools to profuse diarrhea (mild to severe)
- Rectal bleeding
- Fever
- Fatigue with anorexia and weight loss
- Dehydration
- Tachycardia

Management of ulcerative colitis includes any of the following:

- Surgical resection of involved area with probable ileostomy placement
- Dietary modification and support (possible total parenteral nutrition use)
- Anti-inflammatory medications, including steroids
- Activity limitations

- Blood replacement

Related manifestations of ulcerative colitis may include the following:

- Arthritis, ankylosing spondylitis
- Inflammation of the eyes, skin, and mucous membranes
- Hepatitis, bile duct carcinoma

Intestinal Tumors

Benign or metastatic neoplasms of the intestine include colonic adenomas (polyps), villous or papillary adenomas, lipomas, leiomyomas, and lymphoid hyperplasia. Tumors affect motility and absorption functions in the intestine (see Chapter 5, "Cancers of the Body Systems," for further details).

Anorectal Disorders

Disorders of the anus and rectum generally involve inflammation, obstruction, discontinuity from colon, perforations, or tumors. The most common disorders are (1) hemorrhoids, (2) anorectal fistula, (3) anal fissure, (4) imperforate anus, and (5) rectal prolapse. Signs and symptoms include pain with defecation and bloody stools. Management is supportive according to the disorder, and surgical correction is performed as necessary.

Liver And Biliary Disorders

Hepatitis

Hepatic inflammation and hepatic cell necrosis may be acute or chronic and may result from viruses, toxins, alcohol, leukemias, lymphomas, and Wilson's disease (a rare copper metabolism disorder). Viral hepatitis is the most common and can be classified a hepatitis A, B, C, D, or E (i.e., HAV, HBV, HCV, HDV, and HEV, respectively) [10].

Signs and symptoms of hepatitis include the following:

- Abrupt onset of malaise
- Fever

- Anorexia
- Nausea
- Headache
- Abdominal discomfort and pain
- Jaundice
- Itching
- Dark-colored urine

Management of hepatitis includes any of the following:

- Vaccinations
- Fluid and nutritional support
- Removal of precipitating irritants (e.g., alcohol and toxins)
- Anti-inflammatory agents, including corticosteroids
- Antiviral agents

Cirrhosis

Cirrhosis is a disease state that is characterized by hepatic parenchymal cell destruction and necrosis, and regeneration and scar tissue formation. Cirrhosis may result from the following [1]:

- Alcohol or drug abuse
- Viral hepatitis B, C, or D
- Hemochromatosis
- Wilson's disease
- α_1-antitrypsin deficiency
- Biliary obstruction
- Venous outflow obstruction
- Cardiac failure
- Malnutrition
- Cystic fibrosis

- Congenital syphilis

Signs and symptoms of cirrhosis include the following:

- Recent weight loss or gain
- Easily fatigued
- Jaundice
- Ascites
- Lower-extremity edema
- Anorexia, nausea, or vomiting
- Fever
- Decreased urine output (urine dark yellow or amber)
- Associated GI manifestations of esophageal varices, bowel habit changes, and GI bleeding
- Altered mental status

Management of cirrhosis includes the following:

- Supportive care, including IV fluids, blood, colloid (albumin), vitamin and electrolyte replacement, and dietary modifications
- Medical correction, surgical correction, or both of primary etiology or secondary complications as indicated
- Paracentesis
- Supplemental oxygen

Hepatic Encephalopathy and Coma

Acute and chronic liver diseases may lead to neuropsychiatric manifestations that may progress from hepatic encephalopathy to precoma to coma. The majority of neuropsychiatric manifestations are linked to ammonia intoxication from faulty liver metabolism [1].

Signs and symptoms leading to coma may include the following:

- Altered states of consciousness (e.g., lethargy, stupor, confusion, slowed responses)

- Neuromuscular abnormalities (e.g., tremor, dyscoordination, slurred speech, altered reflexes, ataxia, rigidity, Babinski's sign, and impaired handwriting)

- Altered intellectual function (decreased attention span, amnesia, disorientation)

- Altered personality and behavioral changes (euphoria or depression, irritability, anxiety, paranoia, rage)

Management of hepatic encephalopathy and coma may consist of any of the following:

- Correction of electrolyte imbalances

- Supplemental oxygen

- Removal of any precipitating substances

- Gastric lavage or enemas

- Ammonia detoxicants

- Anti-infective agents

- Surgical correction of causal or contributing factors (rare)

Cholecystitis with Cholelithiasis

Cholecystitis is acute or chronic inflammation of the gallbladder. It is associated with obstruction by gallstones in 90% of cases. Gallstone formation (cholelithiasis) is associated with three factors: gallbladder hypomobility, supersaturation of bile with cholesterol, and crystal formation from an increased concentration of insoluble bilirubin in the bile [1].

Signs and symptoms of cholecystitis include the following:

- Severe abdominal pain in right upper quadrant with possible pain referral to right scapula

- Rebound tenderness and abdominal rigidity

- Jaundice

- Anorexia

- Nausea, vomiting, or both

- Fever

Management of cholecystitis includes any of the following:

- Cholecystectomy
- Cholecystostomy (temporary drain placement until obstruction is relieved)
- Gallstone dilution therapy
- Anti-infective agents
- Pain management
- IV fluids
- Insertion of nasogastric tube

Pancreatic Disorders

Pancreatitis

Pancreatitis is an autodigestive process of the pancreas that results from intrapancreatic digestive enzyme activation. The inflammatory response may be acute or chronic. The exact trigger to this process is unknown, but contributing factors are the following [1]:

- Alcohol and drug abuse
- Gallstones
- Trauma
- Endoscopic retrograde cholangiography
- Metabolic disorders
- Vasculitis
- Pancreatic obstruction
- Penetrating peptic ulcer
- Genetic predisposition
- Renal failure
- Hepatitis

- Medications

- Postoperative sequelae from abdominal or cardiothoracic surgery

Signs and symptoms of pancreatitis include the following:

- Steady, dull abdominal pain in the epigastrium, left upper quadrant or periumbilical area often radiating to back, chest, and lower abdomen

- Nausea, vomiting, and abdominal distention

- Fever, tachycardia, and hypotension (in acute cases)

- Jaundice

- Abdominal tenderness or rigidity

- Diminished or absent bowel sounds

- Associated pulmonary manifestations, such as pleural effusions and pneumonitis

- Decreased urine output

- Weight loss

Management of pancreatitis includes any of the following:

- Pain management

- IV fluid replacement

- Nutritional support

- Surgical correction or resection of obstructions

- Antacids

- Nasogastric suctioning

- Supplemental oxygen and mechanical ventilation (as indicated)

- Invasive monitoring (in more severe cases)

Management

General management of GI disorders may consist of any of the following: pharmacologic therapy, nutritional support, dietary modifications, and surgical procedures. Nutritional support and dietary modifications are beyond the scope of this book. This section focuses on pharmacologic therapy and surgical procedures. A discussion of physical therapy intervention is also included.

Pharmacologic Therapy

Medications used to treat GI disorders can be broadly categorized as (1) those that control gastric acid secretion and (2) those that normalize gastric motility (see the Chapter 8 Appendix).

Surgical Procedures

Surgical intervention is indicated in GI disorders when medical intervention is insufficient. The location and extent of incisions depend on the exact procedure. The progress of laparoscopic technology, however, has reduced many postoperative complications from procedures that, at one time, required large abdominal incisions. Postoperative complications may arise from incisional pain, leading to reduced ventilatory and cough ability, as well as bed rest deconditioning (see Appendix V for further descriptions of operative considerations).

The following are the common surgical procedures and their definitions [1]:

Appendectomy	Removal of appendix
Cholecystectomy	Removal of the gallbladder
Colectomy	Resection of a portion of the colon with the name of the section removed being added to the procedure title (e.g., transverse colectomy is resection of the transverse colon.)
Colostomy	A procedure used to divert stool from a portion of the diseased colon. The involved segment is removed or bypassed with a loop or end of the colon being brought through a small opening in the abdominal wall,

forming a stoma. An external, plastic pouch is placed over the stoma in which the patient's stool collects. Patients are instructed on proper care and emptying of their colostomy pouch. This procedure can be performed in the ascending, transverse, and sigmoid portions of the colon, with sigmoid colostomies being the most commonly performed.

Gastrectomy	Removal of a portion (partial) or all (total) of the stomach
Ileostomy	A procedure similar to a colostomy that is performed in areas of the ileum (distal portion of the small intestine). A continent ileostomy is another method of diverting stool; however, instead of draining into an external pouch, a nipple valve that is surgically created allows stool to be drained into more distal and functioning portions of the intestine.
Resection and reanastomosis	The removal (resection) of a nonfunctioning portion of the GI tract and the reconnection (reanastomosis) of proximal and distal GI portions that are functional. The name of the procedure will then include the sections that are resected or reanastomosed—for example, a pancreaticojejunostomy is the joining of the pancreatic duct to the jejunum after a dysfunctional portion of the pancreas is resected [20, 21].
Whipple procedure (pancreatico-duodenectomy)	Consists of "en bloc" removal of the duodenum, a variable portion of the distal stomach and the jejunum, gallbladder, common bile duct, and regional lymph nodes. This removal is followed by pancreaticojejunostomy and gastrojejunostomy. This procedure is indicated for the patient with chronic pancreatitis or pancreatic cancer [20, 21].

Clinical tip

Before any mobility treatment, the physical therapist should ensure that the colostomy pouch is securely closed and adhered to the patient.

Physical Therapy Intervention

The following are general goals and guidelines for the physical therapist when working with the patient who has GI dysfunction. These guidelines should be adapted to a patient's specific needs.

The primary physical therapy goals for this patient population are similar to those of other patients in the acute care setting: (1) To optimize functional mobility, (2) to maximize activity tolerance and endurance, and (3) to prevent postoperative pulmonary complications.

General guidelines include, but are not limited to, the following:

1.   The patient's nutritional status will affect his or her participation and activity tolerance. Consultation with the nutritionist is helpful in gauging the appropriate activity prescription, which is based on the patient's caloric intake. It is difficult to improve the patient's strength or endurance if his or her caloric intake is insufficient for the energy requirements of exercise.

2.   Patients who are status post surgical procedures with pain from abdominal incisions have difficulty performing deep breathing and coughing, performing bed mobility, and standing in a full upright position. Effective pain management before physical therapy intervention, along with diligent position changes, instruction on incisional splinting during deep breathing and coughing, and early mobilization, will help prevent pulmonary complications and deconditioning from developing.

References

1. Broadwell DC. Gastrointestinal System. In JM Thompson, JE Hirsch, GK MacFarland, et al. (eds), Clinical Nursing Practice. St. Louis: Mosby, 1986;1105.

2. Koopmeiners MB. Screening for Gastrointestinal System Disease. In WG Boissonnault (ed), Examination in Physical Therapy Practice. New York: Churchill Livingstone, 1991;105.

3. Laparoscopy and Laparoscopic Surgery. In GL Eastwood, C Avunduk, Manual of Gastroenterology (2nd ed). Boston: Little, Brown, 1994;27.

4. Imaging Studies. In GL Eastwood, C Avunduk, Manual of Gastroenterology (2nd ed). Boston: Little, Brown, 1994;42.

5. Kapelman B. Approach to the Patient with Liver Disease. In DB Sachar, JD Waye, BS Lewis (eds), Pocket Guide to Gastroenterology. Baltimore: Williams & Wilkins, 1991;90.

6. Chobanian SJ. Dysphagia. In MM van Ness, SJ Chobanian (eds), Manual of Clinical Problems in Gastroenterology. Boston: Little, Brown, 1994;3.

7. Castell DO. Esophageal Motility Disorders and Angina. In MM van Ness, SJ Chobanian (eds), Manual of Clinical Problems in Gastroenterology. Boston: Little, Brown, 1994;5.

8. Wong RKH. Achalasia. In MM van Ness, SJ Chobanian (eds), Manual of Clinical Problems in Gastroenterology. Boston: Little, Brown, 1994;10.

9. Richter JE. Gastroesophageal Reflux. In MM van Ness, SJ Chobanian (eds), Manual of Clinical Problems in Gastroenterology. Boston: Little, Brown, 1994;14.

10. Johnson DA. Barrett's Esophagus. In MM van Ness, SJ Chobanian (eds), Manual of Clinical Problems in Gastroenterology. Boston: Little, Brown, 1994;28.

11. Gage TP. Esophageal Rings, Webs and Diverticula. In MM van Ness, SJ Chobanian (eds), Manual of Clinical Problems in Gastroenterology. Boston: Little, Brown, 1994;32.

12. Shay SS, van Ness MM. Infectious Esophagitis. In MM van Ness, SJ Chobanian (eds), Manual of Clinical Problems in Gastroenterology. Boston: Little, Brown, 1994;35.

13. Miller WO, van Ness MM. Esophageal Varices. In MM van Ness, SJ Chobanian (eds), Manual of Clinical Problems in Gastroenterology. Boston: Little, Brown, 1994;195.

14. Jones DM. Upper Gastrointestinal Bleeding. In MM van Ness, SJ Chobanian (eds), Manual of Clinical Problems in Gastroenterology. Boston: Little, Brown, 1994;45.

15. Lawson JM, Johnson DA. Acute and Chronic Gastritis. In MM van Ness, SJ Chobanian (eds), Manual of Clinical Problems in Gastroenterology. Boston: Little, Brown, 1994;48.

16. Lawson JM, Johnson DA. Gastric Ulcer. In MM van Ness, SJ Chobanian (eds), Manual of Clinical Problems in Gastroenterology. Boston: Little, Brown, 1994;51.

17. Humphries TJ. Duodenal Ulcer. In MM van Ness, SJ Chobanian (eds), Manual of Clinical Problems in Gastroenterology. Boston: Little, Brown, 1994;69.

18. Dubois A. Disorders of Gastric Emptying. In MM van Ness, SJ Chobanian (eds), Manual of Clinical Problems in Gastroenterology. Boston: Little, Brown, 1994;57.

19. Collen MJ. Zollinger-Ellison Syndrome. In MM van Ness, SJ Chobanian (eds), Manual of Clinical Problems in Gastroenterology. Boston: Little, Brown, 1994;66.
20. Chronic Pancreatitis. In GL Eastwood, C Avunduk, Manual of Gastroenterology (2nd ed). Boston: Little, Brown, 1994;309.
21. Pancreatic Cancer. In GL Eastwood, C Avunduk, Manual of Gastroenterology (2nd ed). Boston: Little, Brown, 1994;313.

Appendix 8-A:
Gastrointestinal System
Medications

Table 8-A.1. Gastric Acid Medications and Their Side Effects

Type of Medication	Generic Name (Brand Name)	Side Effects
Antacids	Numerous over-the-counter and prescription drugs (e.g., TUMS, Rolaids)	Constipation Diarrhea
H_2-receptor blockers	Cimetidine (Tagamet) Famotidine (Pepcid) Nizatidine (Axid) Ranitidine (Zantac)	Headache Dizziness Mild nausea, diarrhea, or constipation

Source: Data from CD Ciccone. Gastrointestinal Drugs. In CD Ciccone (ed), Pharmacology in Rehabilitation (2nd ed). Philadelphia: FA Davis, 1996;390.

Table 8-A.2. Gastric Motility Medications and Their Side Effects

Type of Medication	Generic Name (Brand Name)	Side Effects
Antidiarrheal	Kaolin (Kaopectate, Kao-Tin) Pectin (Kapectolin) Bismuth salicylate (Pepto-Bismol) Diphenoxylate (Diphenatol, Lomotil) Loperamide (Imodium)	Nausea Abdominal discomfort Constipation Drowsiness, fatigue Dizziness
Laxatives	Methylcellulose (Citrucel, Cologel) Psyllium (Fiberall, Metamucil) Bisacodyl (Dulcolax) Castor oil (Purge) Phenolphthalein (Correctol, Ex-Lax, Feen-A-Mint) Glycerin (Sani-Supp) Lactulose (Chronulac) Magnesium hydroxide (Phillips' Milk of Magnesia) Magnesium sulfate (Epsom salts) Sodium phosphate (Fleet Enema) Docusate (Colace, Disonate) Mineral oil (Agoral, Nujol)	Nausea Cramps Spastic colitis Fluid and electrolyte imbalances Dehydration

Source: Data from CD Ciccone. Gastrointestinal Drugs. In CD Ciccone (ed), Pharmacology in Rehabilitation (2nd ed). Philadelphia: FA Davis, 1996;393.

9

Genitourinary System

Jaime C. Paz

Introduction

The regulation of fluid and electrolyte levels by the genitourinary system is very important in cellular and cardiovascular function. Imbalance of fluids, electrolytes, or both can lead to blood pressure changes or impaired metabolism and can ultimately influence the patient's activity tolerance (see Appendix II). Genitourinary structures can also cause pain that is referred to the abdomen and back. To help differentiate neuromuscular and skeletal dysfunction from systemic dysfunction, physical therapists need to be aware of pain referral patterns from these structures (Table 9-1). The objectives for this chapter are to provide the following:

1. A basic understanding of the structure and function of the genitourinary system

2. Information about the clinical assessment of the genitourinary system, including physical examination and diagnostic studies

3. A basic understanding of the various diseases and disorders of the genitourinary system

4. Information about the management of genitourinary disorders, including dialysis therapy and surgical procedures

Table 9-1. Segmental Innervation and Pain Referral Areas of the Urinary System

Structure	Segmental Innervation	Possible Pain Referral
Kidney	T10–L1	Lumbar spine (ipsilateral flank) Upper abdomen
Ureter	T11–L2, S2–S4	Groin Upper and lower abdomen Suprapubic region Scrotum Medial and proximal thigh Thoracolumbar region
Urinary bladder	T11–L2, S2–S4	Sacral apex Suprapubic region Thoracolumbar region

Source: Reprinted with permission from WG Boissonnault, C Bass. Pathological origins of trunk and neck pain: part I. Pelvic and abdominal visceral disorders. J Orthop Phys Ther 1990;12:194.

5. Guidelines for physical therapy intervention in patients with genitourinary diseases and disorders

Structure and Function

The genitourinary system consists of two kidneys, two ureters, one urinary bladder, and one urethra. The genitourinary system also includes the reproductive organs: the prostate gland, testicles, and epididymis in males and the uterus, fallopian tubes, ovaries, vagina, external genitalia, and perineum in females. Of these reproductive organs, only the prostate gland is discussed in this chapter.

The anatomy of the genitourinary system is shown in Figure 9-1. An expanded, frontal view of the kidney is shown in Figure 9-2. The structural and functional unit of the kidney is called the nephron. The nephron is located in the renal cortex and the medulla and has two parts: a renal corpuscle and a renal tubule. There are approximately 1 million nephrons in each kidney. Urine is formed in the nephron

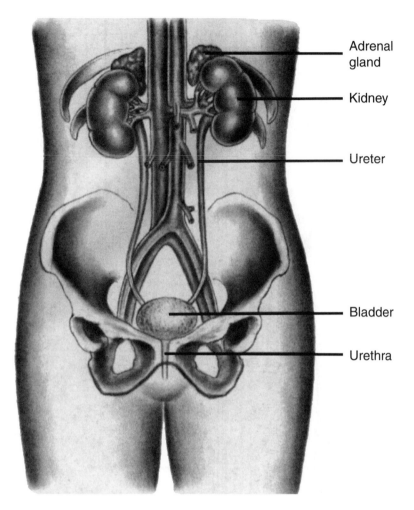

Figure 9-1. *Components of the genitourinary system without reproductive organs shown. (Reprinted with permission from JM Thompson, GK McFarland, JE Hirsch, et al. Mosby's Clinical Nursing [3rd ed]. St. Louis: Mosby–Year Book, 1993;894.)*

through a process consisting of glomerular filtration, tubular reabsorption, and tubular secretion [1].

The following are the primary functions of the genitourinary system [1, 2]:

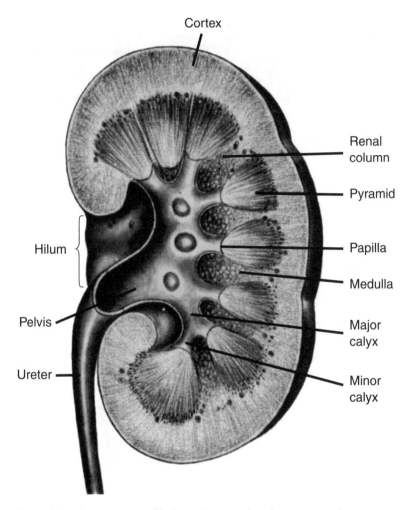

Figure 9-2. *Cross section of kidney. (Reprinted with permission from JM Thompson, GK McFarland, JE Hirsch, et al. Mosby's Clinical Nursing [3rd ed]. St. Louis: Mosby–Year Book, 1993;894.)*

- Excretion of cellular waste products (e.g., urea, creatinine, and ammonia) through urine formation and micturition (voiding)

- Regulation of blood volume by conserving or excreting fluids

- Electrolyte regulation by conserving or excreting minerals

Table 9-2. Urine Abnormalities

Abnormality	Etiology
Glycosuria (presence of glucose)	Elevated blood glucose levels result in glycosuria, which is a sign of diabetes.
Proteinuria (presence of protein)	Proteinuria indicates a kidney disease that allows passage of proteins into the urine. Proteins are usually too large to be filtered; therefore, permeability has abnormally increased.
Hematuria (presence of blood and red blood cells)	Hematuria can indicate urinary tract bleeding or kidney disease that results in increased permeability to red blood cells.
Bacteriuria (presence of bacteria)	Bacteriuria can indicate urinary tract infection. Urine is generally cloudy in appearance, with the possible presence of white blood cells.
Ketonuria (presence of ketones)*	Ketonuria can result from diabetes or a high-protein diet.

*Ketones are formed from protein and fat metabolism, and trace amounts in the urine are normal.
Source: Adapted from VC Scanlon, T Sanders. Essentials of Anatomy and Physiology (2nd ed). Philadelphia: FA Davis, 1995;416.

- Acid-base balance regulation (H^+ [acid] and HCO_3 [base] ions are conserved or excreted to maintain homeostasis)

- Arterial blood pressure regulation (sodium excretion and renin secretion to maintain homeostasis)

- Erythropoietin secretion

- Gluconeogenesis (formation of glucose)

Neural Regulation

The brain stem controls micturition through the autonomic nervous system. Parasympathetic fibers stimulate voiding, whereas sympathetic fibers inhibit it. The internal urethral sphincter of the bladder and the external urethral sphincter of the urethra control flow of urine. Urine abnormalities are summarized in Table 9-2 [2].

Clinical Assessment

Evaluation of the genitourinary system involves the integration of physical findings with laboratory data.

Physical Examination

History

Performing a patient interview; completion of a health questionnaire regarding pain location and behavior and other signs and symptoms (e.g., changes in urinary patterns); or both provide a good screening tool for possible genitourinary system pathology. Renal and urinary pains can vary according to their structural origins; however, they are generally described as pain that is colicky, wavelike, or burning, or occurring as dull aches in the abdomen, back, or buttocks [3].

A description of micturition patterns or changes in voiding habits should also be noted and are listed below [2, 3]:

- Dysuria, which is pain with voiding (can indicate a urinary tract infection)

- Incontinence (an inability to control voiding; can indicate sphincter and autonomic dysfunction)

- Hematuria (can indicate serious pathology or traumatic Foley catheterization [In either case, the physician should be notified.])

- Urinary urgency (can indicate bladder, urethral, or prostate infection)

- Increase in urinary frequency, especially at night (can indicate obstruction from prostate enlargement)

- Decreased force of urinary flow (can indicate obstruction in the urethra or prostate enlargement)

Clinical tip

If the patient has a history of urinary incontinence, a condom catheter (for males) or adult diapers (for males and females) can be applied before mobility treatment to aid in completion of the session.

Observation

The presence of abdominal or pelvic distention, incisions, scars, tubes, drains, and catheters should be noted when performing patient inspection because these may reflect current pathology and recent interventions. The physical therapist must handle external tubes and drains carefully during positioning or functional mobility treatments.

Clinical tip

- Securing tubes and drains with a pin or a clamp to a patient's gown during a mobility session can help prevent accidental displacement.

- Moving tubes and drains out of the way during bed mobility prevents the patient from possibly rolling onto them.

Palpation

The kidneys and a distended bladder are the only palpable structures of the genitourinary system. Distention or inflammation of the kidneys results in sharp or dull pain (depending on severity) with palpation [2].

Diagnostic Tests*

Urinalysis

Urine specimens can be collected by having the patient void into a sterile specimen container, bladder catheterization, or suprapubic aspiration of bladder urine. Urinalysis is performed to assess the following [3]:

- Urine color, clarity, and odor

- Specific gravity, osmolarity, or both (concentration of urine ranges from 300 [dilute] to 1,200 [concentrated] mOsm/kg)

- pH (4.5–8.0)

---

*Normal values may vary according to institutions; therefore, the physical therapist should check the back of the medical record for the facility's normal ranges.

- Presence of glucose, ketones, proteins, and related substances

- Sediment, consisting of cells, crystals, casts, bacteria or other microorganisms, enzymes, and electrolytes

---

Clinical tip

If the patient is having a 24-hour urine catch (to measure hormone and metabolite levels), the physical therapist should have the patient use the predesignated receptacle if the patient needs to urinate during a physical therapy session. This will ensure that the collection is not interrupted.

Creatinine Tests

Two measurements of creatine (a muscle metabolism end product) are performed: measurements of plasma creatinine and creatinine clearance. The normal range of plasma creatinine is 0.7–1.3 mg/dl. Increased levels indicate decreased renal function. The normal range of creatinine clearance is 75–125 ml/min. Creatinine clearance specifically tests glomerular filtration rate. Decreased clearance (indicated by elevated levels) indicates decreased renal function [4].

Blood Urea Nitrogen

As an end product of protein metabolism, increased blood urea nitrogen (BUN) levels indicate decreased renal function or fluid intake and increased catabolism and protein intake. Normal BUN levels are 5–20 mg/dl. BUN should be correlated with plasma creatinine levels to implicate renal dysfunction (e.g., acute renal failure) because BUN level can be affected by a variety of factors that affect protein metabolism. Alterations in BUN and creatinine level can lead to alteration in the patient's mental status [4].

Clinical tip

Noting BUN and creatinine levels on a daily basis for any changes may help explain changes in the patient's mental status, participation in physical therapy sessions, or both.

Radiographic Examination

Kidneys, Ureters, and Bladder X-ray

An x-ray of the kidneys, ureters, and bladder (KUB) to visualize the structures and determine the position, shape, size, and number of macroscopic (gross) renal, ureteral, and bladder structures and surrounding bones is an initial screening tool for genitourinary disorders. For example, renal calculi (kidney stones) can be detected on KUB x-ray. The renal and calculi will then require further evaluation.

Pyelography

Radiopaque dyes are used to radiographically examine the urinary system. Two types of tests are performed: excretory urography (intravenous pyelography) and retrograde urography.

In excretory urography, radiopaque dye is injected intravenously and is excreted through the urine. During the circulation of the dye through the genitourinary system, sequential radiographs are taken to evaluate the size, shape, and location of urinary tract structures and to evaluate renal excretory function.

In retrograde urography, a catheter or cystoscope is passed into the bladder and directed proximally into the ureters before injecting the dye. Radiographic information gathered from this test includes renal pelvis anatomy. This test is performed when an obstruction or trauma is suspected. This procedure is usually performed in conjunction with a cystoscopic examination.

Additional indications for retrograde urography include the evaluation of the following [3]:

- Hypertension
- Renal disease
- Masses
- Cysts
- Ureteral obstructions
- Retroperitoneal tumors
- Renal trauma
- Bladder abnormalities

Renal Arteriography and Venography
With renal arteriography and venography, radiopaque dye is injected
into the renal artery (arteriography) or vein (venography) through a
catheter, which is inserted into the femoral or axillary artery or
femoral vein. Arterial and venous blood supply to and from the kidneys can then be assessed radiographically. Indications for arteriography include renovascular hypertension and trauma, palpable renal
masses, and suitability of renal donors. Indications for venography
include renovascular hypertension, renal vein thrombosis, and renal
cell carcinoma [5].

Bladder Examination: Cystoscopy and Panendoscopy

In cystoscopy, a flexible, fiberoptic scope is passed through the urethra into the bladder to examine the bladder neck, urothelial lining,
and ureteral orifices. Cystoscopy is indicated for assessment of hematuria and dysuria, as well as for tumor or polyp removal. Panen-
doscopy is a similar procedure to cystoscopy that is used to view the
prostatitic urethra (in males), external urinary sphincters, and anterior urethra [4, 5].

Urodynamic Studies

Uroflowmetry
In uroflowmetry, voiding is analyzed graphically to determine the rate,
time, and volume of urinary flow so that ureteral, urethral, and bladder function can be assessed and described [5].

Urethral Pressure Studies
In urethral pressure studies, a catheter is used to measure urethral resistance to urinary outflow to help assess bladder disorders [5].

Cystometry
Cystometry is used to evaluate bladder filling and storage and expulsion and micturition. A catheter is inserted into the bladder to inject
a radiopaque material. This process is followed by radiographic
viewing [5].

Radioisotope Studies

Renography
In renography, a radioisotope is injected intravenously and allowed to
circulate through the urinary system and be excreted in the urine. A
renogram (graphic record) is taken to assess renal blood flow, glomerular filtration, and tubular secretion [4].

Renoscan

In a renoscan, an external scanning device, such as a scintillator, outlines the kidney after intravenous radioisotope injection. Decreased areas of kidney function do not show up on the scan [4].

Nuclear Cystogram (Radionuclide Cystogram)

In a nuclear cystogram, radioisotope material and normal saline are injected into the bladder through a catheter to assess bladder function. This procedure requires less radiation than cystography but does not provide the same anatomic detail [5].

Ultrasonography Studies

Ultrasound is used (1) to evaluate kidney size and shape; (2) to determine the presence of kidney stones, cysts, and prerenal collections of blood, pus, lymph, urine, and solid masses; and (3) to identify the presence of a dilated collecting system [5].

Computed Tomography

Indications for computed tomography of the genitourinary system include defining renal parenchyma abnormalities and differentiating solid mass densities as either cystic or hemorrhagic. Kidney size and shape, as well as the presence of cysts, abscesses, masses, hematomas, and collecting system dilation, can also be assessed with computed tomography [3].

Magnetic Resonance Imaging

Detection of renal masses and differentiation of simple cysts from complicated hemorrhagic masses are the most useful indications for magnetic resonance imaging of the genitourinary system [5].

Biopsies

Renal Biopsy

In a renal biopsy, a small portion of renal tissue is obtained percutaneously or surgically to assist in the evaluation of persistent proteinuria, nephrotic syndrome, and unexplained hematuria, as well as to assess controlled pharmacologic trials [5].

Bladder, Prostate, Urethral Biopsies

Bladder, prostate, and urethral biopsies involve taking tissue specimens from the bladder, prostate, and urethra with a cystoscope, panendoscope, or needle aspiration via the transrectal or transperineal approach. Examination of pain, hematuria, and suspected neoplasm are indications for these biopsies [5].

Pathophysiology

Renal System Dysfunction

Acute Renal Failure

Acute renal failure (ARF) can result from a variety of causes and is defined as a sudden, rapid deterioration in renal function that results in decreased urine output. The mortality of ARF is more than 50% [6]. The etiologies of ARF can be categorized as prerenal, renal, or postrenal. Prerenal ARF is caused by a decrease in renal blood flow from dehydration, hemorrhage, shock, burns, or trauma. Renal ARF involves primary damage to kidneys and is caused by glomerulonephritis, acute pyelonephritis, renal artery or vein occlusion, bilateral renal cortical necrosis, nephrotoxic substances, or blood transfusion reactions. Postrenal ARF involves obstruction distal to the kidney and is caused by acute urinary tract obstruction [6, 7]. The following are five stages of ARF of all etiologies [6, 7]:

1. *Onset* is the time from the precipitating event to the onset of decreased urine output, or oliguria.

2. *Oliguric or anuric (no urine) phase* occurs when urine output is less than 400 ml in 24 hours, which can last 8–15 days, with prognosis worsening as the duration increases.

3. *Diuretic phase* is the period from the time urine output is less than 400 ml in 24 hours to the time the BUN level stops rising.

4. The *late or recovery period* is the time between falling to stabilizing (i.e., within normal range) BUN levels.

5. The *convalescent phase* occurs when urine output and BUN levels are stable within normal ranges. This phase may last several months and may ultimately progress to chronic renal failure (CRF).

Complications of ARF include the following:

- Acidosis
- Hyperkalemia
- Infection
- Hyperphosphatemia

- Hypertension
- Anemia
- Hypovolemia
- Hypokalemia

Management of ARF includes any of the following:

- Treatment of primary etiology
- Hydration (intravenous fluids and osmotics [proteins])
- Diuretics
- Hemodialysis
- Transfusions and blood products
- Nutritional support
- Anti-infective agents

Chronic Renal Failure

CRF is an irreversible reduction in renal function that occurs as a slow, insidious process from the permanent destruction of nephrons. The renal system has considerable functional reserve, and as many as 50% of the nephrons can be destroyed before symptoms occur. CRF can result from primary renal disease or other systemic diseases. Primary renal diseases that cause CRF are polycystic kidney disease, chronic glomerulonephritis, chronic pyelonephritis, hypernephroma, and chronic urinary obstruction. Systemic diseases that cause CRF are hypertensive nephropathy, diabetic nephropathy, gouty nephropathy, lupus nephritis, renal amyloidosis, myeloma kidney, nephrocalcinosis, and hereditary nephropathy. Complications of CRF are similar to those of ARF.

Management of CRF may consist of any of the following [6, 7]:

- Peritoneal dialysis or hemodialysis for fluid and electrolyte balancing
- Nutritional support
- Anticonvulsant agents
- Antihypertensive agents
- Diuretics

- Anti-infective agents
- Antacids
- Antiemetic agents
- Renal transplantation

Pyelonephritis

Pyelonephritis is an acute or chronic inflammatory response in the kidney, particularly the renal pelvis, from bacterial, fungal, or viral infection. It can be classified as acute or chronic.

Acute Pyelonephritis

Predisposing factors for acute pyelonephritis include kidney stones, chronic urine reflux from the ureter to the kidney (vesicoureteral reflux), pregnancy, neurogenic bladder, catheter or endoscope insertion, and female sexual trauma [7]. Spontaneous resolution of acute pyelonephritis may occur in some cases without intervention.

Signs and symptoms of acute pyelonephritis may include the following [7, 8]:

- Sudden onset of fever and chills
- Tenderness with deep palpatory pressure of one or both costovertebral areas
- Flank or groin pain
- Urinary frequency
- Dysuria, hematuria, pyuria (presence of white blood cells [leukocytes])

Management of acute pyelonephritis may consist of any of the following [7, 8]:

- Organism-specific anti-infective agents
- Hydration

Chronic Pyelonephritis

Chronic pyelonephritis is recurrent or persistent inflammation and scarring of one or both kidneys as a result of autoimmune infection. Chronic pyelonephritis can also result from kidney stones or acute pyelonephritis and may lead to chronic renal failure. Specific etiologies are difficult to diagnose [7, 8].

Signs and symptoms of chronic pyelonephritis include the following:

- Hypertension

- Mild and vague dysuria, urinary frequency, and flank pain

- Renal insufficiency (decreased urine output) possibly progressing to failure

- Pyuria (white blood cells in the urine)

Management of chronic pyelonephritis includes any of the following:

- Treatment of primary etiology (if diagnosed)

- Anti-infective agents (either short or prolonged course)

Glomerulonephritis

Glomerulonephritis is an inflammation of the glomerular portion of the kidney that can result from immunologic abnormalities, drug or toxin effects, vascular disorders, or systemic disorders. Definitive etiology may be difficult to ascertain in some cases. Glomerulonephritis can be classified according to cause, pathologic lesions, disease progression, or clinical presentation. This section discusses the common types of glomerulonephritis [7].

Poststreptococcal Glomerulonephritis

Poststreptococcal glomerulonephritis occurs most commonly in children. Group A- and β-hemolytic streptococci are the causative pathogens that lead to the damage of surface proteins in the glomeruli [7, 8]. (Other bacterial organisms, viruses, and parasites may also cause poststreptococcal glomerulonephritis, but are less common.)

Signs and symptoms of poststreptococcal glomerulonephritis include the following:

- Acute onset of edema

- Oliguria

- Mild to moderate proteinuria

- Anemia

- Cola-colored urine with red blood cell casts
- Hypertension

Management of poststreptococcal glomerulonephritis includes any of the following:

- Antibiotics
- Antihypertensive agents
- Diuretics
- Fluid and electrolyte support (as needed)
- Hemodialysis

Rapidly Progressive Glomerulonephritis

Rapidly progressive glomerulonephritis (RPGN) is also known as subacute, crescentic, or extracapillary glomerulonephritis. It involves glomerular inflammation that progresses to renal failure in weeks to months [1]. This disease primarily affects adults who are in their 50s and 60s and has a relatively poor prognosis. Causes of RPGN can include acute or subacute infection from β-hemolytic streptococci or from other bacteria, viruses, or parasites. It can also be caused by multisystem or autoimmune disease [7, 8].

Signs and symptoms of RPGN include the following:

- Rapid, progressive reduction in renal function
- Severe oliguria
- Anuria, with irreversible renal failure

Management of RPGN includes any of the following:

- Anti-inflammatory agents (e.g., prednisone)
- Plasmapheresis
- Anticoagulation treatment
- Hemodialysis
- Renal transplantation

Immunoglobulin A Neuropathy (Berger's Disease)
Immunoglobulin (Ig) A neuropathy is an abnormality of immune regulation that can result in deposits of IgA complexes within the glomeruli and influence the filtration process. Fifty percent of cases progress to renal failure within 20 years of onset [7, 8].

Signs and symptoms of IgA neuropathy include the following:

- Hematuria

- Proteinuria

- Oliguria

Management of IgA neuropathy includes the administration of any of the following:

- Steroidal anti-inflammatory agents

- Cytotoxic agents

- Phenytoin (shown to lower serum IgA levels)

Chronic Glomerulonephritis
Chronic glomerulonephritis is the culmination of a variety of any or all glomerular diseases that progress to renal failure after a number of years. Scarring and obliteration of the glomeruli along with vascular sclerosis of arteries and arterioles occur [7, 8].

Signs and symptoms of chronic glomerulonephritis include the following:

- Uremia

- Proteinuria

- Hypertension

- Azotemia

Management of chronic glomerulonephritis includes any of the following:

- Treatment of primary disease or dysfunction

- Administration of steroidal anti-inflammatory agents

- Administration of anti-infective agents
- Dialysis
- Administration of cytotoxic agents

Other types of glomerulonephritis are minimal change disease (lipoid nephrosis), focal segmental glomerulonephrosis, membranous nephropathy, and membranoproliferative glomerulonephritis (slowly progressive glomerulonephritis) [5]. These are not discussed in this chapter because they have similar clinical manifestations as the types of glomerulonephritis discussed above.

Nephrotic Syndrome

Nephrotic syndrome is a group of symptoms characterized by an increased permeability of the glomerular basement membrane that results in increased excretion of protein molecules. The following conditions can lead to nephrotic syndrome [6, 7]:

- Glomerulonephritis
- Diabetes mellitus
- Infections
- Circulatory diseases
- Allergen or drug reactions
- Pregnancy
- Renal transplantation

Physical findings of nephrotic syndrome include the following:

- Hypoalbuminemia
- Generalized edema
- Hyperlipidemia
- Lipiduria (lipid casts or free fat droplets in urine)
- Vitamin D deficiency

Management of nephrotic syndrome includes any of the following:

- Treatment of underlying disease

- Dietary modifications (e.g., normal protein, low fat, salt restrictions)

- Diuretics

- Administration of steroidal anti-inflammatory agents

- Albumin replacement

Interstitial Nephritis

Infections, urinary tract obstruction, and reactions to medications can result in inflammatory interstitial tissue damage, which is referred to as *interstitial nephritis*. Scarring from the inflammatory process leads to reduced kidney function that can progress to chronic renal failure. Early detection is helpful in treating the inflammatory response, and caution is warranted with over-the-counter analgesic use, particularly acetaminophen [6].

Physical findings of interstitial nephritis include the following [6]:

- Polyuria

- Nocturia

- Pyuria

- Mild hematuria

- Mild proteinuria

Management of interstitial nephritis includes any of the following:

- Fluid and nutritional support

- Dialysis (as indicated)

- Surgery to relieve obstructions (if present)

- Anti-infective agents

Nephrolithiasis

Nephrolithiasis is a condition characterized by renal calculi (kidney stones) that form in the renal pelvis and can result from infections or obstructions in the urinary tract. They occur more commonly in men. Many factors contribute to stone formation and include high urinary concentration of stone-forming substances (listed below); presence of crystal growth facilitators; and urine pH, which affects solubility. There are three primary types of kidney stones, which are categorized according to the stone-forming substances: calcium oxalate, struvite (composed of magnesium, ammonium, and phosphate), and uric acid [6, 7].

Signs and symptoms of kidney stones include the following:

- Pain in the flank or groin, depending on the stone location (pain increases as the stone passes through the ureters.)

- Hematuria

- Fever

- Variable urine pH

- Variable levels of serum calcium, chloride, phosphate, carbon dioxide, uric acid, and creatinine

Management of kidney stones includes any of the following:

- Analgesics

- Hydration and diuretics

- Anti-infective agents

- Reduction in dietary consumption of predisposing factors, such as calcium

- Surgery (as a last resort)

Diabetic Nephropathy

Diabetic nephropathy is characterized by systemic vascular changes that occur with diabetes. An example of a systemic vascular change is lesions to the arterioles and glomeruli that result in scarring (sclerosis) of the glomeruli and ultimately in reduced kidney function. Pyelonephritis and necrosis of the renal papillae are often associated with diabetic nephropathy. All insulin-dependent diabetic patients are likely to develop this nephropathy. Morbidity and mortality are high [6].

Signs and symptoms of diabetic nephropathy include the following:

- Proteinuria, oliguria, anuria

- Fever

- Hypertension

- Peripheral edema

Management of diabetic nephropathy includes any of the following:

- Dialysis

- Insulin (requirements adjusted accordingly)

- Anticonvulsive agents

- Antihypertensive agents

- Diuretics

- Anti-infective agents

- Antacids

- Nutritional support

- Renal transplantation as a last resort (usually has a poor outcome)

Nephrosclerosis

Nephrosclerosis is damage to the renal vasculature and glomeruli resulting from prolonged systemic hypertension. Nephrosclerosis leads to decreased renal function. Renal damage is usually slow but can be rapid depending on the extent of systemic hypertension [6].

Signs and symptoms of nephrosclerosis include the following [5, 6]:

- Hypertension

- Nocturia

- Oliguria progressing to anuria

- Fever

Management of nephrosclerosis includes any of the following:

- Antihypertensive agents

- Diuretics

- Dialysis

- Nutritional modification and support

- Renal transplantation

Renal Vascular Abnormalities

Renal Artery Stenosis or Occlusion

Renal artery stenosis is a narrowing of the renal artery lumen; renal artery occlusion is blockage of the renal artery lumen. Renal artery stenosis or occlusion can result from any or all of the following: atherosclerotic disease, subacute bacterial endocarditis, emboli from mitral valve stenosis, or mural thrombi that develop after myocardial infarction. Decreased renal perfusion results in renovascular hypertension as a result of increased renin production [6].

Signs and symptoms of renal artery stenosis or occlusion include the following:

- Microscopic hematuria
- Flank or upper abdominal pain
- Hypertension
- Renal artery bruits

Management of renal artery stenosis or occlusion includes any of the following:

- Anticoagulation agents
- Analgesics
- Antihypertensive agents
- Dialysis
- Surgery (bypass grafting or angioplasty)

Renal Vein Thrombosis

Renal vein thrombosis is the accumulation of plaque in the renal vein. Renal vein thrombosis can be caused by dehydration, sepsis, or a hypercoagulable state. Sudden occlusion of the renal vein results in renal infarcts [6].

Signs and symptoms of renal vein thrombosis include the following [5, 6]:

- Flank pain

- Gross hematuria

- Proteinuria

- Oliguria

Renal vein thrombosis can be managed with anticoagulation agents.

Urinary Tract Dysfunction

Cystitis

Bacteria, viruses, fungi, chemical agents, and radiation exposure are causative agents that can lead to cystitis, which is an inflammation of the bladder wall. Cystitis and urinary tract infections are not synonymous but are associated. Cystitis can be associated with prostatitis or pyelonephritis, or it can occur alone. Those at greater risk of developing cystitis are people who are sexually active or those who have an indwelling catheter, urinary tract obstructions, diabetes mellitus, neurogenic bladders, or poor hygiene [8].

Signs and symptoms of cystitis include the following:

- Urinary frequency and urgency

- Dysuria

- Hematuria (in more serious cases)

- Suprapubic pain, low back pain, or both

Management of cystitis includes any of the following:

- Anti-infective agents

- Increased fluid intake

Urinary Calculi

Urinary calculi are stones that can form anywhere in the urinary tract outside of the kidneys. Formation of stones, symptoms, and management are similar to that of kidney stones (see "Nephrolithiasis" for further details on the formation and clinical presentation of kidney stones) [9].

Neurogenic Bladder

A neurogenic bladder is characterized by bladder paralysis that occurs with central nervous system disruption at the cortical or spinal cord level, resulting in urinary flow disturbances. Lesions above the sacral level of the spinal cord result in loss of voluntary control of voiding; lesions below the sacral level result in the loss of both voluntary and involuntary control of voiding. Neurogenic bladders may lead to infection, especially when there is associated bladder distention and urine retention, catheter placement, or stone formation, which is caused by bone resorption from physical immobility [7].

Symptoms of neurogenic bladders with infection are difficult to assess because altered sensation from neurologic disturbance often masks pain or other symptoms. The patient may report a burning sensation with voiding, however [7].

Management consists of addressing the neurologic disturbance (as able) and providing anti-infective agents for any associated infection. Table 9-3 provides a summary of the different types of urinary incontinence.

Prostate Disorders

Benign Prostatic Hypertrophy

Benign prostatic hypertrophy (BPH) is a benign, progressive enlargement of the prostate gland. Almost all men older than age 50 develop BPH, which is associated with the normal aging process. Concern arises when enlargement interferes with normal voiding patterns. Acute urinary retention and urinary tract infection are the primary complications of BPH [10].

Signs and symptoms of BPH include the following:

- Palpable prostate gland lobes with digital rectal examination
- Decreased force of urinary stream
- Straining to void
- Postvoid dribble
- Urinary frequency with incomplete emptying

Management of BPH includes any of the following:

Table 9-3.   Types of Urinary Incontinence

Type	Description	Common Causes
Stress	Loss of urine that occurs involuntarily in situations associated with increased intra-abdominal pressure, such as with laughing, coughing, or exercise	Weakness in the bladder outlet region, or urethral sphincter, or pelvic floor muscles
Urge	Leakage of urine that occurs after a sensation of bladder fullness is perceived	Cystitis, urethritis, tumors, stones, outflow obstructions, stroke, dementia, and parkinsonism
Overflow	Leakage of urine from mechanical forces or urinary retention from an overdistended bladder	Obstruction by prostate, stricture, or cystocele A noncontractile bladder, as occurs in diabetes mellitus or spinal cord injury A neurogenic bladder, as occurs in multiple sclerosis or other lesions above the sacral portion of the spinal cord
Functional	The inability to void because of cognitive or physical impairments, psychological unwillingness, or environmental barriers	Depression, anger, hostility, dementia, and other neurologic disorders

Source: Adapted from Disorders of Micturition and Obstruction of the Genitourinary Tract. In BL Bullock. Pathophysiology: Adaptations and Alterations in Function (4th ed). Philadelphia: Lippincott, 1996;648.

- Surgery (Transurethral resection of the prostate [TURP] is the most common; however, suprapubic or retropubic prostatectomy [open removal of the prostate] can also be performed.)

- Anti-infective agents (if there is associated infection)

- Intermittent self-catheterization

Prostatitis

Prostatitis is an inflammation of the prostate gland. It can be divided into four categories: (1) acute bacterial, (2) chronic bacterial, (3) non-bacterial, and (4) prostatodynia (presence of prostatitis symptoms without physical findings).

Signs and symptoms of prostatitis include the following [9]:

- Increased urinary frequency
- Urgency to void
- Painful urination (dysuria)
- Bladder irritability
- Difficulty initiating a stream

Management of prostatitis includes any of the following:

- Surgery (open resection of the prostate or TURP)
- Anti-infective agents
- Antipyretics
- Dietary modifications (alcohol, chili powder, and other hot spices can aggravate symptoms)

Management

The management of various genitourinary disorders are discussed earlier in the specific pathophysiology sections. This section expands on dialysis therapy and surgical procedures. Guidelines for physical therapy intervention for patients who have genitourinary dysfunction are also discussed.

Renal Failure Interventions

There are three methods to help manage fluid and electrolyte balance when renal function is interrupted: (1) continuous arteriovenous hemofiltration (CAVH), (2) hemodialysis, and (3) peritoneal dialysis.

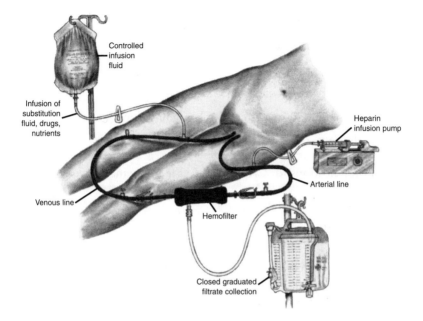

Figure 9-3. *Schematic of continuous arteriovenous hemofiltration. (Reprinted with permission from JM Thompson, GK McFarland, JE Hirsch, et al. Mosby's Clinical Nursing [3rd ed]. St. Louis: Mosby–Year Book, 1993;935.)*

Continuous Arteriovenous Hemofiltration

Figure 9-3 demonstrates the set-up of CAVH, which is frequently used in the critical care setting to stabilize and manage patients with fluid and electrolyte imbalances. The femoral artery and vein are common sites for vascular access. Pressure gradients between the arterial and venous system along with oncotic pressures help drive the hemofiltration process, which mimics the urine formation process in the renal glomerulus. Heparin is infused to help prevent clotting in the hemofilter and tubing. Medications and nutrition can also be administered through the circuit [6]. (Continuous venovenous hemofiltration is another form of this procedure, but is not discussed in this chapter.)

Indications for CAVH include the following:

- Unresponsiveness to diuretic therapy
- Cardiovascular instability

- Parenteral nutrition
- Cerebrovascular disease
- Coronary artery disease
- Uncomplicated acute renal failure
- Acute renal failure with multiple organ failure
- Inability to tolerate hemodialysis

Contraindications for CAVH include the following:

- Hypercatabolic state
- Hyperkalemia
- Poisoning
- Shock
- Low colloid oncotic pressure
- Congestive heart failure
- Severe arthrosclerosis
- Low blood flow (i.e., mean arterial pressure less than 60 mm Hg)

Hemodialysis

Figure 9-4 schematically demonstrates the hemodialysis process. Kidney functions that are controlled by dialysis include (1) fluid volume, (2) electrolyte balance, (3) acid-base balance, and (4) filtration of nitrogenous wastes. The patient's blood is mechanically circulated through semipermeable tubing that is surrounded by a dialysate solution in the artificial kidney. Vascular access is either through cannula insertion or through an internal arteriovenous fistula, which is surgically created in the forearm. The dialysate fluid contains electrolytes similar to those in normal blood plasma to permit diffusion of electrolytes into or out of the patient's blood [4, 6].

Indications for hemodialysis include the following:

- Acute poisoning
- Acute and chronic renal failure
- Severe states of edema

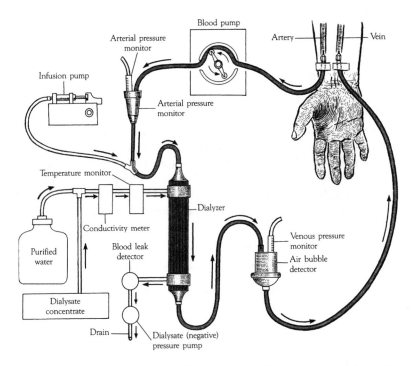

Figure 9-4. *Schematic of hemodialysis. (Reprinted with permission from JM Thompson, GK McFarland, JE Hirsch, et al. Mosby's Clinical Nursing [3rd ed]. St. Louis: Mosby–Year Book, 1993;938.)*

- Hepatic coma
- Metabolic acidosis
- Extensive burns with prerenal azotemia
- Transfusion reactions
- Postpartum renal insufficiency
- Crush syndrome

Contraindications for hemodialysis include the following [6]:

- Associated major chronic illnesses
- No vascular access

- Hemorrhagic diathesis
- Age extremes
- Poor compliance with treatment regimen

Peritoneal Dialysis
Figure 9-5 demonstrates the process of peritoneal dialysis. The process involves using the peritoneal cavity as a semipermeable membrane between dialysate fluid and the blood vessels in the abdominal cavity. Dialysate fluid is usually instilled and drained manually into the peritoneum to help with fluid and electrolyte balance [6].

The following are indications for peritoneal dialysis [4, 6]:

- Need for less rapid treatment
- Staff and equipment for hemodialysis are not available
- Inadequate vascular access for hemodialysis
- Shock
- Status post cardiac surgery (e.g., coronary artery bypass grafting)
- Severe cardiovascular disease
- Patient refusal of blood transfusions

The following are contraindications for peritoneal dialysis:

- Peritonitis
- Abdominal adhesions
- Recent abdominal surgery

Clinical tip

- Mobility treatments are contraindicated while a patient is undergoing any form of dialysis.

- Pulmonary hygiene treatments can be performed during dialysis; however, this depends on the hemodynamic stability of the patient, and is at the discretion of the nurse or

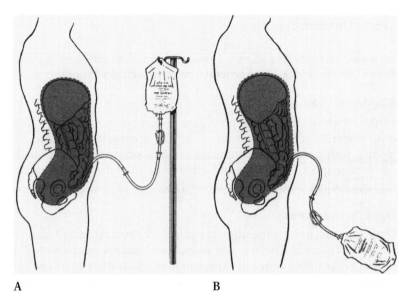

Figure 9-5. *Peritoneal dialysis diagram. A. Inflow. B. Outflow (drains to gravity). (Reprinted with permission from JM Thompson, GK McFarland, JE Hirsch, et al. Mosby's Clinical Nursing [3rd ed]. St. Louis: Mosby–Year Book, 1993;944.)*

physician. Extreme caution should be taken with the access site to prevent accidental disruption.

• The dialysis nurse is generally nearby to monitor the procedure and is a valuable source of information regarding the patient's hemodynamic stability.

• Activity tolerance can be altered when fluid and electrolyte levels are unbalanced. In general, patients are more fatigued at the end of a dialysis session but are more refreshed the day after dialysis.

• Fluid and electrolyte imbalance can also alter the hemodynamic responses to activity; therefore, careful vital sign and symptom monitoring should always be performed.

Surgical Interventions

Surgical interventions for genitourinary system disorders are discussed below. See Appendix V for general operative considerations.

Bladder Neck Suspension

Bladder neck suspension is a procedure used in women to help restore urinary continence by increasing urethral resistance. It is indicated for women with stress incontinence as a result of pelvic relaxation. Bladder neck suspension is contraindicated in cases of urethral sphincter damage leading to stress incontinence [9].

Open Prostatectomy

Open prostatectomy is the surgical removal of a prostate gland with or without its capsule. Five types of surgical approaches can be used: (1) transcoccygeal, (2) perineal, (3) retropubic, (4) transvesical, and (5) suprapubic. This procedure is contraindicated if the prostate is small and fibrous. The suprapubic and retropubic approaches of this procedure are contraindicated in the presence of cancer [9].

Open Urologic Surgery

Open urologic surgery is a large category of surgical procedures that are beyond the scope of this chapter but includes the following [9]:

- Nephrectomy (kidney removal)

- Partial nephrectomy (partial kidney removal)

- Nephrolithotomy (renal incisions for kidney stone removal)

- Pyelolithotomy (removal of the kidney stone from the pelvis of the kidney)

- Ureterolithotomy (removal of a urinary stone from the ureter)

- Cystectomy (bladder removal)

Percutaneous Nephroscopic Stone Removal

Percutaneous nephroscopic stone removal involves the removal of stones formed in the urinary tract under fluoroscopic monitoring, which allows for visualization of percutaneous nephrostomy tube placement. Depending on the size of the stone, stones may need to be broken up, then removed with a basket. Small fragments can be flushed through the system mechanically or physiologically. Considerations for this procedure include controlling septicemia before removal of the stones [9].

Transurethral Resection

Transurethral resection (TUR) refers to the surgical approach performed when managing bladder tumors, bladder neck fibrosis, and prostatic hyperplasia. The most common type of TUR is a TURP, which this section focuses on. TURP is indicated for obstructive BPH. Involved tissues are resected with a resectoscope that is inserted through the urethra. Excision and coagulation of tissue is accompanied by continuous irrigation. Contraindications for TURP include the presence of urinary tract infection and a prostate gland weighing more than 40 g. TURP is contraindicated with conditions that interfere with positioning for the procedure, such as irreversible scrotal hernia or ankylosis of the hip [9].

Urinary Diversion

Impeded urinary flow by obstruction can be resolved by diverting urine through a stoma at any level of the urinary tract. There are three types of diversions: (1) supravesical, (2) ureteroenterocutaneous, and (3) continent urinary diversion [9].

Supravesical Diversion

A supravesical diversion is one in which the urine is diverted at the level of the kidney by nephrostomy, pyelostomy, or ureterostomy.

In nephrostomy, a catheter is placed through the renal pelvis and into the renal calyces to temporarily drain urine. It should be noted that complications, such as stone formation, infection, hemorrhage, and hematuria, are associated with long-term nephrostomy tube placement.

Pyelostomy is urine drainage by catheter placement or stoma creation in the renal pelvis. Ureterostomy is the diversion of obstructions in the ureters with a tube placement or stoma creation. The ureter may also be anastomosed to the skin to form a cutaneous ureterostomy. These are difficult to manage, because urinary reflux and infections are common [9].

Ureteroenterocutaneous Diversions

In ureteroenterocutaneous diversions, segments of small and large bowel distal to the jejunum are used as a conduit to bridge the gap from the ureter to the skin when the bladder must be removed or bypassed [3]. Bladder carcinoma and severe neuropathic bladder dysfunction are common indications for this procedure.

Continent Urinary Diversion

Continent urinary diversions are internal urine reservoirs that are surgically constructed from segments of small intestine. This eliminates the need for external appliances and allows more control for the patient. The internal reservoir is connected to an abdominal stoma and patients perform intermittent self-catheterizations through the stoma [9].

Physical Therapy Intervention

The following are general goals and guidelines for the physical therapist when working with patients who have genitourinary dysfunction. These guidelines should be adapted to a patient's specific needs.

The primary physical therapy goals in this patient population are similar to those of other patients in the acute care setting. These goals are to (1) optimize functional mobility, (2) maximize activity tolerance and endurance, and (3) prevent postoperative pulmonary complications.

General guidelines include, but are not limited to, the following:

• Fluid and electrolyte imbalances in patients with genitourinary dysfunction affect activity tolerance. Appendix II describes the clinical presentation of various fluid and electrolyte imbalances that can affect physical therapy intervention. Assessing laboratory values before evaluation or treatment helps in deciding which particular signs and symptoms to monitor as well as in determining the parameters of the session.

• Patients who are status post surgical procedures with abdominal incisions are less likely to perform deep breathing and coughing because of incisional pain. Diligent position changes, instruction on incisional splinting during deep breathing, and coughing, along with early mobilization, help prevent the development of pulmonary complications.

References

1. Scanlon VC, Sanders T. Essentials of Anatomy and Physiology (2nd ed). Philadelphia: FA Davis, 1995;416.
2. Bullock BL. Normal Renal and Urinary Excretory Function. In BL Bullock (ed), Pathophysiology: Adaptations and Alterations in Function (4th ed). Philadelphia: Lippincott, 1996;616.

3. McLinn DM, Boissonnault WG. Screening for Male Urogenital System Disease. In WG Boissonnault (ed), Examination in Physical Therapy Practice: Screening for Medical Disease. New York: Churchill Livingstone, 1991;121.

4. Richard CJ. Urinary Function. In GA Harkness, JR Dincher (eds), Medical Surgical Nursing: Total Patient Care (9th ed). St. Louis: Mosby, 1996;760.

5. Thompson FD, Woodhouse CRJ. Disorders of the Kidney and Urinary Tract. London: Edward Arnold, 1987.

6. Renal System. In JM Thompson, GK McFarland, JE Hirsch, et al. (eds), Mosby's Manual of Clinical Nursing Practice (2nd ed). St. Louis: Mosby, 1989;1021.

7. Huether SE. Alterations of Renal and Urinary Tract Function. In KL McCance, SE Huether (eds), Pathophysiology: The Biologic Basis for Disease in Adults and Children (2nd ed). St. Louis: Mosby, 1994;1212.

8. Bullock BL. Immunologic, Infectious, Toxic and Other Alterations in Function. In BL Bullock (ed), Pathophysiology: Adaptations and Alterations in Function (4th ed). Philadelphia: Lippincott. 1996;633.

9. Genitourinary System. In JM Thompson, GK McFarland, JE Hirsch, et al. (eds), Mosby's Manual of Clinical Nursing Practice (2nd ed). St. Louis: Mosby, 1989;1086.

10. Bullock BL. Disorders of Micturition and Obstructions of Genitourinary Tract. In BL Bullock (ed), Pathophysiology: Adaptations and Alterations in Function (4th ed). Philadelphia: Lippincott. 1996;646.

10

Infectious Diseases

Jaime C. Paz

Introduction

A patient may be admitted to the hospital setting with an infectious process or may develop one as a complication from the medical environment, postsurgical environment, or both. Although an infectious process can have a primary site of origin, it may result in diffuse systemic effects that may limit the patient's mobility and activity tolerance. Therefore, a basic understanding of these infectious processes is useful in designing, implementing, and modifying physical therapy treatment programs. The physical therapist may also provide treatment to patients who have disorders resulting from altered immunity. These disorders are mentioned in this chapter because immune system reactions can be similar to those of infectious disease processes (see Chapter Appendix 10-A for discussions of three common disorders of altered immunity: systemic lupus erythematosus, sarcoidosis, and amyloidosis). The objectives of this chapter are to provide a basic understanding of the following:

1. Clinical assessment of infectious diseases and altered immune disorders, including physical examination and laboratory studies

2. Various infectious disease processes, including etiology, clinical presentation, and management

3.   More commonly encountered altered immune disorders, including etiology, clinical presentation, and management

4.   Precautions and guidelines that a physical therapist should use when treating a patient with an infectious process or altered immunity

Definition of Terms

The following terminology is commonly used in reference to infectious processes:

Antibody	A highly specific protein that is manufactured in response to antigens and that defends against subsequent infection [1]
Antigen (immunogen)	An agent that is capable of producing antibodies when introduced into the body of a susceptible person [1]
Carrier	A person who harbors an infectious agent that can cause a specific disease but who demonstrates no evidence of the disease [1]
Colonization	The process of a group of organisms living together; the host can carry the microorganism without being symptomatic [1, 2]
Communicable (contagious)	The ability of an infective organism to be transmitted from person to person, either directly or indirectly [1]
Disseminated	Distributed over a considerable area [3]
Host	The person whom the infectious agent invades and from whom it gathers its nourishment [1, 2]
Immunocompromised immune system	An immune system that is incapable of responding to pathogenic organisms and tissue damage [2]
Immunosuppression	The prevention of formation of an immune response [2]

Opportunistic infection	An infectious process that develops in immunosuppressed individuals (opportunistic infections do not normally develop in individuals with intact immune systems.) [1]
Pathogen	An organism capable of producing a disease [2]
Subclinical infection	A disease or condition that does not produce clinical symptoms or the time period before the appearance of disease-specific symptoms [1, 2]

Clinical Assessment

Assessment of infectious diseases in a patient consists of combining information gathered from physical examination and laboratory studies.

Physical Examination

When an infectious process is suspected, a physical examination is performed to serve as a screening tool for the differential diagnosis and to help determine if or which tests are required to identify a specific pathogen. The following are components of the physical examination:

1. **Patient interview.** Potential contributing factors of the infection are sought out, such as exposure to infectious individuals or recent travel to foreign countries. Also, a qualitative description of the symptomatology is discerned, such as onset or nature of symptoms (e.g., a nonproductive versus a productive cough).

2. **Vital sign assessment.** Measurement of heart rate and blood pressure helps in determining whether an infectious process is occurring (infections result in an increased metabolic rate, which presents as an increased heart rate). Blood pressure may also be elevated when metabolism is increased, or blood pressure can be decreased secondary to vasodilation from inflammatory responses in the body.

3. **Temperature curve.** Monitoring the patient's temperature over time (both throughout the day and daily) provides information regarding the progression (a rise in temperature) or a regression (a fall in temperature) of the infectious process. A fall in body temper-

ature from a relatively elevated temperature may also signify a response to a medication.

4. **Observation of symptoms.** Infectious processes have distinct symptoms. Observing these symptoms can assist with the inclusion and exclusion of potential sources of infection.

Laboratory Studies

Most of the evaluation process for diagnosing an infectious disease is based on laboratory studies. These studies are performed to (1) isolate the microorganisms from various body fluids or sites; (2) directly examine specimens by microscopic, immunologic, or genetic techniques; or (3) assess specific antibody responses to the pathogen [4].

Leukocyte Count

Leukocyte, or white blood cell (WBC), count is measured to determine if an infectious process is present. An increase in the number of WBCs, which is required for phagocytosis (cellular destruction of microorganisms), indicates an infectious process in the body. A decreased WBC count at baseline can indicate altered immunity, whereas a decreased WBC count relative to a previously high count (i.e., becoming more within normal limits) can indicate a resolution of an infectious process. The normal range for a complete WBC count is 4,500–11,000/µl. Percentages of the five types of WBCs (i.e., lymphocytes, monocytes, neutrophils, basophils, and eosinophils) can also be calculated [5, 6] (see Chapter 6, Table 6-7, for further description of complete blood counts).

Microbiology

In microbiology studies, specimens from suspected sources of infection (e.g., sputum, urine, feces, or wounds) are collected by sterile technique and analyzed by culture, sensitivity, or Gram's stain.

Culture

A culture consists of placing a specimen in one or more growth media to help identify the organism that may be responsible for the infectious process. Different microorganisms grow in a variety of environments, such as different pH levels and oxygen contents (aerobic vs. anaerobic). After microorganisms grow, further examination by Gram's staining and sensitivities can be performed [5, 6].

Sensitivity

Sensitivity* refers to the effectiveness of antibiotic therapy against a microorganism. A microorganism is referred to as "sensitive" to an antibiotic when its growth is inhibited by that antibiotic. Conversely, a microorganism is referred to as "resistant" to an antibiotic when its growth is not inhibited by that antibiotic [6].

Gram's Stain

Gram's stain is a microscopic study used to differentiate types of bacteria. A specimen is placed on a microscope slide and the following four-step process is performed:

1. A violet stain is applied.

2. An iodine solution is applied.

3. The specimen is decolorized with alcohol or acetone.

4. Safranin is applied to counterstain (pink) the specimen.

The results of Gram's stain can be pink or violet, indicating the presence of gram-negative or gram-positive bacteria, respectively [6].

Cytology

Cytology is a complex method of studying cellular structures, functions, origins, and formations. Cytology assists with the differential diagnosis of infectious processes or malignancy, as certain abnormal characteristics found in the cells can help differentiate between an infection or a malignancy [6]. It is beyond the scope of this chapter, however, to describe all of the processes involved in studying cellular structure dysfunction.

Body Fluid Examination

Pleural Tap

A pleural tap, or thoracentesis, is the process by which a needle is inserted through the chest wall into the pleural cavity to collect pleural fluid for examination of possible malignancy, infection, inflammation, or any combination of these. A thoracentesis may also be performed to drain excessive pleural fluid in large pleural effusions [5].

**C & S* is an abbreviation referring to culture and sensitivity testing.

Gastric Lavage

A gastric lavage is the suctioning of gastric contents through a nasogastric tube to examine the contents for the presence of sputum in patients suspected of having tuberculosis. The assumption is that patients swallow sputum while they sleep. If sputum is found in the gastric contents, appropriate sputum analysis should be performed to help confirm the diagnosis of tuberculosis [5].

Peritoneal Fluid Analysis

Peritoneal fluid analysis, or paracentesis, is the aspiration of peritoneal fluid with a needle. It is performed to (1) determine the composition of ascitic fluid (which can be a manifestation of an infectious disease), (2) assist in the diagnosis of hepatic or systemic diseases, and (3) help detect the presence of abdominal trauma [5].

Other Studies

Imaging with plain x-rays, computed tomography scans, and magnetic resonance imaging scans can also help identify areas with infectious lesions. In addition, the following diagnostic studies can also be performed to help with the differential diagnosis of the infectious process. For a description of these studies refer to the chapter indicated.

- Sputum analysis (see Chapter 2, "Diagnostic Studies")

- Cerebrospinal fluid (see Chapter 4, "Lumbar Puncture")

- Urinalysis (see Chapter 9, "Diagnostic Studies")

- Wound cultures (see Chapter 7, "Wound Assessment and Acute Care Management of Wounds")

Pathophysiology

Pertussis

Pertussis, or whooping cough, is an acute bacterial infection of the mucous membranes of the tracheobronchial tree. It occurs most commonly in children younger than 1 year of age and in children and adults of lower socioeconomic populations. The defining characteristics are violent cough spasms that end with an inspiratory "whoop" followed by the expulsion of clear tenacious secretions. Symptoms may last 1–2 months. Pertussis is transmitted through airborne particles.

Management of pertussis may consist of any of the following [5]:

- Anti-infective and anti-inflammatory medications

- Bronchopulmonary hygiene with endotracheal suctioning as needed

- Supplemental oxygen, assisted ventilation, or both

- Fluid and electrolyte replacement

- Respiratory isolation for 3 weeks after the onset of coughing spasms or 7 days after antimicrobial therapy

Histoplasmosis

Histoplasmosis is a pulmonary and systemic infection that is caused by infective spores (fungi) in the soil. The spores form lesions within the lung parenchyma that can be spread to other tissues. Infants, immunosuppressed individuals, and chronically debilitated individuals are most severely affected. Different clinical forms of histoplasmosis are (1) acute, benign respiratory disease, which results in flu-like illness and pneumonia; (2) acute disseminated disease, which can result in septic-type fever; (3) chronic disseminated disease, which involves lesions in the bone marrow, spleen, and lungs; and (4) chronic pulmonary disease, which manifests as progressive emphysema. Clinical symptoms are representative of the affected areas. Histoplasmosis is transmitted by inhalation of the infective spores. No human-to-human transmission has been documented.

Management of histoplasmosis may consist of the following [5, 7]:

- Anti-infective agents

- Corticosteroids

- Antihistamines

- Supportive care appropriate for affected areas in the different forms of histoplasmosis

Influenza

Influenza is an acute, generalized disease associated with upper and lower respiratory tract infections that result from influenza viruses A,

B, or C and their mutagenic strains. Signs and symptoms of the disease include (1) a severe cough, (2) abrupt onset of fever and chills, (3) headache, (4) backache, (5) myalgia, (6) prostration (exhaustion), (7) coryza (nasal inflammation with profuse discharge), and (8) mild sore throat. Gastrointestinal signs and symptoms of nausea, vomiting, abdominal pain, and diarrhea can also present in certain cases. The disease is usually self-limiting, lasting 1–2 weeks. Bacterial pneumonia can occur as a complication of influenza infection, especially in the elderly and chronically diseased individuals. Influenza is transmitted by aerosolized mucous droplets.

Management of influenza may consist of the following [1, 2, 5]:

- Anti-infective agents
- Antipyretic agents
- Adrenergic agents
- Antitussive agents
- Active immunization by vaccines
- Supportive care with IV fluids and supplemental oxygen as needed

Legionellosis

Legionellosis is an acute bacterial infection resulting in patchy pulmonary infiltrate(s) and consolidation. It is transmitted by inhalation of aerosolized organisms from infected water sources. Legionellosis is commonly referred to as legionnaire's disease. Signs and symptoms include high fever, malaise, myalgia, headache, and nonproductive cough. There is a high risk for respiratory failure and death from legionellosis. The disease is rapidly progressive during the first 4–6 days of illness, with complications that include renal failure, bacteremic shock, and respiratory failure.

Management of legionellosis may consist of the following [1, 5]:

- Anti-infective agents
- Supplemental oxygen with or without assisted ventilation
- Temporary renal dialysis
- IV fluid and electrolyte replacement

Tuberculosis

Tuberculosis is a chronic pulmonary and extrapulmonary infectious disease caused by the tubercle bacillus. The bacilli can remain quiescent in the body for years and become opportunistic when a person becomes ill or immunocompromised. Tuberculosis is transmitted through airborne *Mycobacteria*. Skin testing, using either the Mantoux or purified protein derivative (PPD) test, helps to confirm the diagnosis.*

Signs and symptoms associated with pulmonary tuberculosis include (1) an initial nonproductive cough; (2) mucopurulent secretions that present later; and (3) hemoptysis, dyspnea at rest or with exertion, adventitious breath sounds at lung apices, pleuritic chest pain, hoarseness, and dysphagia, all of which may occur in the later stages.

Extrapulmonary tuberculosis occurs more rarely but can affect the meninges, blood vessels, kidneys, bones, joints, larynx, skin, intestines, lymph nodes, peritoneum, or eyes. Symptoms that manifest are representative of the particular organ system involved.

The populations at higher risk for acquiring tuberculosis include (1) the elderly; (2) Native Americans, Eskimos, and blacks (in particular if they are homeless or economically disadvantaged); (3) incarcerated individuals; (4) immigrants from Southeast Asia, Ethiopia, Mexico, and Latin America; (5) malnourished individuals; (6) infants and children younger than 5 years of age; (7) those with decreased immunity (e.g., from acquired immunodeficiency syndrome [AIDS] or after chemotherapy); and (8) those with diabetes mellitus, end-stage renal disease, or both [3].

Management of tuberculosis may consist of the following [1, 2, 5]:

- Anti-infective agents

- Corticosteroids

- Surgical intervention to remove cavitary lesions (rare) or to correct hemoptysis, spontaneous pneumothorax, abscesses, intestinal obstruction, ureteral stricture, or any combination of these

- Respiratory isolation until antimicrobial therapy is initiated

---

*A person who has been exposed to the tubercle bacillus will demonstrate a raised and reddened area 2–3 days after being injected with the protein derivative of the bacilli.

- Blood and body fluid precautions if extrapulmonary disease is present
- Skin testing (i.e., Mantoux test and PPD)
- Vaccination for prevention

Clinical tip

- Facilities often provide specialized masks to wear around patients on respiratory precautions for tuberculosis. The masks are impermeable to the airborne mycobacterium. Always check with the nursing staff or physician before working with these patients to determine which mask to wear.

- Patients who are suspected of but not diagnosed with tuberculosis are generally placed on "rule-out tuberculosis" protocol, in which case respiratory precautions should be observed.

Poliomyelitis

Poliomyelitis is an acute systemic viral disease that affects the central nervous system. Polioviruses are a type of enteroviruses that multiply in the intestinal tract. Vaccination has greatly reduced the number of cases in recent times. Clinical presentation can range from subclinical infection, to nonfebrile illness (24–36 hours), to aseptic meningitis, to paralysis (after 4 days), and possibly to death. If paralysis occurs, it is generally asymmetric and involves muscles of respiration, swallowing, and the lower extremities. Poliomyelitis is transmitted by the fecal-oral route.

Management of poliomyelitis may consist of any of the following [5]:

- Active immunization (vaccination) for prevention
- Analgesics and antipyretics
- Enteric precautions for 7 days after the onset of the disease
- Supplemental oxygen, assisted ventilation, or both
- Bronchopulmonary hygiene

- Intravenous (IV) fluids and nasogastric feedings
- Bed rest
- Contracture prevention with positioning and range of motion

Postpoliomyelitis Syndrome

Postpoliomyelitis syndrome occurs many years after an attack of paralytic poliomyelitis. It results in muscle fatigue and decreased endurance. Muscle atrophy and fasciculations may also be present. Older or critically ill patients who have had a previous diagnosis of paralytic poliomyelitis are most susceptible to the development of this syndrome [8].

Meningitis

Meningitis is an inflammation of the meninges, which cover the brain and spinal cord, that results from acute infection by bacteria, viruses, fungi, or parasitic worms. The route of transmission is primarily inhalation of infected airborne mucous droplets released by infected individuals. The more common types of meningitis are (1) meningococcal meningitis, which is bacterial in origin and occurs in epidemic form; (2) *Hemophilus* meningitis, which is the most common form of bacterial meningitis; (3) pneumococcal meningitis, which occurs as an extension of a primary bacterial upper respiratory tract infection; and (4) viral (aseptic or serous) meningitis, which is generally benign and self-limiting.

Bacterial meningitis is more severe than viral meningitis. Complications of bacterial meningitis include hydrocephalus, arthritis, myocarditis, pericarditis, neuromotor and intellectual deficits, and blindness and deafness from cranial nerve dysfunction.

Management of any form of meningitis may consist of the following [5]:

- Anti-infective agents
- Analgesics
- Immunologic agents
- Mechanical ventilation (as needed)
- Blood pressure maintenance with IV fluid and vasopressors (e.g., dopamine)
- Intracranial pressure control

Encephalitis

Encephalitis is an inflammation of the tissues of the brain and spinal cord resulting from infection by ameba or viruses. The most common types of encephalitis are amebic meningoencephalitis, mosquito-borne viral encephalitis, and infectious viral encephalitis. Amebic meningoencephalitis is transmitted in water and can enter a person's nasal passages while he or she is swimming. Amebic meningoencephalitis cannot be transmitted from person to person. Mosquito-borne viral encephalitis is transmitted by infectious mosquito bites and cannot be transmitted from person to person. Infectious viral encephalitis is transmitted by direct contact of droplets from respiratory passages or other infected excretions. It can occur as a sequela from other viral diseases such as measles, mumps, rubella, and chickenpox.

Clinical presentation of encephalitis may include any of the following:

- Fever

- Signs of meningeal irritation (e.g., severe frontal headache, nausea, vomiting, dizziness, nuchal rigidity)

- Altered level of consciousness, irritability, bizarre behaviors (if the temporal lobe is involved)

- Seizures (mostly in infants)

- Aphasia

- Focal neurologic signs

- Weakness

- Altered deep tendon reflexes

- Ataxia, spasticity, tremors, or flaccidity

- Hyperthermia

- Alteration in antidiuretic hormone secretion

Management of encephalitis may consist of the following [5]:

- Anti-infective agents

- Mechanical ventilation

- Tracheostomy (as indicated)

- Sedation
- IV fluid and electrolyte replacement
- Nasogastric tube feedings

Acute Bacterial Gastroenteritis and Acute Viral Gastroenteritis

Many forms of acute bacterial gastroenteritis and acute viral gastroenteritis exist, including those caused by *Escherichia coli*, *Shigella* (causes bacterial dysentery), and *Clostridium difficile*. The primary manifestations of any form of gastroenteritis are "crampy" abdominal pain, nausea, and diarrhea, all of which vary in severity and duration according to the type of infection. Gastroenteritis is generally a self-limiting infection. It is transmitted by ingestion of contaminated food, water, or both or by direct and indirect fecal-oral transmission.

Management of acute gastroenteritis may consist of the following [5, 7]:

- Anti-infective agents
- IV fluid and electrolyte replacement
- Antiemetic agents (if nausea and vomiting occur)

Clinical tip

Strict contact and enteric precautions should be observed with patients who have a diagnosis of *C. difficile* infection.

Water-Borne and Food-Borne Salmonella Infections

Infection by *Salmonella* bacteria can initially present with symptoms similar to gastroenteritis but can also progress to septicemia. Two types of systemic infection can manifest: paratyphoid fever or typhoid fever, the latter being more severe. Signs and symptoms associated with typhoid fever include a sustained, high fever; headache; myalgia; diarrhea or constipation; abdominal discomfort and distention; and a dulled facial expression. Complications that can occur with *Salmonella* infection are endocarditis, meningitis, psychosis, myocarditis, pneumonia, pyelonephritis, osteomyelitis, cholecystitis, and hepatitis. *Salmonella* is transmitted by the ingestion of contaminated food or water.

Management of a *Salmonella* infection may consist of the following [5]:

- Anti-infective agents
- Corticosteroids
- IV fluid and electrolyte replacement
- Bed rest
- Hyperalimentation
- Avoidance of antispasmodics, laxatives, and salicylates
- Typhoid vaccination
- Food- and water-handling precautions to assist with transmission prevention

Rheumatic Fever

Rheumatic fever is a clinical sequela occurring in 2.8% of patients with group-A streptococcal infection of the upper respiratory tract. It occurs primarily in children 5–12 years old. An altered immune reaction to the infection is suspected, but the etiology is unknown. Rheumatic fever is characterized by nonsuppurative inflammatory lesions occurring in any or all of the connective tissues of the heart, joints, subcutaneous tissues, and central nervous system [5, 9].

Cardiac manifestations can include pericarditis, myocarditis, left-sided endocarditis, and valvular stenosis and insufficiency. All of these conditions can lead to significant morbidity or death.

Management of rheumatic fever follows the treatment for streptococcal infection. The secondary complications mentioned above are then managed specifically. The general intervention scheme may include the following [5, 9]:

- Prevention of streptococcal infection
- Anti-infective agents
- Antipyretic agents
- Corticosteroids
- Bed rest

- IV fluids (as needed)

- Secretion precautions 24 hours after initiation of antibiotic therapy

Mononucleosis

Mononucleosis is an acute viral disease that has several causes; the more common causes are the Epstein-Barr virus (EBV) and cytomegalovirus (CMV). The disease is characterized by lymph node hyperplasia that results in fever, exudative pharyngitis, lymphadenopathy, and splenomegaly. Complications that may occur from mononucleosis are hepatitis, pneumonitis, and central nervous system involvement. Mononucleosis is transmitted generally through saliva from symptomatic or asymptomatic carriers (the Epstein-Barr virus can remain infective for 18 months in the saliva).

Management of mononucleosis may consist of the following [5]:

- Corticosteroids

- Bed rest during the acute stage

- Saline throat gargle

- Aspirin or acetaminophen for sore throat and fever

Cytomegalovirus Infection

CMV infection is a common viral infection that is either asymptomatic or symptomatic. If CMV infection is symptomatic, one clinical presentation can be mononucleosis in adults. CMV is a member of the herpesvirus group and can be found in all body secretions, including saliva, blood, urine, semen, cervical secretions, and breast milk. CMV infection results in an inflammatory response with focal tissue destruction, areas of calcification, and hyperplasia of the reticuloendothelial system. CMV is transmitted by prolonged contact with infected body secretions. Transmission can also occur congenitally or perinatally.

Management of CMV infection may consist of the following [5]:

- Antiviral agents

- Corticosteroids
- Immune globulins
- Blood transfusions for anemia or thrombocytopenia
- Antipyretics

Toxoplasmosis

Toxoplasmosis is a systemic protozoan infection in which tissue cysts and calcifications form that can impair organ function in the spleen, liver, brain, lung, myocardium, and eyes. Clinical manifestations can range from subclinical infection, to severe generalized infection, to death. Toxoplasmosis is transmitted through the ingestion of infected food, or it can occur congenitally.

Management of toxoplasmosis may consist of the following [5]:

- Anti-infective agents
- Vitamins (folic acid)

Necrotizing Cellulitis

Necrotizing cellulitis, or erysipelas, is an acute, rapidly progressive inflammatory reaction of the superficial lymph vessels that is frequently associated with previous respiratory or systemic infections by group A *Streptococcus* or with preexisting lymph obstruction. The infection may remain localized in the dermis, spread to the subcutaneous tissue, or be disseminated into the bloodstream. The primary manifestations are fever with an abrupt onset of hot, stinging, and itchy skin and painful, red, thickened lesions that have firm, raised palpable borders in the affected areas. Management of necrotizing cellulitis consists of administration of anti-infective agents [5].

Osteomyelitis

Osteomyelitis is an acute infection of the bone that can occur as either acute hematogenous osteomyelitis or acute contagious osteomyelitis. Both of these types can potentially progress to chronic osteomyelitis.

Acute hematogenous osteomyelitis is a blood-borne infection that generally results from *Staphylococcus aureus* infection (80%) [1] and occurs mostly in infants; children (in the metaphysis of growing long bones); or patients undergoing long-term intravenous therapy, hyperalimentation, hemodialysis, or corticosteroid or antibiotic therapy. Patients who are malnourished, obese, diabetic, or have chronic joint disease are also susceptible to osteomyelitis.

Acute contagious osteomyelitis is an extension of concurrent infection in adjacent tissues to the bony area. Trauma resulting in compound fractures and tissue infections is a common example. Prolonged orthopedic surgery, wound drainage, or both also predispose patients to osteomyelitis.

Clinical presentation of both types of acute osteomyelitis includes (1) pain, (2) tenderness, (3) swelling, and (4) warmth in the affected area. Fever is present with hematogenous osteomyelitis. Appropriate antibiotic therapy is the general treatment course [1, 7].

Chronic osteomyelitis is an extension of the acute cases discussed above. It results in marked bone destruction, draining sinus tracts, pain, deformity, and the potential of limb loss. Chronic osteomyelitis can also result from infected surgical prostheses or infected fractures. Debridement of dense formations (sequestra) may be a necessary adjunct to the antibiotic therapy.

Clinical tip

Clarify weight-bearing orders with the physician if the lower extremities are involved when performing gait training with patients who have any form of osteomyelitis.

Sepsis

Sepsis is a general term that describes three progressive infectious conditions: bacteremia, septicemia, and shock syndrome (or septic shock).

Bacteremia is a generally asymptomatic condition that results from bacterial invasion of blood from contaminated needles, catheters, monitoring transducers, or perfusion fluid. Bacteremia can also occur from a preexisting infection from another body site. Bacteremia can resolve spontaneously or progress to septicemia.

Septicemia is a symptomatic extension of bacteremia, with clinical presentations that are representative of the infective pathogen and the organ system(s) involved. Sites commonly affected are the brain, endo-cardium, kidneys, bones, and joints. Renal failure and endocarditis may also occur.

Shock syndrome is a critical condition of systemic tissue hypoper-fusion that results from microcirculatory failure (i.e., decreased blood pressure or perfusion). Bacterial damage of the peripheral vascular sys-tem is the primary cause of the tissue hypoperfusion.

Management of sepsis may consist of any of the following [5]:

- Removal of suspected infective sources (e.g., lines or tubes)

- Anti-infective agents

- Blood pressure assistance with adrenergic agents and cortico-steroids

- Blood transfusions

- IV fluids

- Cardiac glycosides

- Supplemental oxygen or mechanical ventilation

- Anticoagulation

Nosocomial Infection

Nosocomial infection is a general term that refers to an infection that is acquired in the hospital setting. A nosocomial infection can result from (1) contact with infected individuals, (2) contact with contaminated environment (lines, tubes, or needles), or (3) microor-ganisms that are normally present in a patient and become oppor-tunistic. Patients that are most susceptible to these infections are those with chronic disease, malnutrition, dehydration, body fluid stasis, traumatized tissue, leukopenia, preexisting infection, or immunosuppression or immunocompromise. Common nosocomial infections occur in the urinary tract, surgical wounds, and the lower respiratory tract (e.g., pneumonia). Bacteremia and septicemia (described in the previous section, "Sepsis") are also forms of noso-comial infections. Clinical manifestations and management of noso-comial infections vary according to the pathogen and organ system involved [5].

Methicillin-Resistant Staphylococcus Aureus Infection

Methicillin-resistant *S. aureus* (MRSA) is a strain of *Staphylococcus* that is resistant to antibiotics such as penicillins (methicillin is a form of penicillin), cephalosporins, and aminoglycosides. The following patients are at risk for developing MRSA infection:

- Patients who are debilitated, elderly, or both

- Patients who are hospitalized for prolonged time periods

- Patients who have multiple surgical or invasive procedures, an indwelling cannula, or both

- Patients who are taking multiple antibiotics, antimicrobial treatments, or both

- Patients who are undergoing treatment in critical care units

MRSA is generally transmitted by person-to-person contact or person-to-object-to-person contact. MRSA can survive for prolonged periods of time on inanimate objects such as telephones, bed rails, and tray tables, unless such objects are properly sanitized. Hospital personnel can be primary carriers of MRSA, as the bacterium can be colonized in healthy adults. Management of MRSA is difficult and may consist of combining local and systemic antibiotics, as well as applying whole body antiseptic solutions. Prevention of MRSA infection is, therefore, the primary treatment strategy and consists of the following [9, 10]:

- Placing patients with MRSA infection on isolation or contact precautions

- Use of gloves, gowns (gowns are institution dependent), or both

- Strict hand washing regulations before and after patient care

- Disinfection of all contaminated objects

Vancomycin-Resistant Enterococci Infection

Vancomycin-resistant enterococci (VRE) infection is a relatively new infectious process that is resistant to vancomycin, aminoglycosides, and ampicillin and occurs in certain patient populations. Patients at risk of developing VRE infection are those who fall into any of the following categories [11]:

- Critically ill patients with severe underlying disease or immuno-suppression

- Patients in intensive care units, oncology wards, or transplant wards

- Patients who are status post intra-abdominal or cardiothoracic surgeries

- Patients with indwelling urinary or central venous catheters

- Patients who have a prolonged hospital stay

- Patients who received multiantimicrobial therapy, vancomycin therapy, or both

The infection can develop as endogenous enterococci (which are normally found in the gastrointestinal or the female reproductive tract) become opportunistic in the above patient populations. Transmission of the infection can also occur by (1) direct patient-to-patient contact, (2) indirect contact through asymptomatic hospital personnel who can carry the opportunistic strain of the microorganism, or (3) contact with contaminated equipment or environmental surfaces.

Management of VRE infection is difficult, and treatment options are limited to a combination of antimicrobial agents and experimental compounds that have unproved efficacy. The best intervention plan is to prevent the spread of the infectious process. Strategies for preventing VRE infection include the following [11]:

- The controlled use of vancomycin

- Timely communication between the microbiology laboratory and appropriate personnel to initiate contact precautions as soon as VRE is detected

- Implementation of screening procedures to detect VRE infection in hospitals where VRE has not yet been detected (i.e., by randomly culturing potentially infected items or patients)

- Preventing the transmission of VRE by placing patients in isolation or grouping patients with VRE together, wearing gown and gloves (which need to be removed inside the patient's room), and washing hands immediately after working with an infected patient

- Designating commonly used items, such as stethoscopes and rectal thermometers, to be used only with VRE patients

- Disinfecting any item that has been in contact with VRE patients with the hospital's approved cleaning agent

---

Clinical tip

Equipment that is used during physical therapy treatments for VRE patients, such as assistive devices, cuff weights, or goniometers, should be left in the patient's room and not be taken out until the infection is resolved. If there is an equipment shortage, thorough cleaning of the equipment is necessary before using the equipment with other patients.

Human Immunodeficiency Virus Infection

Human immunodeficiency virus is a retrovirus that preferentially infects the (1) helper T cells (T4) of the immune system, (2) epithelial cells, and (3) cells in the central nervous system. The infection is progressive and can be categorized by various stages. Two classification systems of HIV infection exist: the Centers for Disease Control (CDC) system, which has four categories of the infection according to signs and symptoms, and the Walter Reed staging system, which has six categories of the infection grouped according to the quantity of helper T cells and characteristic signs, such as the presence of an HIV antigen or antibody [12].

HIV infection can progress to AIDS, which is characterized by severe immunologic deficiency, opportunistic infectious diseases, Kaposi's sarcoma, and non-Hodgkin's lymphoma. The Centers for Disease Control further extends its definition of AIDS to any patient with a positive serologic (antibody) or virologic test for HIV and the presence of any of the following diseases:

- Disseminated histoplasmosis

- Isosporiasis with diarrhea lasting more than 1 month

- Bronchial or pulmonary candidiasis

HIV can be transmitted in blood, semen, or vaginal secretions, by sexual, perinatal, or contaminated blood or blood product contact. A glycoprotein (CD4) on the surface of the T4 cell serves as the receptor site for HIV, with active replication destroying the host cells. The result is a decrease in the number of T4 cells and resultant immunodeficiency [1].

There are five laboratory tests used according to the physician's discretion to detect HIV infection [13]:

1. **Enzyme-linked immunosorbent assay (ELISA) test.** This procedure tests for the presence of antibodies to HIV proteins in the patient's serum. A sample of the patient's blood is exposed to an HIV viral envelope obtained from a culture. Any antibodies present will attach to the HIV.

2. **Western blot test.** This test detects the presence of HIV proteins in the blood and is used as a confirmatory tool for a positive ELISA test.

3. **HIV culture.** This test is a difficult and time-consuming procedure that requires special test facilities in order to produce a live virus from the patient's blood or infected cells.

4. **p24 antigen assay.** This procedure detects the viral antigen from the patient's blood or infected cells so that the treatment effects of antiviral agents can be evaluated.

5. **Polymerase chain reaction for HIV nucleic acid.** This highly specific and extremely sensitive test is used to detect HIV in high-risk patients before the development of antibodies, as well as to help confirm a positive ELISA test result.

To determine the status of HIV and AIDS progression, a T4-cell count is performed. In this count, the absolute number of T4 cells is an index of the immune capability of the patient. According to the Walter Reed classification system, a T4 count of 400 cells/μl serves as the marker to begin classifying the stages of HIV infection. A normal T4 count is 650–1,200 cells/μl [13]. The ratio of T4 cells to suppressor T8 cells is also used as an indicator of cell-mediated immunity, with the normal ratio of T4 to T8 equaling 0.9–2.7 [14]. In those with HIV infections, the ratio is often less than 1.0 [12].

Many systemic effects of HIV infection arise from opportunistic infections and can influence physical therapy intervention. Opportunistic infections that affect the pulmonary system are summarized in Table 10-1; neurologic complications are summarized in Table 10-2. Cardiac complications from HIV infection include pericarditis, cardiac tamponade, marantic (thrombotic) endocarditis, dilated cardiomyopathy, *Mycobacterium avium intracellulare* infection, and cryptococcal endocarditis [12]. Refer to Chapter 1 for a description of pericarditis, endocarditis, dilated cardiomyopathy, and concomitant physical therapy considerations.

Management

Physical Therapy Intervention

The following are general physical therapy goals and guidelines to be used when working with patients who have infectious disease processes, as well as disorders of altered immunity. These guidelines should be adapted to a patient's specific needs.

The primary physical therapy goals in this patient population are similar to those of patient populations in the acute care setting: (1) to optimize the patient's functional mobility, (2) to maximize the patient's activity tolerance and endurance, and (3) to maximize ventilation and gas exchange in the patient who has pulmonary involvement.

General physical therapy guidelines include, but are not limited to, the following:

- The best modes of preventing the transmission of infectious diseases are to adhere to the standard precautions established by the Centers for Disease Control and to follow proper hand-washing techniques. Facilities' warning or labeling systems for biohazards and infectious materials may vary slightly. Be sure to check the patient's medical record or signs posted on doors and doorways for indicated precautions. Table 10-3 provides an outline of the types of protective equipment that should be worn with specific precautions.

- Patients who have infectious processes will have an elevated metabolic rate, which will probably manifest as a high resting heart rate. Because of this, the activity intensity level should be modified or more frequent rest periods should be incorporated during physical therapy treatment to enhance activity tolerance.

Table 10-1. Opportunistic Infections in Human Immunodeficiency Virus Infection

Pathogen	Description	Clinical Presentation	Medications Used
Mycobacterium tuberculosis	Tuberculosis may result from activation of previously dormant bacilli from earlier exposure.	Fever Lymphadenitis Initial nonproductive cough that progresses to production of muco-purulent secretions Dyspnea	Isoniazid Rifampin Pyrazinamide Ethambutol
Mycobacterium avium intracellulare	This pathogen is the most common isolated cause of infection among all patients with acquired immunodeficiency syndrome (AIDS).	Wasting syndrome (fever, weight loss, and cachexia) Chronic diarrhea Progressive anemia Chronic malabsorption syndrome	Clarithromycin Ciprofloxacin Rifampin Ethambutol Amikacin Ansamycin
Cytomegalovirus	Infection may present as severe pneumonia in patients with human immunodeficiency virus infection.	Shortness of breath Dyspnea on exertion Dry, nonproductive cough Increased heart and respiratory rates Hypoxemia	DHPG-gancidozia
Pneumocystis carinii	*Pneumocystis carinii* is part of normal human flora and is usually benign except in cases of immunodeficiency.	Progressive dyspnea Tachypnea Persistent, nonproductive cough Fatigue	Prophylaxis: Aerosolized pentamidine AZT Treatment: Pentamidine

| *P. carinii* pneumonia is the most common cause of death in patients with AIDS. | Trimethoprim-sulfamethoxazole
Bactrim
Dapsone
Septra
Cotrimoxazole |

Source: Data from ML Galantino. Pulmonary Complications of HIV. In ML Galantino (ed), Clinical Assessment and Treatment of HIV: Rehabilitation of Chronic Illness. Thorofare, NJ: Slack, 1992;80.

Table 10-2. Neurologic Complications of Human Immunodeficiency Virus Infection

Complication	Clinical Presentation	Medications Used
Cerebral lymphoma Cerebral lymphoma is generally uncommon in the normal population. It is usually multifocal with diffuse brain infiltration.	Memory loss Confusion Lethargy Headache Seizures	Radiation therapy to entire cerebrum Chemotherapy
Cerebral toxoplasmosis Cerebral toxoplasmosis is the most common intracranial infection in patients with acquiredimmunodeficiency syndrome (AIDS). The infection is potentially curable if treatment is started early.	Hemiparesis Ataxia Aphasia Seizures Severe headaches Confusion Lethargy Fever	Pyrimethamine sulfonamides
Cryptococcal meningitis Cryptococcal meningitis is the most common fungal infection in the central nervous system. Complete resolution of this disease is unusual.	Headache Nausea Neck stiffness Altered level of consciousness	Antifungal therapy with: Amphotericin B Flucytosine (oral)
Cytomegalovirus (CMV) CMV may be clinically asymptomatic. Encephalitis is nonspecific and nonuniform in presentation.	Retinitis cerebral vasculitis	DHPG gancidozia

Herpes simplex virus type I The medial, temporal, and inferior frontal lobes are most commonly involved. Biopsy is required for definitive diagnosis.	Hemorrhagic encephalitis Aphasia Seizures Hemiparesis Blindness	Ara-A
Herpes zoster infection (HZV) HZV occurs in 5–10% of patients with HIV. HZV may develop in the asymptomatic stage of HIV infection.	Disseminated skin lesions Meningoencephalitis Transverse myelitis herpes zoster Ophthalmicus with vasculitis and contralateral hemiparesis Blindness	Acyclovir
Progressive multifocal leukoencephalopathy (PML) PML is an unusual demyelinating disease in the brain caused by a papovavirus.	Mental dysfunction Hemiparesis Aphasia Ataxia Cortical blindness	Nonspecific drug therapy (dependent on presentation)
AIDS dementia complex (ADC) ADC is also referred to as HIV encephalitis or subacute encephalopathy. Dementia may be the first sign of HIV infection.	Progressive cognitive loss Motor and behavioral dysfunction Apathy Social withdrawal Deterioration in handwriting Unsteady gait Paraparesis Urinary and fecal incontinence	Antiviral therapy, usually with AZT

Table 10-2. *Continued*

Complication	Clinical Presentation	Medications Used
HIV myopathy Autoimmunity and complications of AZT therapy are suggested causes of HIV myopathy.	Proximal muscle weakness that is symmetric and often in the face and neck	Corticosteroids
Peripheral neuropathy	Presentations vary depending on the type*	Tricyclic antidepressants Anticonvulsants Non-narcotic and narcotic analgesics
Polymyositis	Subacute proximal weakness	Immunosuppressants
Vacuolar myelopathy Vacuolar myelopathy is a specific pathologic abnormality found in patients with AIDS. No treatment has been reported to stop or reverse the disease progression.	Weakness Spasticity ataxia Urinary and fecal incontinence May be accompanied by dementia	Antivirals

*Six presentations of peripheral neuropathy include acute demyelinating peripheral neuropathy, chronic inflammatory peripheral neuropathy, mononeuritis multiplex peripheral neuropathy, progressive inflammatory peripheral neuropathy, sensory ataxic neuropathy, and distal symmetric peripheral neuropathy.

Source: Adapted from E Obbens, ML Galantin. Summary of Nervous System Disorders Associated with HIV. In ML Galantino (ed), Clinical Assessment and Treatment of HIV: Rehabilitation of Chronic Illness. Thorofare, NJ: Slack, 1992;87–94.

Table 10-3. Protective Equipment Used for Standard Precautions

Type of Precaution	Mask	Gown	Gloves	Glasses or Face Shield
Blood and body fluid	—	X	X	X
Contact	X	X	X	—
Drainage and secretions	—	X	X	—
Enteric	—	X	X	—
Respiratory	X	—	—	—
Strict	X	X	X	—
Tuberculosis	X	X	—	—

X = protective device indicated; — = protective device not indicated.
Source: Reprinted with permission from WT Kuntz. The Acute Care Setting. In EA Hillegass, HS Sadowsky (eds), Essentials of Cardiopulmonary Physical Therapy. Philadelphia: Saunders, 1994;613.

- Monitoring the temperature curve and WBC count of patients with infectious processes helps determine the appropriateness of physical therapy intervention. There will be times when the infectious process flares, and rest, rather than activity, is indicated. Clarification with the physician or nurse before physical therapy intervention is helpful in making this decision.

References

1. Smeltzer SC, Bare BG. Brunner and Suddarth's Textbook of Medical-Surgical Nursing (7th ed). Philadelphia: Lippincott, 1992.
2. Thomas CL. Taber's Cyclopedic Medical Dictionary (17th ed). Philadelphia: Davis, 1993.
3. Goodman CC, Snyder TEK. Differential Diagnosis in Physical Therapy: Musculoskeletal and Systemic Conditions. Philadelphia: Saunders, 1995.
4. Gorbach SL, Bartlett JG, Blacklow NR. Infectious Diseases. Philadelphia: Saunders, 1992.
5. Thompson JM, McFarland GK, Hirsch JE, et al. Mosby's Manual of Clinical Nursing (2nd ed). St. Louis: Mosby, 1989.
6. Anderson KN. Mosby's Medical, Nursing, and Allied Health Dictionary (4th ed). St. Louis: Mosby, 1994.
7. Rytel MW, Mogabgab WJ. Clinical Manual of Infectious Diseases. Chicago: Year Book, 1984.
8. Berkow R, Fletcher AJ. Merck Manual of Diagnosis and Therapy (16th ed). Rahway, NJ: Merck Research Laboratories, 1992.

9. Black JM, Matassarin-Jacobs E. Luckmann and Sorenen's Medical-Surgical Nursing: A Psychophysiologic Approach (4th ed). Philadelphia: Saunders, 1993.
10. Shovein J, Young MS. MRSA: Pandora's box for hospitals. Am J Nurs 1992;2:49.
11. The Hospital Infection Control Practices Advisory Committee. Special communication: Recommendations for preventing the spread of vancomycin resistance. Am J Infect Control 1995;23:87.
12. Galantino ML. Clinical Assessment and Treatment of HIV: Rehabilitation of a Chronic Illness. Thorofare, NJ: Slack, 1992.
13. Chandrasoma P, Taylor CR. Concise Pathology (2nd ed). East Norwalk, CT: Appleton & Lange, 1995.
14. Bullock BL. Pathophysiology: Adaptations and Alterations in Function (4th ed). Philadelphia: Lippincott, 1996.

Appendix 10-A:
Disorders of Altered Immunity

Systemic Lupus Erythematosus

Systemic lupus erythematosus (SLE) is a chronic connective tissue disorder thought to be the result of an abnormal immune response to a variety of factors. A definitive cause is unknown; however, there is evidence to support theories of both viral and genetic etiologies of abnormal immune responses. SLE is characterized by a systemic, remitting and relapsing clinical presentation. Women and nonwhite individuals, ages 20–40 years, are most afflicted with SLE. Prognosis for 10-year survival after diagnosis is 90% [1]. The most common cause of death in SLE is renal failure and the second most common is CNS dysfunction.

Clinical presentation of SLE may include the following:

- Stiffness and pain in hands, feet, and large joints
- Red, warm, and tender joints
- Butterfly rash on face
- Renal disease or failure
- Fever, fatigue, anorexia, and weight loss
- Raynaud's phenomenon
- Headache, seizures, organic brain syndrome

- Hemolytic anemia
- Thrombocytopenia
- Leukopenia

Management of SLE may consist of corticosteroid therapy, dialysis, and renal transplantation [1, 2].

Sarcoidosis

Sarcoidosis is a systemic disorder that primarily affects the lungs and is characterized by granulomatous tissue formation in the affected areas. The definitive etiology is unknown, although an alteration in the immune mechanisms is suspected. The age of onset is 20–35 years. It occurs more commonly in women and nonwhite individuals. Sarcoidosis may have periods of progression and remission.

Clinical presentation of sarcoidosis may include the following:

- Bilateral hilar lymphadenopathy on chest x-ray
- Interstitial pneumonitis
- Pulmonary fibrosis
- Eye and skin lesions
- Fever, fatigue, and weight loss
- Hepatosplenomegaly
- Hypercalcemia
- Arthralgia, arthritis

Management of sarcoidosis usually consists of steroid therapy [1, 2].

Amyloidosis

Amyloidosis is a metabolic disorder characterized by deposition of amyloid (a type of protein) in various tissues and organs. Amyloidosis is classified according to protein type and tissue distribution. The etiology of amyloidosis is not fully understood; however, relation to a disordered reticuloendothelial system and abnormal immunoglobulin synthesis have been shown.

Clinical signs and symptoms are representative of the affected areas. The following areas may be affected:

- Tongue

- Heart

- Gastrointestinal tract

- Liver

- Spleen

- Kidney

- Peripheral nerves

- Pancreas

- Cerebral vessels

- Skin

In general, the deposition of protein in these areas will result in firmer, less distensible tissues that compromise organ function.

Management of amyloidosis consists of controlling any primary disease process that may promote deposition of amyloid into the tissues [1, 3].

References

1. Bullock BL. Pathophysiology: Adaptations and Alterations in Function (4th ed). Philadelphia: Lippincott, 1996.
2. Chandrasoma P, Taylor CR. Concise Pathology (2nd ed). East Norwalk, CT: Appleton & Lange, 1995.
3. Goodman CC, Snyder TEK. Differential Diagnosis in Physical Therapy: Musculoskeletal and Systemic Conditions. Philadelphia: Saunders, 1995.

11

Endocrine System

Jaime C. Paz

Introduction

The endocrine system consists of endocrine glands, which secrete hormones into the bloodstream, and target cells for those hormones. Target cells are the principal sites of action for the endocrine glands. Figure 11-1 displays the location of the primary endocrine glands.

The endocrine system has direct effects on cellular function and metabolism throughout the entire body, with symptoms of endocrine or metabolic dysfunction mimicking those of muscle fatigue. It is therefore important for the physical therapist to be able to distinguish between the source (endocrine versus musculoskeletal) of these symptoms to optimally care for the patient. For example, complaints of weakness and muscle cramps can result from either hypothyroidism or inappropriate exercise intensity. If the therapist is aware of the patient's endocrine history, inquiring about a recent medication adjustment may be more appropriate than adjustment of the patient's exercise parameters. The objectives of this chapter are to provide a basic understanding of the following:

1. Normal and abnormal functions of the endocrine system, including the thyroid, pituitary, adrenal, and parathyroid glands

2. Clinical assessment of the function of the thyroid, pituitary, adrenal, and parathyroid glands

3. Management of endocrine system dysfunction

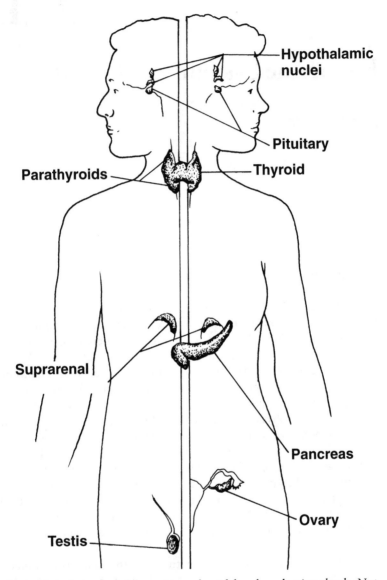

Figure 11-1. *Location of the major male and female endocrine glands. Not shown are the liver, gastrointestinal tract, pineal gland, thymus, and placenta, all of which secrete hormones. (Reprinted with permission from JS Boissonnault, D Madlon-Kay. Screening for Endocrine System Disease. In WG Boissonnault [ed], Examination in Physical Therapy: Screening for Medical Disease. New York: Churchill Livingstone, 1991;156.)*

4. Physical therapy guidelines for working with patients who have endocrine system dysfunction

Clinical Assessment

Screening for Metabolic and Endocrine Dysfunction

The following questions help provide a systematic method to differentiate the patient's symptoms and complaints to a specific endocrine gland. Full integration of the patient's signs and symptoms with laboratory data by the physician is, however, necessary to accurately assess the disorder. Physical therapists can use these questions to help guide their evaluations and organize inquiries for the medical team regarding treatment parameters. For instance, if the questions lead the therapist to suspect pituitary involvement, seeking clarification from the physicians regarding the appropriateness of physical therapy intervention may be necessary [1].

1. Pituitary

   a. Are menses regular? (If they are irregular, hypopituitarism may be suspected.)

   b. Has there been a change in vision? (Large pituitary tumors can result in vision loss.)

2. Adrenal

   a. Is there skin darkening? (Chronic primary adrenal insufficiency results in hyperpigmentation.)

   b. Is there weight loss, nausea, vomiting, or syncope? (These are suggestive of adrenal insufficiency.)

   c. Have there been episodes of tachycardia, headaches, and sweating? (These are suggestive of pheochromocytoma.)

3. Thyroid

   a. Is there a change in the patient's neck size? (This can indicate the presence of goiter or hyperthyroidism.)

   b. What is the room-temperature preference of the patient? (60°F suggests hyperthyroidism, whereas 80°F suggests hypothyroidism.)

4. Parathyroid

   a. Is there a history of thyroid surgery? (This is the usual cause of hypoparathyroidism.)

   b. Are kidney stones, polyuria, and constipation present? (This could indicate hypercalcemia from hypoparathyroidism.)

5. Pancreas

   a. Is there nocturia or noctidipsia (urination or drinking at night, respectively)? (Both of these can suggest diabetes mellitus.)

   b. Has there been a weight loss or gain and increased appetite? (These also suggest diabetes.)

General Assessment of Endocrine Function

Measurement of endocrine function can be performed by examining (1) the endocrine gland itself, using imaging techniques, or (2) levels of hormones or hormone-related substances in the bloodstream or urine. When reviewing the medical record, it is important for the physical therapist to know that high or low levels of endocrine substances can indicate endocrine dysfunction. A common method for assessing levels of hormone is radioimmunoassay [2]. Radioimmunoassay is an immunologic technique for comparing levels of radiolabeled hormone with unlabeled hormone, which compete for binding sites on a given antibody.

Another method of evaluation, referred to as *provocative testing*, can be classified into either suppression or stimulation tests. Stimulation tests are used for testing endocrine hypofunction; suppression tests are useful in endocrine hyperfunction diagnoses [3]. The most widely used endocrine tests are discussed in this chapter. Clinicians should refer to their particular institution's laboratory values (generally located in the back of the clinical record) for normal ranges of hormone or hormone-related substances referenced in their setting.

Clinical tip

An imbalance of hormone levels may affect the patient's tolerance to activity. Familiarity with the endocrine tests and values can help the clinician gauge the intended treatment

Table 11-1. Target Sites and Actions of Thyroid Gland Hormones

Hormone(s)	Target Site(s)	Action(s)
Thyroxine (T4) and triiodothyronine (T3)	Systemic	Metabolic rate, growth, and development
Thyrocalcitonin	Bone	Inhibits bone resorption Lowers blood levels of calcium

Source: Data from BF Fuller. Anatomy and Physiology of the Endocrine System. In CM Hudak, BM Gallo (eds), Critical Care Nursing: A Holistic Approach (6th ed). Philadelphia: Lippincott, 1994;75; and M Hartog (ed). Endocrinology. Oxford: Blackwell Scientific, 1987;23.

parameters (i.e., type, duration, and intensity) for the next session(s).

Thyroid Gland

Function

Table 11-1 summarizes the target sites and actions of the thyroid gland hormones.

Thyroid Tests

Thyroid hormones T4 and T3 circulate throughout the bloodstream either bound to proteins (approximately 99%) or unbound, in which case they are metabolically active by themselves. Thyroxine-binding globulin is the major thyroid transport protein. Serum levels of T4 and T3 are usually measured by radioimmunoassay. Table 11-2 describes the tests used to measure thyroid hormones and their normal laboratory values. Table 11-3 summarizes other tests used to measure thyroid function.

Clinical tip

- Low levels of thyroid hormones T3 or T4 may result in weakness, muscle aching, and stiffness. Based on this information, the physical therapist may decide to alter treatment

Table 11-2. Thyroid Hormone Tests

Hormone	Test Description	Normal Value
Serum thyroxine (T4)	Radioimmunoassay (RIA) measurement	5–12 µg/dl
Serum triiodothyronine (T3)	RIA measurement	90–190 ng/dl
Thyroid-stimulating hormone (TSH) TSH levels are directly influenced by T4 levels through a negative feedback loop.	Radioisotope and chemical labeling measurement	0.4–6.0 µU/ml
Thyrotropin-releasing hormone (TRH) TRH augments the function of TSH in patients with hypothyroidism.	Intravenous administration of TRH to patients to determine if TSH levels rise	Normal rise in men and women is 6 µU/ml above baseline TSH levels. Normal rise in men older than 40 years is 2 µU/ml above baseline. (Hypothyroidism is indicated by increased response to TRH, and hyperthyroidism is indicated by no response to TRH.)

Source: Data from WM Burch (ed). Endocrinology for the House Officer (2nd ed). Baltimore: Williams & Wilkins, 1988;1.

parameters by decreasing the treatment intensity to optimize activity tolerance, minimize patient discomfort, or both.

• Patients may be on bed rest or precautions after radionuclide studies. The physical therapist should refer to the physician's orders after testing to clarify the patient's mobility status.

Table 11-3. Thyroid Function Tests

Test	Description
Triiodothyronine resin uptake (T3U)	T3U indirectly measures the number of unoccupied protein binding sites for T4 and T3 by using radioisotopes. T3U qualifies levels of bound versus unbound T4 and T3.
Thyroidal 24-hour radioactive iodine uptake	Radioactive iodine is used to mark thyroid function and the percentage of total administered radioactivity taken up by the thyroid in 24 hours is calculated. Normal radioactive iodine uptake is 10–30%. (Hypothyroidism results in reduced uptake.)
Thyroid imaging or scan	Intravenous administration of radionuclides allows imaging or scanning of particular areas of the thyroid gland. Increased or decreased uptake of the radionuclide can help diagnose dysfunction.
Ultrasound	Nodules of the thyroid gland that are palpable or suspected may be delineated as cystic or solid lesions by ultrasound.
Needle biopsy	Fine needle aspiration of thyroid cells may help diagnose a suspected neoplasm.

Source: Data from WM Burch (ed). Endocrinology for the House Officer (2nd ed). Baltimore: Williams & Wilkins, 1988;1; and M Hartog (ed). Endocrinology. Oxford: Blackwell Scientific, 1987;25.

Thyroid Disorders

Disorders of the thyroid gland result from a variety of causes and can be classified as either hyper- or hypothyroidism.

Hyperthyroidism

Hyperthyroidism, or thyrotoxicosis, is characterized by excessive sympathomimetic and increased catabolic activity resulting from overexposure of tissues to thyroid hormones. The most common causes of hyperthyroidism are outlined in Table 11-4.

General signs and symptoms of hyperthyroidism include the following [1]:

Table 11-4. Common Causes of Hyperthyroidism

Cause	Description
Graves' disease	Graves' disease is a familial, autoimmune disorder responsible for approximately 80% of hyperthyroid cases. Distinguishing features include diffuse thyroid enlargement, ophthalmopathy, and pretibial myxedema (thickening, redness, and puckering of skin in the front of the shins).
Thyroiditis	Inflammation of the thyroid gland can be acute, subacute, or chronic, each with various causes. Pain may or may not be present on palpation.
Toxic multinodular goiter	Areas of the enlarged thyroid gland (goiter) become autonomous and unresponsive to thyroid-stimulating hormones.
Toxic thyroid adenoma	Solitary, benign follicular adenomas that function autonomously will result in hyperthyroidism if the adenoma nodule is greater than 4 cm in diameter.
Exogenous hyperthyroidism	Ingestion of excessive amounts of thyroid hormone or iodine preparation can be classified as iatrogenic hyperthyroidism, factitious hyperthyroidism, or iodine-induced hyperthyroidism.
Excessive production of thyroid-stimulating hormones	Pituitary tumors can result in the overproduction of thyroid-stimulating hormones, which then results in hyperthyroidism (rare occurrence).
Ectopic thyroid hormone production	Thyroid hormone can be produced from the ovaries or from metastatic follicular thyroid carcinoma (rare occurrence).

Source: Data from WM Burch (ed). Endocrinology for the House Officer (2nd ed). Baltimore: Williams & Wilkins, 1988;126.

- Nervousness, irritation, and emotional lability

- Fatigue and weakness

- Dyspnea

- Palpitations, atrial fibrillation, and tachycardia (heart rate of more than 90 beats per minute at rest)

- Increased perspiration

- Heat intolerance
- Increased appetite
- Hyperdefecation and weight loss
- Menstrual dysfunction
- Presence of goiter
- Moist and warm hands
- Smooth and velvety skin
- Tremor
- Lid lag, retraction, or both
- "Plumber's nails" (onycholysis)
- Thyroid bruit

Management of hyperthyroidism may consist of any of the following [4, 5]:

- Pharmacologic management with
    Antithyroid drugs of the thionamide series (e.g., propylthiouracil [PTU], methimazole [Tapazole])
    Beta-adrenergic blockers (e.g., propranolol [Inderal])
    Iodine (e.g., potassium or sodium iodide [Strong Iodine, Lugol's Solution])
    Corticosteroids
- Radioiodine-131
- Surgical thyroidectomy

Hypothyroidism

Hypothyroidism is the insufficient exposure of peripheral tissues to thyroid hormones. It affects growth and development, as well as many cellular processes. In the majority of cases, hypothyroidism is caused by decreased thyroid hormone production rather than the failure of tissues to respond to thyroid hormones. *Primary hypothyroidism* refers to thyroid gland dysfunction, whereas *secondary hypothyroidism* refers to pituitary disease resulting in reduced thyroid-stimulating hormone (TSH) levels.

The following are the causes of primary and secondary hypothyroidism [4]:

- Maldevelopment, hypoplasia, or aplasia of the thyroid gland
- Inborn deficiencies of biosynthesis or action of thyroid hormone
- Hashimoto's thyroiditis (autoimmune inflammation)
- Lymphatic thyroiditis (autoimmune inflammation that has hyperthyroid symptoms)
- Hypopituitarism or hypothalamic disease
- Severe iodine deficiency
- Thyroid ablation from surgery, radiation of cervical neoplasms, or radioiodine therapy for hyperthyroidism
- Drug toxicity (from amiodarone, antithyroids, or lithium)

General signs and symptoms of hypothyroidism vary according to the degree of thyroid deficiency. Signs and symptoms include the following [1]:

- Marked cold intolerance
- Weakness, muscle cramps, and aching and stiffness
- Hoarseness
- Decreased hearing
- Paresthesia
- Mild weight gain with normal appetite
- Constipation and ileus (decreased motility)
- Rough, scaly, dry, and cool skin and decreased perspiration
- Somnolence and slowness of thought
- Pallid and yellow-tinted skin
- Nonpitting edema of eyelids, hands, and feet
- Slow relaxation time of deep tendon reflexes
- Bradycardia

- Cardiac failure

- Pericardial effusion

- Hypertension

- Coma and respiratory failure in severe cases

- Bilateral carpal tunnel syndrome

Management of hypothyroidism typically consists of lifelong thyroid hormone replacement. Medications commonly used to treat hypothyroidism are the following [5]:

- Natural thyroid hormones (e.g., thyroid USP [Decloid, Thyrar, Thryrocrine, ThryroTeric], thyroglobulin [Proloid])

- Synthetic thyroid hormones (e.g., levothyroxine [Cytolen, Levoid, Levothroid, Synthroid sodium], liothyronine [Cytomel, Cytomine], and liotrix [Euthroid, Thyrolar])

- Adenohypophyseal hormones (e.g., TSH [TSH, Thytropar] and thyrotropin-releasing hormone [protirelin])

Clinical tip

Properly managed hyper- or hypothyroidism should not affect physical therapy intervention or activity tolerance. If the signs or symptoms mentioned above are present during physical therapy evaluation, treatment, or both, consultation with the medical team is indicated to help differentiate the etiology of the physical findings. See "Screening for Metabolic and Endocrine Dysfunction" for more screening information.

Pituitary Gland

Function

Table 11-5 summarizes the target sites and actions of the pituitary gland.

Table 11-5. Target Sites and Actions of Pituitary Gland Hormones

Hormone(s)	Target Site(s)	Action(s)
Anterior lobe		
Growth hormone	Systemic	Growth of bones, muscles, and other organs
	Liver	Formation of somatomedin
Thyrotropin	Thyroid	Growth and secretion activity of the thyroid gland
Adrenocorticotropin	Adrenal cortex	Growth and secretion activity of the adrenal cortex
Follicle-stimulating hormone	Ovaries	Development of follicles and secretion of estrogen
	Testes	Development of seminiferous tubules and spermatogenesis
Luteinizing or interstitial cell–stimulating hormone	Ovaries	Ovulation, formation of corpus luteum, and secretion of progesterone
	Testes	Secretion of testosterone
Prolactin or lactogenic hormone	Mammary glands	Secretion of milk
Melanocyte-stimulating hormone	Skin	Pigmentation
Posterior lobe		
Antidiuretic hormone	Kidney	Reabsorption of water and water balance
Oxytocin	Arterioles	Blood pressure regulation
	Uterus	Contraction
	Breast	Expression of milk

Source: Adapted from BF Fuller. Anatomy and Physiology of the Endocrine System. In CM Hudak, BM Gallo (eds), Critical Care Nursing: A Holistic Approach (6th ed). Philadelphia: Lippincott, 1994;875.

Pituitary Tests

Individual pituitary hormone levels can be measured (1) by random blood samples; (2) by blood samples before and after the administration of specific releasing substances, such as serum TSH, during a thyrotropin-releasing hormone test (see Table 11-2); or (3) by blood samples before and after the administration of specific stimuli acting directly on the pituitary or via the hypothalamus, such as serum growth hormone (GH), serum cortisol, and plasma adrenocorticotropic hormone (ACTH). Pituitary function can also be evaluated by (1) thyroid function tests, which are an indirect assessment of TSH secretion from the pituitary, and (2) plain x-rays or computed tomography with contrast to highlight a pituitary tumor [6].

Pituitary Disorders

Dysfunction of the pituitary-hypothalamic system generally results from hyper- or hyposecretion of tropic hormones. Hypersecretion of pituitary hormones (hyperpituitarism) is most commonly due to benign pituitary tumors. Hyposecretion of pituitary hormones (pituitary insufficiency) can result from pituitary disease, diseases affecting the hypothalamus or surrounding structures, or disturbance of blood flow around the hypothalamus and pituitary [7].

Hyperpituitarism

The overproduction of the pituitary hormones prolactin, GH, ACTH, and antidiuretic hormone (ADH) is discussed below.

Growth Hormone Overproduction

The most common presentation of excessive GH secretion is acromegaly in adults or gigantism in children.

Signs and symptoms of acromegaly include the following [1]:

- Enlargement of hands and feet
- Paresthesia of hands
- Sweating
- Headaches
- Joint pains, osteoarthritis
- Diabetes mellitus
- Coarse facial features with furrowed brows
- Carpal tunnel syndrome
- Greasy skin
- Hypertension

Management of acromegaly may consist of any of the following: surgical resection of lesion (if excess GH secretion is from a tumor); external irradiation, internal irradiation, or both; or bromocriptine administration.

Clinical tip

Given the multisystem effects in patients with acromegaly, activity progression should proceed cautiously with a focus on energy conservation and joint protection techniques.

Adrenocorticotropic Hormone Overproduction

An increase in ACTH production by the pituitary gland results in increased levels of serum cortisol, which is a glucocorticoid secreted by the adrenal glands. Glucocorticoids are involved with carbohydrate, protein, and fat metabolism; therefore, excess cortisol levels affect these cellular processes. Any clinical syndrome that results in glucocorticoid excess is called Cushing's syndrome. Cushing's disease, however, is specific to pituitary lesions that cause bilateral adrenal hyperplasia and will not be discussed in this chapter [1].

Signs and symptoms of Cushing's syndrome include the following [6]:

- Rounding and redness of face

- Weight gain (particularly in the torso)

- Easy bruising, thinning of the skin, and presence of striae and darker pigmentation

- Proximal muscle weakness

- Backache

- Depression

- Hirsutism

- Oligomenorrhea or amenorrhea

- Diabetes mellitus

- Short stature (in children)

- Osteoporosis (radiographically confirmed)

• Hypertension

• Peripheral edema

Management of Cushing's syndrome may consist of any of the following: surgical resection of pituitary lesion or hypertrophied adrenal glands, radiation or chemotherapy for the lesion, or medical management with ketoconazole.

Clinical tip

Management of weakness, myopathy, pain, edema, and osteoporosis should be the focus of physical therapy intervention and be complementary to the medical management of the patient. Blood pressure changes during activity should be monitored given the possibility of hypertension. Caution should also be taken to avoid bruising during mobility. Refer to "Diabetes Mellitus" for further activity considerations.

Antidiuretic Hormone Overproduction
The syndrome of inappropriate secretion of ADH (SIADH) is a condition of fluid and electrolyte imbalance resulting in hyponatremia (reduced sodium levels). In this condition, ADH is secreted when it should be inhibited. Several etiologies of SIADH exist, including head trauma, central nervous system neoplasms, pulmonary diseases, certain endocrinopathies, and some pharmacologic agents (e.g., morphine and barbiturates) [5]. A mild condition of SIADH is usually asymptomatic, but more severe cases can result in headaches; nausea; confusion; intracellular edema, which is present before peripheral edema is noticeable; and cerebral edema that leads to coma (in severe cases).

Management of SIADH may consist of any of the following: treatment of the underlying cause, fluid restriction, or administration of diuretics.

Clinical tip

The physical therapist should be aware of fluid restriction guidelines for patients with SIADH, especially because activity during physical therapy may increase the patient's thirst. These guidelines are often posted at the patient's bedside.

Hypopituitarism

The most common causes of primary (pituitary directly affected) or secondary (hypothalamus or pituitary stalk affected) hypopituitarism are listed in Table 11-6. Symptoms, physical findings, and management depend on the extent of the disorder and the specific hormone and target cells affected. Patients with complete pituitary hormone deficiency (panhypopituitarism) present with the following [6]:

- Hypogonadism
- Dilutional hyponatremia
- Diabetes insipidus (DI)
- Short stature (in children)
- Hypothyroidism
- Glucocorticoid deficiency

Management of panhypopituitarism may consist of any of the following: replacement therapy with thyroxine, glucocorticoids, and GH for children; desmopressin for diabetes insipidus; androgen therapy for men; or estrogen therapy for women younger than 50 years of age.

Diabetes Insipidus

DI involves the excretion of a large volume (i.e., greater than 30 ml/kg/day) of dilute urine (hypotonic polyuria). DI may result from pituitary, renal, or psychogenic disorders. Pituitary DI (i.e., central, cranial, or neurogenic DI) involves the failure to synthesize or release vasopressin (ADH). Renal, or nephrogenic, DI is a deficiency of vasopressin receptors in the renal collecting ducts. Psychogenic or dipsogenic DI involves a large intake of fluid that may suppress ADH secretion [4–6].

Signs and symptoms of DI may be transient or permanent and include the following [4, 5]:

- Polyuria
- Thirst (especially for cold or iced drinks)
- Polydipsia
- Constipation
- Weight loss

Table 11-6. Causes of Hypopituitarism

Primary hypopituitarism

Pituitary tumors
    Intrasellar and parasellar regions

Infarction or ischemic necrosis
    Ischemia or necrosis occurring postpartum (Sheehan's syndrome)
    Shock
    Sickle cell anemia
    Carotid artery aneurysm or thrombosis
    Diabetes mellitus

Inflammatory disease
    Meningitis (tuberculosis, fungal, malarial)
    Pituitary abscess

Infiltrative disorders
    Hemochromatosis

Idiopathic
    Selective hormone deficiency
    Isolated growth hormone deficiency
    Isolated adrenocorticotropic hormone deficiency
    Isolated thyroid-stimulating hormone deficiency
    Hypogonadotropic hypogonadism
    Multiple hormone deficiency

Iatrogenic
    Surgical destruction
    Irradiation to sella turcica or nasopharynx

Secondary hypopituitarism

Destruction of stalk
    Trauma
    Compression by mass
    Surgical transection

Hypothalamic disease
    Inflammation (sarcoidosis, eosinophilic granuloma)
    Trauma
    Hormone-induced (high glucocorticoids)
    Tumors
    Toxic (vincristine)
    Behavior
        Starvation
        Anorexia nervosa

Source: Reprinted with permission from WM Burch. Endocrinology (3rd ed). Baltimore: Williams & Wilkins, 1994;97.

- Dry skin with decreased turgor

- Central nervous system presentations (e.g., irritability, mental dull-ness, ataxia, hyperthermia, and coma) if access to water is interrupted

Management of DI may consist of pharmacologic treatment, such as the following: vasopressin (Aqueous Pitressin, Pitressin Tannate in oil), lypressin nasal solution (Diapid Nasal Spray, synthetic lysine), desmo-pressin (DDAVP), synthetic arginine, chlorpropamide, clofibrate, car-bamazepine, or a combination of thiazides and mild salt depletion (for nephrogenic DI) [4, 5].

Adrenal Gland

Function

Table 11-7 summarizes the target sites and actions of the adrenal gland.

Adrenal and Metabolic Tests

Adrenal Tests

There are three primary types of hormones secreted by the adrenal cor-tex: glucocorticoids, androgens (i.e., estrogens, progesterone, and testosterone), and mineralocorticoids. Evaluation of each type of hor-mone is listed below [6].

Anatomic investigation of the adrenal glands may also provide insight into possible adrenal dysfunction. The most useful methods of investigation are computed tomography scan, radioisotope scan using seleno-cholesterol, ultrasound, arteriogram, adrenal venogram (allows measurements of hormone levels), and intravenous pyelogram (see Chapter 9, "Diagnostic Studies") [6].

Glucocorticoids

Glucocorticoids can be evaluated by testing serum cortisol levels, 24-hour urinary corticosteroids, or ACTH. Altered glucocorticoid levels affect protein and carbohydrate metabolism.

- Serum cortisol levels. Serum cortisol levels are measured by radioimmunoassay. For accuracy, notation should be made as to the time of day the serum was drawn because levels are highly depen-

Table 11-7. Target Sites and Actions of Adrenal Gland Hormones

Hormone(s)	Target site(s)	Action(s)
Cortex		
Mineralocorticoids (aldosterone)	Kidney	Reabsorption of sodium Elimination of potassium
Glucocorticoids (cortisol)	Systemic	Metabolism of carbohydrate, protein, and fat Response to stress Anti-inflammation
Sex hormones	Systemic	Preadolescent growth spurt
Medulla		
Epinephrine	Cardiac and smooth muscle, glands	Emergency functions Simulates the action of the sympathetic system
Norepinephrine	Organs innervated by sympathetic nervous system	Chemical transmitter substance Increases peripheral resistance

Source: Adapted from BF Fuller. Anatomy and Physiology of the Endocrine System. In CM Hudak, BM Gallo (eds), Critical Care Nursing: A Holistic Approach (6th ed). Philadelphia: Lippincott, 1994;875.

dent on the diurnal rhythm of secretion (i.e., maximum levels at 6–8 AM and minimum levels at night).

• Twenty-four–hour urinary corticosteroids. Analysis of urine over a 24-hour period to determine the urinary levels of corticosteroids will provide a rough outline of cortisol output.

• ACTH. Various assays are used to measure ACTH levels. ACTH levels are usually examined concomitantly with cortisol levels.

Androgens
Individual androgen levels can be measured by radioimmunoassay in the serum or by metabolic products (17-ketosteroids) in the urine. High concentrations of androgens may result in the following changes in females [1]:

• Hirsutism, which is excessive hair growth in skin zones considered male in distribution (i.e., upper lip, side burns, chin, neck, chest, and lower abdomen)

- Amenorrhea, which is the absence of menstruation in women older than 16 years of age or the absence of menses for longer than 6 months in women of childbearing age who had been previously menstruating

- Voice change

- Increased muscle mass

Mineralocorticoids

Mineralocorticoids can be evaluated by testing either serum electrolyte levels or plasma renin activity and aldosterone levels [6]. Abnormalities of serum electrolyte levels, such as an increased potassium level, provide a valuable screening tool for mineralocorticoid secretion disorders. Aldosterone is the primary mineralocorticoid and is controlled by the renin-angiotensin system. A rise in serum potassium and angiotensin II results in aldosterone secretion, which helps to balance fluid and electrolyte levels. Blood samples of aldosterone are usually taken first in the early morning while the patient is still recumbent and then again after 4 hours of being awake and active.

Metabolic Tests: Glucose Tolerance Test

A glucose tolerance test is the primary method of establishing the diagnosis of diabetes mellitus. It is performed only on subjects who have been on an unrestricted diet containing at least 300 g of carbohydrates per day and who have been physically active for 3 days before testing. Normal glucose values are (1) fasting glucose level of less than 115 mg/dl and (2) 2-hour plasma glucose level of less than 140 mg/dl.

To perform the test, a 75-g glucose load is given to the subject in the morning after a 10-hour fast. Blood glucose levels are then measured at 0, 30, 60, 90, and 120 minutes after the glucose administration. The subject must remain inactive and refrain from smoking throughout the duration of the test [1].

Adrenal Disorders

Adrenal Insufficiency

Autoimmune dysfunction can lead to destruction of the adrenal cortex (i.e., primary adrenal insufficiency or Addison's disease). Additionally, ACTH deficiency can lead to atrophy of the adrenal cortex (secondary adrenal insufficiency). The net result is an impaired adrenal system with decreased levels of glucocorticoids (cortisols), mineralocorticoids (aldosterone), and androgens. Aldosterone deficiency causes fluid and electrolyte imbalance primarily as a result of increased water excretion that leads to dehydration. Cortisol deficiency results in decreased gluconeogenesis (glucose production), which in turn alters cellular metabolism. Decreased gluconeogenesis also results in hypoglycemia and decreased ability to respond to stress [8].

The following are symptoms and physical findings common to adrenal insufficiency [1]:

- Weakness
- Fatigue
- Anorexia
- Nausea
- Vague abdominal pain
- Vomiting
- Salt craving in less than 20% of patients
- Weight loss
- Hyperpigmentation
- Hypotension

Management of adrenal insufficiency typically consists of pharmacologic intervention with any of the following steroids: hydrocortisone (Cortisol, Compound F), hydrocortisone acetate, prednisone (Deltasone), dexamethasone (Decadron, Dexasone), or fludrocortisone (Florinef) [5].

Pheochromocytoma
Pheochromocytoma is a rare adrenomedullary disorder caused by a tumor of the chromaffin cells in the adrenal medulla, which results in excess secretion of the catecholamines, epinephrine, and norepinephrine. The occurrence is more common in women 35–60 years of age.

Signs and symptoms of pheochromocytoma may include the following [1, 8]:

- Hypertension, palpitations, tachycardia, and postural hypotension
- Excessive perspiration

- Nervousness and emotional outbursts or instability
- Headache
- Elevated blood glucose levels and glucosuria

Management of pheochromocytoma may consist of surgical excision of the tumor or pharmacologic intervention with one of the following medications: alpha-adrenergic blocking agents (e.g., phentolamine [Regitine], phenoxybenzamine [Dibenzyline]), beta-adrenergic blocking agents (e.g., propranolol [Inderal]), or tyrosine inhibitors (alphamethlyparatyrosine [AMPT]) [5].

Metabolic Disorders

Diabetes Mellitus

Diabetes mellitus is a syndrome with metabolic, vascular, and neural components that originates from glucose intolerance that in turn leads to hyperglycemic states (increased plasma glucose levels). Hyperglycemia can result from insufficient insulin production, ineffective receptive cells for insulin, or both. Insulin promotes storage of glucose as glycogen in muscle tissue and the liver. Deficiency of insulin leads to increased levels of plasma glucose. The diagnosis of diabetes is based on the following three factors [1, 9]:

1. Multiple fasting plasma glucose levels that are greater than 140 mg/dl

2. Elevated plasma glucose levels (greater than 200 mg/dl) in response to an oral glucose tolerance test of a 75-g glucose load

3. Random plasma glucose levels above 200 mg/dl combined with symptoms of polydipsia, polyphagia, and polyuria

The two primary types of diabetes mellitus are insulin-dependent (IDDM), or type I, and non–insulin-dependent (NIDDM), or type II. Other forms of glucose intolerance disorders exist but are not discussed in this text.

Insulin-Dependent Diabetes Mellitus

IDDM is an autoimmune disorder that has a genetic-environmental etiology that leads to the selective destruction of pancreatic B cells. This destruction results in decreased or absent insulin secretion [9, 10]. Other etiologies for IDDM (type I diabetes) exist but are not discussed in this text.

Signs and symptoms of IDDM can include the following [9]:

- Hyperglycemia
- Polydipsia
- Polyuria
- Polyphagia
- Weight loss
- Fatigue

Management of IDDM may consist of any of the following: insulin administration; diet modification based on caloric content, proportion of basic nutrients and optimal sources, and distribution of nutrients in daily meals; meal planning; or exercise [10].

Clinical tip

- Hypoglycemia may occur during exercise or up to 24 hours afterward because of an inability to regulate insulin levels. To help prevent this, the patient should consume extra carbohydrates before and during exercise (e.g., 10 g of carbohydrates per 30 minutes of activity), and the nurse may also decrease the dose or rate of insulin infusion.

- Circulation of insulin that is injected into an exercising limb is enhanced as a result of increased blood flow and temperature. The injection into the exercising limb may therefore lead to hypoglycemia. Insulin can be injected into the abdomen to help prevent this process.

- Insulin is necessary to modulate lipolysis and hepatic (liver) glucose production during exercise. Performing exercise without adequate insulin can lead to hyperglycemia and ketogenesis.

- The physical therapist should inquire about the patient's blood glucose levels before and after exercise to assist in physical therapy planning.

- Coordinating physical therapy sessions with meals and insulin injections may help optimize exercise tolerance.

- Keeping graham crackers close by when working with diabetic individuals is helpful in case hypoglycemia does occur with activity.

Non–Insulin-Dependent Diabetes Mellitus

NIDDM is more common in the United States than IDDM and generally occurs after 40 years of age. Type II diabetes is significantly linked to obesity. Obesity results in decreased ability of B cells in the pancreas to respond to elevated plasma glucose levels with the appropriate insulin secretion [9, 10]. Other etiologies for type II diabetes exist but are not discussed in this text.

Signs and symptoms of NIDDM may be similar to those of IDDM but can also include the following:

- Recurrent infections and prolonged wound healing

- Genital pruritus

- Visual changes

- Paresthesias

Management of NIDDM may consist of any of the following [10]:

- Weight loss through dietary and behavior modification

- Exercise

- Insulin administration (if other measures are not effective)

- Pharmacologic intervention with sulfonylureas (which increase insulin production and effectiveness) listed below:
      Tolbutamide (Orinase, Oramide)
      Tolazamide (Tolinase, Ronase, Tolamide)
      Chlorpropamide (Diabinese)
      Acetohexamide (Dymelor)
      Glyburide (DiaBeta, Micronase)
      Glipizide (Glucotrol)

Complications of Diabetes Mellitus

Patients with diabetes mellitus, despite management, can still develop organ and organ system damage linked to lesions of the small and large blood vessels. Complications can manifest 2–15 years after diagnosis.

They can be classified as (1) microangiopathy (microvascular disease), which causes retinopathy, nephropathy, and foot ischemia; (2) macroangiopathy (macrovascular disease), which accelerates widespread atherosclerosis; or (3) neuropathy [10]. Another complication from diabetes that is not directly linked to vascular damage is ketoacidosis.

Ketoacidosis. The metabolic syndrome of diabetes mellitus gradually progresses from mild to moderate glucose intolerance to fasting hyperglycemia to ketosis and finally to ketoacidosis. Most patients do not progress to the ketotic state but have the potential to do so if proper treatment is not administered [7].

Diabetic ketoacidosis is the end result of ineffective levels of circulating insulin, which leads to elevated levels of ketone bodies in the tissues. This state of an elevated level of ketone bodies is referred to as ketosis. Decreased insulin levels lead to uncontrolled lipolysis (fat breakdown), which increases the levels of free fatty acids in the liver and ultimately leads to an overproduction of ketone bodies. Ketone bodies are acids, and if they are not buffered properly by bases, a state of ketoacidosis occurs. Ketoacidosis almost always results from uncontrolled diabetes mellitus; however, it may also result from alcohol abuse [7].

The following are signs and symptoms of diabetic ketoacidosis [7]:

- Polyuria
- Polydipsia
- Weakness and lethargy
- Myalgia
- Headache
- Anorexia
- Nausea, vomiting
- Abdominal pain
- Dyspnea
- Hypothermia
- Acute abdomen
- Stupor (coma)
- Hypotonia

- Dehydration
- Uncoordinated movements
- Hyporeflexia
- Fixed, dilated pupils
- Deep and sighing respirations (Kussmaul's)
- Acetone-smelling ("fruity") breath

Management of diabetic ketoacidosis may consist of any of the following: insulin administration, hydration, electrolyte (sodium, potassium, and phosphorus) replacement, or supplemental oxygen or mechanical ventilation [9].

Nephropathy. See Chapter 9 for a discussion of nephropathy.

Diabetic Foot. Foot lesions in diabetics are common and multifactorial in nature. Lesions may result from any combination of the following [10]:

- Loss of sensation from sensory neuropathy
- Skin atrophy from microangiopathy
- Decreased blood flow from macroangiopathy
- Autonomic neuropathy resulting in abnormal blood distribution that may cause bone demineralization and Charcot's joint (disruption of the midfoot)

Proper foot care in diabetic individuals helps prevent complications, such as poor wound healing, which can progress to tissue necrosis and ultimately lead to amputation. Table 11-8 describes patient information regarding diabetic foot care.

Coronary Artery Disease. See Chapter 1, "Myocardial Ischemia," for a discussion of coronary artery disease.

Stroke. See Chapter 4, "Cerebrovascular Accident," for a discussion of stroke.

Peripheral Vascular Disease. See Chapter 6, "Atherosclerosis," for a discussion of peripheral vascular disease.

Infection. Individuals with diabetes are at a higher risk for infection because of (1) decreased sensation (both vision and touch); (2) poor

Table 11-8. Diabetic Foot Care

Do	Don't
Inspect feet daily for abrasions, blisters, and cuts. Use a mirror if soles cannot be seen. If vision is poor, another person should check feet.	Smoke.
	Wash feet in cold or hot water. The water temperature should be lukewarm (approximately 85–95°F)
Wash feet daily with lukewarm water and soap. Carefully dry, especially between the toes.	Use a heating pad, heating lamp, or hot water bottles to warm the feet.
Apply hand cream or lanolin to feet (dry areas). Be careful not to leave cream between the toes.	Use razor blades or scissors to cut corns or calluses. Have a podiatrist per.-form this procedure.
	Use over-the-counter medications on corns or calluses.
Wear clean socks or stockings daily.	Cross legs when sitting.
Cut nails straight across and file down edges with an emery board.	Wear girdles or garters.
	Walk barefoot.
Wear comfortable shoes that fit and don't rub. A wide toe-box is recommended.	Wear shoes without socks or stockings.
Inspect the inside of shoes for any objects, tacks, or torn linings before putting on the shoes.	Wear sandals with thongs between the toes.
Make sure a physician checks feet at each visit.	Wear socks or stockings with raised seams.

Source: Data from WM Burch (ed). Endocrinology for the House Officer (2nd ed). Baltimore: William & Wilkins, 1988;59.

blood supply, which leads to tissue hypoxia; (3) hyperglycemic states, which promote rapid proliferation of pathogens that enter the body; (4) decreased immune response from reduced circulation, which leaves white blood cells unable to get to affected area; (5) impaired white blood cell function, which leads to abnormal phagocytosis; and (6) chemotaxis [9].

Diabetic Neuropathy. The exact link between neural dysfunction and diabetes is unknown; however, the vascular and metabolic changes that occur with diabetes can promote destruction of myelin sheaths and therefore interfere with normal nerve conduction.

Neuropathies can be manifested as (1) focal mononeuropathy and radiculopathy (disorder of single nerve or nerve root), (2) symmetric sensorimotor neuropathy, associated with disabling pain and depression, or (3) autonomic neuropathy. Generally, sensory deficits occur in a "glove-and-stocking" pattern, with loss of pinprick and light touch sensations in these areas. Sensory deficits are greater than motor deficits. Foot ulcers and footdrop are common manifestations of diabetic neuropathies. Table 11-9 outlines the signs and symptoms of the different types of diabetic neuropathy [6, 9, 10].

Hypoglycemia (Hyperinsulinism)

Hypoglycemia is a state of decreased blood sugar levels. Excess serum insulin results in decreased blood sugar levels, which leads to symptoms of hypoglycemia. Causes of this imbalance of insulin and sugar levels can be grouped as (1) fasting, (2) postprandial, or (3) induced. Fasting hypoglycemia occurs before eating and can be caused by (1) an insulin-producing islet cell tumor, (2) an extrapancreatic neoplasm, or (3) leucine. It can also occur in infants with diabetic mothers. Postprandial hypoglycemia occurs after eating and can be caused by (1) reactive hypoglycemia, (2) early diabetes mellitus, or (3) rapid gastric emptying. Hypoglycemia can also be induced by external causes, such as exogenous insulin or miscellaneous drugs [5].

Signs and symptoms of hypoglycemia may include the following:

- Tachycardia and hypertension
- Hunger
- Weight changes
- Tremor
- Headache
- Mental dullness, confusion, and amnesia
- Seizures
- Paralysis and paresthesias
- Dizziness

Table 11-9. Signs and Symptoms of Diabetic Neuropathy

Classification of Diabetic Neuropathy	Subjective Complaints Commonly Found in Physical Therapy Evaluation	Signs Commonly Found in Physical Therapy Evaluation
Symmetric polyneuropathies		
Peripheral sensory polyneuropathy	Paresthesias Numbness, coldness, tingling (mainly in feet) Pain, often disabling, worse at night	Absent ankle jerk Impairment of vibration sense in feet Foot ulcers (often over metatarsal heads)

Peripheral motor neuropathy	Complaints of weakness	Bilateral
		  Interosseous muscle atrophy
		  Claw or hammer toes
		  Decreased grip strength
		  Decreased manual muscle test grades

Autonomic neuropathy	Diarrhea after meals Bladder problems Distal anhidrosis (symmetric) Impotence Dysphagia	Orthostatic hypotension Elevated resting heart rate Peripheral edema
Focal and multifocal neuropathies		
Cranial neuropathy	Pain behind or above the eye Headaches Facial pain	Palpebral ptosis Inward deviation of one eye

Table 11-9. *Continued*

Classification of Diabetic Neuropathy	Subjective Complaints Commonly Found in Physical Therapy Evaluation	Signs Commonly Found in Physical Therapy Evaluation
Trunk and limb mononeuropathy	Abrupt onset of cramping or lancinating pain Hyperalgesia with hyperesthesia Cutaneous hyperesthesia of the trunk	Peripheral nerve-specific motor loss Abdominal wall weakness
Proximal motor neuropathy or diabetic amyotrophy	Pain in proximal lower limbs that is worse at night	Asymmetric proximal weakness Atrophy in lower limbs Absent or diminished knee jerk

Source: Reprinted with permission from JS Boissonnault, D Madlon-Kay. Screening for Endocrine System Disease. In WG Boissonnault (ed), Examination in Physical Therapy: Screening for Medical Disease. New York: Churchill Livingstone, 1991;159.

Table 11-10. Primary Tests Used to Evaluate Parathyroid Function

Test	Description
Serum calcium*	Measurements of blood calcium levels (8.5–10.2 mg/dl) indirectly examines parathyroid function. Low calcium levels stimulate parathyroid hormone secretion.
Parathyroid hormone	Radioimmunoassays and urinalysis are used to measure parathyroid hormone levels.

*Parathyroid glands are the primary regulators of serum calcium.
Source: Data from WM Burch. Endocrinology for the House Officer (2nd ed). Baltimore: Williams & Wilkins, 1988.

- Irritability

- Visual disturbance

- Loss of consciousness

Management of hypoglycemia may consist of any of the following: dietary modifications, surgery (e.g., subtotal pancreatectomy, insulinoma resection), or pharmacologic agents (e.g., diazoxide [Hyperstat] or streptozocin [Zanosar]) [5].

Parathyroid Gland

Function

Parathyroid hormone (PTH) is the primary hormone secreted from the parathyroid gland. The target sites are the kidney, intestine, and bone. The actions of PTH are to promote bone resorption, increase calcium absorption, and raise blood calcium levels [11].

Parathyroid Tests

Table 11-10 summarizes the primary tests used to evaluate parathyroid function.

Parathyroid Disorders

Hyperparathyroidism

Hyperparathyroidism is a disorder caused by overactivity of one or more of the parathyroid glands that leads to increased PTH levels, which then increases blood calcium levels, decreases bone mineralization, and decreases kidney function. Hyperparathyroidism can be classified as primary, secondary, or tertiary. Primary hyperparathyroidism usually results from hyperplasia or an adenoma in the parathyroid gland(s). Secondary hyperparathyroidism results from another organ system disorder such as renal failure, osteogenesis imperfecta, Paget's disease, multiple myeloma, or bone metastases. Tertiary hyperparathyroidism occurs when PTH secretion is autonomous despite normal or low serum calcium levels [8].

Signs and symptoms of hyperparathyroidism may include the following [8]:

- Hypercalcemia and hypercalciuria (calcium in urine)

- Bone demineralization and resorption (which causes skeletal changes such as dorsal kyphosis)

- Backache, joint and bone pain, and pathologic fractures

- Kidney stone formation, abdominal pain, peptic ulcer disease

- Nausea, thirst, anorexia, constipation

- Hypertension, dysrhythmias

- Listlessness, depression, and paranoia

- Decreased neuromuscular excitability

Management of hyperparathyroidism may consist of any of the following [5, 8]:

- Parathyroidectomy
- Pharmacologic intervention with the following:
  Diuretic agents (e.g., furosemide [Lasix])
  Phosphates
  Parathyroid agents (e.g., calcitonin [Calcimar, Cibacalcin])
  Bone resorption inhibitors (e.g., mithramycin [Mithracin] and gallium nitrate [Ganite])

- Fluid replacement

- Dietary modification (a diet low in calcium and high in vitamin D)

Hypoparathyroidism

Hypoparathyroidism is a disorder caused by underactivity of one or more of the parathyroid glands that leads to decreased PTH levels. Decreased levels of PTH occur most commonly as a result of damage to the parathyroid glands during thyroid or parathyroid surgery. Damage to the parathyroid glands can occur less commonly from autoimmune dysfunction.

Signs and symptoms of hypoparathyroidism may include the following [8]:

- Hypocalcemia

- Increased neuromuscular irritability (tetany)

- Painful muscle spasms

- Tingling of the fingers

- Laryngospasm

- Dysrhythmias

- Lethargy

- Personality changes

- Thin, patchy hair

- Brittle nails

- Dry, scaly skin

- Convulsions

- Cataracts

Management of hypoparathyroidism may consist of any of the following [5, 8]:

- Dietary modifications that promote a diet high in calcium and low in phosphate

- Pharmacologic intervention with the following:
  PTH

Vitamins
  Dihydrotachysterol (Hytakerol)
  Dihydroxycholecalciferol
  Calciferol (Vitamin D$_2$)
Nutritional supplements
  Calcium gluconate
  Calcium glubionate
  Calcium lactate
  Calcium chloride

Metabolic Bone Disorders

Paget's Disease

Paget's disease is a bone disease of unknown etiology that usually presents after the age of 40 years. The primary feature is thick, spongy bone that is unorganized as a result of excessive osteoclastic and subsequent osteoblastic activity. Some evidence points to an inflammatory or viral origin. Fractures and compression of the cranial nerves (especially the eighth nerve) and spinal cord are complications of Paget's disease.

Paget's disease is generally asymptomatic; however, the following clinical manifestations may present:

- Bone pain that is unrelieved by rest and persists at night

- Bone deformity (e.g., skull enlargement, bowing of leg and thigh)

- Increased warmth of overlying skin of affected areas

Management of Paget's disease may consist of any of the following: administration of calcitonin or diphosphonates, promotion of mobility, or adequate hydration.

Osteoporosis

Osteoporosis is a multifactorial bone disorder that leads to decreased bone volume and trabecular bridging. Trabecular bone (e.g., vertebrae, femoral head, distal radius) is more affected than cortical bone (long bone shafts) [1]. Osteoporosis can be classified as type I or II. Type I osteoporosis occurs in women 51–65 years of age, who may present with a vertebral fracture. Type II (senile) osteoporosis affects both men and women older than 70 years of age, who may present with fractures of both the trabecular and cortical bone.

Risk factors for osteoporosis in women include the following: white or Asian race, petite frame, inadequate dietary intake of calcium, positive family history of osteoporosis, alcohol abuse, cigarette smoking, sedentary lifestyle, reduced bone mineral content (most predictive factor), and early menopause or oophorectomy (ovary removal) [1].

Signs and symptoms of osteoporosis may include the following [1]:

- Back pain (aggravated by movement or weightbearing, relieved by rest)
- Vertebral deformity (kyphosis and anterior wedging)
- Presence of compression fractures

Management of osteoporosis may consist of any of the following: supplementation with calcium, estrogen, or vitamin D; calcitonin supplementation (increases total body calcium), biphosphonate supplementation (inhibits bone resorption); fluoride supplementation (increases bone mass); physical therapy; or fracture management (e.g., acute bed rest followed by early ambulation) [3].

Clinical tip

An abdominal corset can provide additional support for stable vertebral compression fracture(s). Also, using a rolling walker that is adjusted higher than normal can promote a more upright posture. Both of these techniques may also help to decrease back pain in patients with osteoporosis. Gentle exercises to improve the strength of thoracic extensors can also assist with posture and reduced pain.

Osteomalacia

Osteomalacia, or rickets in children, is a disorder characterized by decreased bone mineralization, reduced calcium absorption from the gut, and compensatory hyperparathyroidism. The etiology of osteomalacia stems from any disorder that lowers serum phosphate or calcium levels.

Signs and symptoms of osteomalacia may include the following [6]:

- Softening of cranial vault (in children)

- Swelling of costochondral joints (in children)
- Predisposition to femoral neck fractures (in adults)
- Bone pain and tenderness
- Proximal myopathy
- Waddling gait

Medical management of osteomalacia may consist of treatment of the underlying or predisposing condition or supplementation with calcium and vitamin D.

Management

Clinical management of endocrine dysfunction is discussed earlier in specific endocrine gland and metabolic disorders sections. This section focuses on goals and guidelines for physical therapy intervention.

Physical Therapy Intervention

The following are general physical therapy goals and guidelines for working with patients who have endocrine or metabolic dysfunction. These guidelines should be adapted to a patient's specific needs. Clinical tips are provided throughout the chapter to address specific situations in which the tips may be most helpful.

Goals

The primary physical therapy goals in this patient population are the following: (1) to optimize functional mobility, (2) to maximize activity tolerance and endurance, (3) to prevent skin breakdown in the patient with altered sensation (e.g., diabetic neuropathy), (4) to decrease pain (e.g., in patients with osteoporosis or hyperparathyroidism), and (5) to maximize safety for prevention of falls, especially in patients with altered sensation or muscle function.

Guidelines

Patients with diabetes or osteoporosis represent the primary patient population with which the physical therapist intervenes. Physical therapy considerations for these patients are discussed in the form of clinical tips in earlier sections: "Diabetes" and "Osteoporosis," respectively.

For other patients with endocrine or metabolic dysfunction, the primary physical therapy treatment guidelines are the following:

1. It may be necessary to decrease exercise intensity when the patient's medication regimen is being adjusted to improve activity tolerance. For example, a patient with insufficient thyroid hormone replacement will fatigue more quickly than a patient with adequate thyroid hormone replacement. In this example, knowing the normal values of thyroid hormone and following the laboratory tests will help the therapist gauge treatment intensity.

2. Consult with the clinical nutritionist to help determine the appropriate activity level, based on the patient's caloric intake, since caloric intake and metabolic processes are affected by endocrine and metabolic disorders.

References

1. Burch WM. Endocrinology for the House Officer (2nd ed). Baltimore: Williams & Wilkins, 1988.
2. Bullock BL. Pathophysiology: Adaptations and Alterations in Function (4th ed). Philadelphia: Lippincott, 1996.
3. Diagnostic Procedures. In JM Thompson, GK McFarland, JE Hirsch, et al., Mosby's Manual of Clinical Nursing Practice (2nd ed). St. Louis: Mosby, 1989;1594.
4. Lavin N. Manual of Endocrinology and Metabolism (2nd ed). Boston: Little, Brown, 1994.
5. Allen MA, Boykin PC, Drass JA, et al. Endocrine and Metabolic Systems. In JM Thompson, GK McFarland, JE Hirsch, et al. (eds), Mosby's Manual of Clinical Nursing Practice (2nd ed). St. Louis: Mosby, 1989;876.
6. Hartog M. Endocrinology. Oxford: Blackwell Scientific, 1987.
7. Hershman JM. Endocrine Pathophysiology: A Patient-Oriented Approach (3rd ed). Philadelphia: Lea & Febiger, 1988;225.
8. Black JM, Matassarin-Jacobs E. Luckmann and Sorensen's Medical Surgical Nursing: A Psychophysiologic Approach (4th ed). Philadelphia: Saunders, 1993.
9. McCance KL, Huether SE. Pathophysiology: The Biologic Basis for Disease in Adults and Children (2nd ed). St. Louis: Mosby, 1994;674.
10. Lorenzi, M. Diabetes Mellitus. In PA Fitzgerald (ed), Handbook of Clinical Endocrinology (2nd ed). East Norwalk, CT: Appleton & Lange. 1992;463.
11. Hudak CM, Gallo BM. Critical Care Nursing: A Holistic Approach (6th ed). Philadelphia: Lippincott, 1994;874.

Suggested Reading

Boissonnault JS, Madlon-Kay D. Screening for Endocrine System Disease. In WG Boissonnault (ed), Examination in Physical Therapy: Screening for Medical Disease. New York: Churchill Livingstone, 1991;153.

Smeltzer SC, Bare BG. Brunner and Suddarth's Textbook of Medical-Surgical Nursing (7th ed). Philadelphia: Lippincott, 1992;1074.

I

Medical Record Review

Michele Panik

The medical record is a legal document that chronicles a patient's clinical course during hospitalization and is the primary means of communication between the various health care providers caring for a single patient.

The organization of the medical record can vary from institution to institution; however, the medical record is typically composed of three major sections:

1. **Doctor's order book (DOB).** The DOB is a log of all instructions of the plan of care for the patient, including medications, diagnostic or therapeutic tests and procedures, vital sign parameters, activity level, diet, the need for consultation services, and resuscitation status. The physical therapist's ability to take a verbal order varies according to hospital and departmental policies.

2. **History.** The history portion of the record includes a physician admission note and progress notes (a shortened version of the initial note with emphasis on the physical findings, assessment, and plan), a nursing admission assessment and problem list, consult service notes from physicians and allied health professionals, and operative and procedure notes.

3. **Reports.** A variety of reports are filed chronologically in individual sections in the medical record (e.g., radiologic or laboratory reports).

The following outline summarizes the basic format of the admission (initial) note written by a physician in the medical record. The italicized items indicate the standard information the physical therapist should review before beginning physical therapy intervention.

I. History (subjective information) [1]

    A. Data that identify the patient, including the source and degree of reliability of the information

    B. History of present illness (HPI), including the *chief complaint* and a chronological list of the problems associated with the chief complaint

    C. *Past medical or surgical history* (PMH, PSH) and *risk factors* for disease (e.g., history of smoking)

    D. Family health history (If the family members are deceased, the relation, age, and reason for death should be noted.)

    E. Social history (e.g., *psychosocial support* or *architectural barriers at home*)

    F. *Current medications*, including level of *compliance*

II. The physical examination (objective information). Positive (abnormal) findings are described in detail according to the following outline:

    A. General information, including *vital signs, laboratory findings, mental status,* and appearance

    B. *Head, eyes, ears, nose, throat (HEENT), and neck*

    C. *Chest*

    D. *Heart (Cor)*

    E. *Abdomen*

    F. *Extremities* (musculoskeletal)

    G. *Neurologic*

III. Assessment. The assessment is a statement of the condition and prognosis of the patient in regard to the chief complaint and medical-surgical status. If the etiology of the problem(s) is unclear, differential diagnoses are listed.

IV. Plan. The plan of care includes further observation, tests, laboratory analysis, consultation with additional specialty services or providers, pharmacologic therapies, other interventions, and discharge planning.

References

1. Seidel HM, Ball JW, Dains JE, Benedict GW. Mosby's Guide to Physical Examination (3rd ed). St. Louis: Mosby–Year Book, 1995;823.

II

Fluid and Electrolyte Imbalances

Jaime C. Paz

Many systemic disorders can result in one or more fluid and electrolyte imbalances that can influence physical therapy intervention. Insight into these imbalances can help the therapist decide how to modify the treatment plan (i.e., change treatment parameters, await medical stabilization of the imbalances, or both). Discussion with the physician or nurse helps to confirm these decisions. The most common fluid and electrolyte imbalances are described in Table II.1 in terms of the most common contributing factors; clinical findings, which can influence physical therapy; and the laboratory findings. Figure II.1 demonstrates how the electrolytes are generally schematically represented in the medical record [1].

Table II.1. Electrolyte Imbalances

Electrolyte Imbalance	Definition	Contributing Factors	Clinical Findings	Laboratory/Diagnostic Findings
Hypovolemia	Fluid volume deficit	Vomiting, diarrhea, fever, blood loss, and uncontrolled diabetes mellitus	Weak, rapid pulse; decreased blood pressure; dizziness; thirst; confusion; and muscle cramps	Increased hemoglobin, hematocrit, BUN, and creatinine levels
Hypervolemia	Fluid volume excess	Renal failure, congestive heart failure, and prolonged corticosteroid therapy	Shortness of breath, increased blood pressure, bounding pulse, and presence of cough	Decreased hemoglobin and hematocrit levels
Hyponatremia	Sodium deficit (serum sodium level of <135 mEq/liter)	Diuretic therapy, renal disease, hyperglycemia, and congestive heart failure	Lethargy, confusion, muscle cramps, and muscular twitching	Decreased urine and serum sodium levels
Hypernatremia	Sodium excess (serum sodium level of >145 mEq/liter)	Diabetes insipidus; hyperventilation; and excessive corticosteroid, sodium bicarbonate, or sodium chloride administration	Elevated body temperature, lethargy, irritability, and pulmonary edema	Increased serum sodium and decreased urine sodium levels
Hypokalemia	Potassium deficit (serum potassium level of <3.5 mEq/liter)	Diarrhea, vomiting, gastric suction, corticosteroid therapy, and digoxin therapy	Fatigue, muscle weakness, ventricular fibrillation, paresthesias, leg cramps, and decreased blood pressure	ST depression or prolonged PR interval on ECG

| Hyperkalemia | Potassium excess (serum potassium level of >5.0 mEq/liter) | Renal failure, Addison's disease, burns, and use of potassium-conserving diuretics | Vague muscular weakness, bradycardia, dysrhythmia, flaccid paralysis, paresthesia, irritability, and anxiety | ST depression; tall, tented T waves; or absent P waves on ECG |

BUN = blood urea nitrogen; ECG = electrocardiogram.

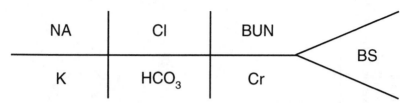

Figure II.1. *Schematic representation of electrolyte levels. (Na = sodium; Cl = chloride; BUN = blood urea nitrogen; BS = blood sugar; K = potassium; HCO₃ = bicarbonate; Cr = creatinine.)*

References

1. Mulvey M. Fluid and Electrolytes: Balance and Disorders. In SC Smeltzer, BG Bare (eds), Brunner and Suddarth's Textbook of Medical-Surgical Nursing (8th ed). Philadelphia: Lippincott, 1996;231.

III-A

Supplemental Oxygen Delivery Systems

Sean M. Collins

Supplemental oxygen delivery systems are indicated in acute conditions when (1) partial pressure of arterial oxygen (PaO_2) is less than 60 mm Hg or (2) when arterial saturation (SaO_2) is below 90%. Tissue hypoxia is commonly assumed to be present at these laboratory levels [1].

The systemic effects of supplemental oxygen delivery systems include the following:

- Supplemental oxygen can decrease cardiac output and myocardial workload [2].

- Small increases in SaO_2 can be related to large increases in PaO_2 (see Chapter 2, Figure 2-9).

- Supplemental oxygen can depress respiratory drive in patients with chronic lung disease [3].

- If the supplemental oxygen is humidified, mucociliary clearance is enhanced.

Physical therapy considerations include the following:

- Close monitoring of SaO_2, PaO_2, and hemodynamic parameters is necessary with patients receiving supplemental oxygen before, during, and after physical therapy intervention [3].

- Ensure that the oxygen tank is sufficiently full before proceeding with activity that requires supplemental oxygen.

See Table III-A.1 for a description of supplemental oxygen delivery systems for the spontaneously breathing patient.

Table III-A.1. Supplemental Oxygen Delivery Systems for Spontaneously Breathing Patients

System	FIO_2	Considerations
Nasal cannula[a]	1 lpm = 24% 2 lpm = 28% 3 lpm = 32% 4 lpm = 36% 5 lpm = 40% 6 lpm = 44%	FIO_2 values are based on constant normal minute volume. Patients must inhale through their nose to get maximum benefit. Nasal cannula is not recommended for patients who are mouth breathers or in situations of respiratory distress.
Standard face mask[a] Simple	5–6 lpm = 35% 6–7 lpm = 45% 7–10 lpm = 55%	The standard face mask is recommended for mouth breathers. Use a properly sized face mask because the exact FIO_2 can fluctuate according to fit of mask. A variation of the simple face mask is the face tent, which is useful for patients who have large jaws or experience discomfort when wearing face masks.
Aerosol	8–15 lpm with range of 28–98%	See Simple face mask, above.
Controlled O_2 delivery (Venturi) mask[b]	Varied lpm flow settings for FIO_2 that are between 24% and 50%	Controlled oxygen delivery masks that have adapters with different size apertures for FIO_2 determination.

System	FiO_2	Considerations
Reservoir system[a]		
Partial rebreathing mask	4–10 lpm with a range of 40–60% for a partial rebreathing mask	A reservoir bag is required with a face mask that provides an adequate seal.
Nonrebreathing mask	and 60–100% for a nonbreathing mask	

FiO_2 = fraction of inspired oxygen; lpm = liter per minute.
[a]Low-flow system of oxygen administration that does not guarantee delivery of the prescribed amount of FiO_2. Delivery of FiO_2 depends on the patient's ventilatory pattern and anatomic dead space [4].
[b]High-flow system of oxygen administration that is more accurate than a low-flow system because FiO_2 does not change with the patient's ventilatory pattern [4].

References

1. Anonymous. ACCP-NHLBI National Conference on Oxygen Therapy. Chest 1984;86:234.
2. DeGautre JP, Demenighetti G, Naeije R, et al. Oxygen delivery in acute exacerbation of chronic obstructive disease. Effects of controlled oxygen therapy. Am Rev Respir Dis 1981;124:26.
3. Marino P. The ICU Book. Philadelphia: Lea & Febiger, 1991.
4. Kersten LD. Oxygen Therapy. In LD Kersten (ed), Comprehensive Respiratory Nursing: A Decision-Making Approach. Philadelphia: Saunders, 1989;600.

III-B

Mechanical Ventilation

Sean M. Collins

Mechanical ventilatory support provides positive pressure to inflate the lungs. Patients with acute illness, serious trauma, exacerbation of chronic illness, or progression of chronic illness may require mechanical ventilation [1].

The following are physiologic objectives of mechanical ventilation [2]:

- Support or manipulate pulmonary gas exchange
- Increase lung volume
- Reduce or manipulate the work of breathing

The following are clinical objectives of mechanical ventilation [2]:

- Reverse hypoxemia and acute respiratory acidosis
- Relieve respiratory distress
- Reverse ventilatory muscle fatigue
- Permit sedation, neuromuscular blockade, or both
- Decrease systemic or myocardial oxygen consumption, and intracranial pressure
- Stabilize the chest wall
- Provide access to tracheal-bronchial tree for pulmonary hygiene
- Provide access for delivery of an anesthetic, analgesic, or sedative medication

The following are indications for mechanical ventilation [2]:

- Partial pressure of arterial oxygen (PaO_2) of less than 50 mm Hg with supplemental oxygen
- Respiratory rate of more than 30 breaths per minute
- Vital capacity less than 10 liters per minute
- Negative inspiratory force of less than 25 cm H_2O
- Protection of airway from aspiration of gastric contents

Process of Mechanical Ventilation

Intubation

Before initiation of mechanical ventilation, an artificial airway should be placed (*intubation*). Intubation is the passage of a tube into the patient's trachea, generally through the mouth (endotracheal tube intubation) or occasionally through the nose (nasotracheal intubation). The process of removing the artificial airway is called *extubation*.

When patients require ventilatory support for a prolonged time period, a tracheostomy is considered. According to one author, it is best to allow 1 week of endotracheal intubation, then if extubation seems unlikely during the next week, tracheostomy should be considered [1]. A tracheostomy tube is inserted directly into the anterior trachea below the vocal cords and is generally performed in the operating room. Benefits of tracheostomy include (1) reduced laryngeal injury, (2) improved oral comfort, (3) decreased airflow resistance, (4) increased effectiveness of airway care, and (5) feasibility of oral feeding and vocalization. If the patient is able to be weaned from ventilatory support, humidified oxygen can be delivered through a tracheostomy mask.

Cuff

Approximately 0.5 in. from the end of an endotracheal or tracheal tube is a cuff (balloon). The cuff is inflated to (1) ensure that all of the supplemental oxygen being delivered by the ventilator via the artificial airway enters the lungs and (2) help hold the artificial airway in place. Cuff inflation pressure should be adequate to ensure that no air is leaking around the tube; however, cuff pressures should not exceed 20 mm Hg. High cuff pressures have been linked to tracheal damage and scarring.

Clinical tip

• A cuff leak should be suspected if the patient is able to phonate or audible sounds come from his or her mouth.

• Cuff leaks can occur if the endotracheal tube is shifted (positional leak) or if the pressure changes in the cuff.

• If a cuff leak is suspected, the respiratory therapist or nurse should be notified. (Physical therapists who specialize in critical or cardiopulmonary care may be able to address this issue according to the facility's guidelines.)

Ventilatory Settings

Ventilatory settings are the parameters that provide the necessary support to meet the patient's individual ventilatory and oxygenation needs [3]. Settings can range from providing total support (no assistance by the patient) to minimal support (near total work performed by the patient). Establishment of the parameters is dependent on the patient's (1) arterial blood gas levels, (2) vital signs, (3) airway pressures, (4) lung volumes, and (5) pathophysiologic condition, including his or her ability to spontaneously breathe [3].

Settings That Affect Oxygenation

Fraction of Inspired Oxygen

Fraction of inspired oxygen (FIO_2) is the percentage of inspired air that is oxygen. At normal lung volumes and flow rates, an FIO_2 of 21% (ambient air) yields a normal oxygen partial pressure of 95–100 mm Hg. Patients who are having difficulty with oxygenation may require an increase in FIO_2 because an increased percentage of oxygen delivered to the alveoli results in a greater driving force of oxygen into the blood [2].

Positive End Expiratory Pressure

Positive end expiratory pressure (PEEP) is the pressure maintained by the mechanical ventilator in the airways at the end of expiration. Normal physiologic PEEP (maintained by sufficient surfactant levels) is considered to be 5 cm H_2O. This value is routinely used as an initial setting for PEEP. The setting is then adjusted, as needed, to maintain functional residual capacity above closing capacity in order to avoid closure of alveoli. Closure of alveoli can result in shunting of blood past the alveoli without gas exchange, which results in decreased oxygenation [2].

Settings That Affect Ventilation

Respiratory Rate
Respiratory rate is set according to the amount of spontaneous ventilatory efforts that the patient makes. Different ventilatory modes, described in "Modes of Ventilation," are prescribed according to the patient's needs. In general, patients who are unable to generate any spontaneous breaths are fully ventilated at respiratory rates of 12–20 breaths per minute [2]. This rate is then adjusted accordingly for those who are able to generate spontaneous breaths.

Tidal Volume
Tidal volume is the amount of volume delivered with each breath. It is adjusted with respiratory rate to control partial pressure of arterial carbon dioxide ($PaCO_2$).

Inspiratory Flow Rate
The inspiratory flow rate is set ideally to match the patient's peak inspiratory demands. If this match is not correct, it can cause the patient discomfort in breathing with the ventilator [2].

Inspiratory-to-Expiratory Ratio
To maximize comfort, the inspiratory-to-expiratory ratio is set with the goal of allowing the ventilator to be as synchronous as possible with the patient's respiratory ratio. In patients who are not spontaneously breathing, this ratio is set according to what is required to maintain adequate ventilation and oxygenation [2].

Modes of Ventilation

Control Mode

The control mode of ventilatory assist or controlled mechanical ventilation (CMV) is characterized by total control of the patient's ventilation. It is indicated for patients who have no respiratory drive or spontaneous breaths. Control mode has a prescribed rate, FiO_2, tidal volume, and flow rate. Inspiratory and expiratory ratios are also predetermined.

Assisted Ventilation

Assisted ventilation (AV) allows the patient to control the breathing pattern and the respiratory rate. The patient initiates each breath by lowering the airway pressure to open a unidirectional valve that is part of a circuit. Once initiated, the ventilator delivers the desired volume. The amount of volume delivered with each breath and the flow rate of inspiration can be manipulated according to the patient's needs [2].

During assisted ventilation, however, the patient's respiratory muscles do not fully rest. The diaphragm still initiates each breath and does not stop when the machine is triggered. If the parameters are not adjusted properly or weaning support is performed too quickly, a patient can experience respiratory muscle fatigue and shortness of breath. Oxygenation and minute volumes, however, are maintained without difficulty. With AV, patients who have very high respiratory rates will trigger the ventilator frequently and can produce respiratory alkalosis and auto PEEP.

Auto PEEP occurs when the lung volumes fail to return to functional residual capacity before the onset of the next inspiration. The process that leads to auto PEEP is referred to as *dynamic hyperinflation* [2]. The primary consequence is increased air trapping, which results in decreased gas exchange and increased work of breathing. Increased air trapping can occur (1) when the minute ventilation is too high, (2) in ventilated patients with obstructive disease, (3) when the endotracheal tube is too narrow or kinked, (4) when there is excess water condensation in the tubes, or (5) with any combination of these.

Intermittent Mandatory Ventilation

Intermittent mandatory ventilation (IMV) delivers breaths intermittently at a set rate per minute with a set volume and flow rate per breath [2]. The patient is allowed to spontaneously breathe in between machine-delivered breaths. It is different from AV in that every attempt to breathe by the patient is not followed by a machine breath. A problem can arise with IMV if the patient tries to exhale during the mechanical inspiratory phase.

Synchronous Intermittent Mandatory Ventilation

Synchronous IMV is similar to AV in that it delivers a breath only when the patient first initiates a breath [2]. Mandatory breaths, however, are delivered by the machine, if the patient does not initiate a breath for a preset period of time.

Pressure Support Ventilation

Pressure-support ventilation (PSV) is similar to IMV because it augments spontaneous breathing. It is similar to AV because it augments every breath. The difference, however, is that the breath delivered is not of a set volume. Instead, it is delivered at a set pressure. The result is that PSV increases the tidal volume and reduces the work of breathing [2]. With PSV, the patient indirectly controls the rate, tidal volume, and minute ventilation. It is also important to note that the inspiratory time in PSV is controlled by the patient, and in AV the inspiratory time is preset.

Pressure-Control Ventilation

Pressure-control (PC) ventilation delivers an airway pressure at a prescribed rate for a predetermined inspiratory time interval [2]. The inspiratory time is usually prolonged, and patients are generally sedated because of discomfort due to the prolonged mechanical inspiration. The total volume is set by lung compliance.

Continuous Positive Airway Pressure

Continuous positive airway pressure (CPAP) is intended to decrease the work of breathing by reducing the airway pressure necessary to generate inspiration throughout the respiratory cycle while the patient is spontaneously breathing [2]. The positive pressure is maintained above atmospheric pressure. CPAP is most commonly used during weaning from the mechanical ventilator or in an attempt to postpone intubation in patients with acute respiratory distress syndrome, chronic obstructive pulmonary disease, refractory hypoxemia, or any combination of these. CPAP can be delivered via an endotracheal tube or a specially designed face mask. These masks are typically uncomfortable, however, and poorly tolerated by patients.

High-Frequency Ventilation

High-frequency ventilation is a relatively rare technique of ventilation that is administered with frequencies of 100–3,000 breaths per minute and consequently small tidal volumes of 1–3 ml/kg. The primary advantage is the dramatic reduction in the pressure in the airways. High-frequency ventilation has shown beneficial results in neonates with acute respiratory distress syndrome [2]. It is contraindicated in patients with obstructive airway disease due to the risk of hyperinflation [2].

Inverse-Ratio Ventilation

Inverse-ratio ventilation is also a rarely used technique that involves the use of an inspiratory-to-expiratory ratio of more than 1 to 1. This can be delivered as a pressure-controlled or volume-cycled mode. The proposed benefit of such a mode is the recruitment of a greater number of lung units during the respiratory pause and longer inspiration [2]. There is a potential risk of generating auto PEEP and dynamic hyperinflation.

Complications of Mechanical Ventilation

The following are possible complications of mechanical ventilation [2, 3]:

- Improper intubation
  Improper intubation can result in esophageal or tracheal tears. If the artificial airway is mistakenly placed in the esophagus and is not detected, gastric distention can occur with the initiation of positive pressure.

- Barotrauma
  Trauma due to high pressures can result in a pneumothorax, especially in patients with emphysema.

- Oxygen toxicity
  Oxygen levels that are too high and maintained for a prolonged time period can result in (1) substernal chest pain that is exacer-

bated by deep breathing, (2) dry cough, (3) tracheal irritation, (4) pleuritic pain with inspiration, (5) dyspnea, (6) nasal stiffness and congestion, (7) sore throat, and (8) eye and ear discomfort.

- Cardiovascular complications   High positive pressures can result in decreased cardiac output from compression of great vessels by overinflated lungs.

Weaning from Mechanical Ventilation

The process of decreasing or discontinuing mechanical ventilation in a patient is referred to as the *weaning process* [3]. This process involves many different techniques. None of these techniques has been proven superior to another; however, there are correct and incorrect ways to wean patients from mechanical ventilation [2].

Five major factors to consider during a patient's wean are the following [3]:

1. Respiratory load and the ability of the neuromuscular system to cope with the load

2. Oxygenation

3. Cardiovascular performance

4. Psychological factors

5. Adequate rest and nutrition

The following are signs of increased distress during a ventilator wean [3]:

- Increased tachypnea (greater than 30 breaths per minute)

- Agitation, panic, diaphoresis, or tachycardia unrelieved by assurance or adjustment of the mechanical ventilation system

- Drop in pH to less than 7.25–7.30 associated with an increasing $PaCO_2$

Physical Therapy Indications

A patient who is mechanically ventilated may require ventilatory support for a prolonged period of time. Patients who require prolonged ventilatory support are at risk for developing pulmonary complications, skin breakdown, joint contractures, and deconditioning from bed rest. Physical therapy intervention, including functional mobility, can help prevent or reverse these complications despite mechanical ventilation.

References

1. Marino P. The ICU Book. Philadelphia: Lea & Febiger, 1991.
2. Slutsky AS. Mechanical ventilation. American College of Chest Physicians' Consensus Conference [see comments]. Chest 1993;104:1833. [Published erratum appears in Chest 1994;106:656.]
3. Gerold KB. Physical therapists' guide to the principles of mechanical ventilation. Cardiopul Phys Ther 1992;3:8.

III-C

Life Support Devices

Sean M. Collins

Life support devices assist with circulation or oxygenation in critically ill patients.

Circulatory Support Devices

Intra-Aortic Balloon Pump

The intra-aortic balloon pump (IABP) consists of a sausage-shaped balloon that is attached to a catheter inserted into the thoracic aorta via the femoral artery. The balloon inflates during ventricular filling (diastole) and deflates during ventricular contraction (systole). This is referred to as *counterpulsation*. The blood in the aorta is then propelled forward into the systemic circulation. The deflation of the balloon just before aortic valve opening decreases afterload and reduces resistance to ejection of blood during systole.

The following are indications for IABP:

- Left ventricular failure

- Unstable angina

- Cardiogenic shock

- Papillary muscle dysfunction

- Ventricular septal defect

- Refractory ventricular dysrhythmias

- Patients awaiting heart transplantation

The ratio of heart beats to counterpulsations of the IABP indicates the amount of circulatory support an individual needs (e.g., 1 to 1 is one counterpulsation to one heart beat; 1 to 8 is one counterpulsation to every eight heart beats; a ratio of 1 to 1 provides maximum circulatory support). Weaning from IABP involves gradually decreasing the number of counterpulsations to heart beats and is usually done to the point at which there is one counterpulsation for every eighth heart beat, as tolerated, before discontinuing the IABP.

The following are complications of IABP:

- Ischemia of the involved limb secondary to occlusion of femoral artery from compression or from thrombus formation

- Slippage of the balloon resulting in occlusion of subclavian or renal arteries

---

Clinical tip

During IABP, the lower extremity in which femoral access is obtained cannot be flexed at the hip.

Ventricular Assist Device

A ventricular assist device (VAD) is an extracorporal pump that pumps 25–50% of the systemic blood flow around a failing ventricle, thereby allowing the myocardium to rest. The following are three types of VAD:

1. A left VAD has surgically placed tubes in the left atrium and aorta that carry the blood surgically placed into the left atrium and aorta.

2. A right VAD has tubes placed into the right atrium and pulmonary artery.

3. A biVAD is used for both right- and left-sided heart failure. Tubes are placed in both atria and both outflow arteries.

VAD is indicated in cases of refractory cardiogenic shock or persistent ventricular failure and for patients awaiting heart transplantation.

Weaning from VAD involves a gradual decrease in flow rates, which allows the patient's ventricle to contribute more to total systemic circulation.

Complications of VAD include (1) thrombosis, (2) bleeding, and (3) infection.

Oxygenation Support Devices: Extracorporal Membranous Oxygenation

Extracorporal membranous oxygenation (ECMO) involves the use of a device external to the body for blood oxygenation. This allows the lungs to rest. ECMO is routinely used for neonates with respiratory failure. The use of ECMO in adults is variable from physician to physician because research has shown mortality rates of 40–90% [1, 2].

The use of ECMO is reserved for patients with reversible cardiac or pulmonary failure who in the acute stage of failure have a 90% mortality risk [2].

ECMO is obtained with the insertion of large catheters that shunt the blood through the oxygenator by either venovenous or venoarterial access.

In weaning from ECMO, blood pressure and cardiac and urinary output are monitored in patients with cardiac failure to determine tolerance to withdrawing ECMO support. In patients with respiratory failure, arterial oxygen partial pressure (PaO_2), carbon dioxide partial pressure ($PaCO_2$), and mixed venous oxygen saturation are monitored. Consistent improvement in these values helps determine the patient's ability to be weaned from ECMO.

Bleeding and infection are possible complications of ECMO.

Physical Therapy Considerations

*   Patients requiring the use of life support devices are on bed rest, and therapy usually consists of bronchopulmonary hygiene and air-

way clearance, along with the prevention of secondary complications of bed rest such as joint contracture and skin breakdown.

- Special care should be taken to avoid disruption of the tubes associated with these devices.

- Range of motion exercises should not be performed on extremities with catheters unless otherwise cleared by the physician.

References

1. Zapol WM, Snider MT, Hill JD, et al. Extracorporeal membranous oxygenation in severe acute respiratory failure: A randomized prospective study. JAMA 1979;242:2193.
2. Anderson H, Steimle C, Shapiro M, et al. Extracorporeal life support for adult cardiorespiratory failure. Surgery 1993;114:161.

IV-A

Peripheral and Central Lines and Intracranial Pressure Monitoring

Sean M. Collins

Peripheral and Central Lines

This appendix provides a basic explanation of lines commonly encountered by the physical therapist in the acute care setting. Lines are categorized by access location: peripherally, centrally, or intracranially.

The two primary uses of peripheral and central lines are the following [1]:

1.   Gaining access to the arterial (intra-arterial) system, the venous (intravenous) system, or both for obtaining blood or infusing fluids, medications, or blood

2.   Monitoring the patient's hemodynamic condition, intracranial pressure (ICP), or both

Peripheral Lines

Peripheral lines refer to lines entering into the circulation through a peripheral vessel (Table IV-A.1). Complications associated with peripheral lines include the following [2]:

- Local complications—Hematoma, cellulitis, thrombosis, phlebitis

Table IV-A.1. Common Locations, Indications, and Monitoring Values of
Peripheral Lines

Access	Location	Indication	Normal Values

Venous
  Intravenous
    line
	External
	  jugular
	Forearm
	Hand
		Administration of
		  drugs and fluids
		Blood transfusion
		Obtaining venous
		  blood
			Not applicable

Arterial			

Arterial line	Radial
	  artery
	Brachial
	  artery
		Monitoring arterial
		  blood pressure
		  directly with
		  digital display
		Access for arterial
		  blood gas
		  measurements
			BP = $\dfrac{100–140}{60–80}$
			MAP = 82–102
			Arterial blood gas
			  measurements
			PaO_2 = 80–100
			  mm Hg
			$PaCO_2$ = 35–45
			  mm Hg
			pH = 7.35–7.45

BP = blood pressure (systolic/diastolic) in mm Hg average for normal adults (see
Chapter 1 for further detail); MAP = mean arterial pressure (systolic + 2(diastolic)/3)
in mm Hg; PaO_2 = partial pressure of oxygen in mm Hg; $PaCO_2$ = partial pressure of
carbon dioxide mm Hg.
Source: Data from P Marino. The ICU Book. Philadelphia: Lea & Febiger, 1991.

- Systemic complications—Sepsis, pulmonary thrombosis, catheter
  fragment emboli, air embolism

Central Lines

Central lines enter through a peripheral vessel and travel to the heart
(Table IV-A.2). Complications associated with central lines include the
following [2]:

- Thrombosis or phlebitis into deep iliac veins or vena cava

- Possible loss of limb from arterial cannulation

- Compromised airway from hematoma

Table IV-A.2. Common Locations, Indications, and Monitoring Values of Central Lines

Name	Location	Indication	Normal Values
Central venous line	Subclavian or internal jugular vein Femoral vein	Monitoring central venous pressure Administering drugs, fluids, TPN Blood transfusions Obtaining venous blood	CVP = 0–8
Swan-Ganz catheter (PA line)	Subclavian or internal jugular vein	Calculation of the following: RVPs PA mean wedge pressure PCWP Left ventricular end diastolic pressure CO CI	RAP = 0–8 RVP = 20–25 4–8 PAP = 20–25 6–12 PCWP = 6–12 CO = 4–5 CI = 2.5–3.5
		PAP (systolic/diastolic)	
Percutaneous intracardiac cathether	Forearm vein to right atrium	Administration of drugs,* fluids, TPN Blood transfusions Obtaining venous blood	Not applicable

PA = pulmonary artery; CVP = central venous pressure in mm Hg; RAP = right atrial pressure in mm Hg; RVP = right ventricle pressure (systolic/diastolic) in mm Hg; PAP = pulmonary artery pressure (systolic/diastolic) in mm Hg; PCWP = pulmonary capillary wedge pressure, CO = cardiac output in liters/min, CI = cardiac index (CO/body surface area) in liters/min/m^2; TPN = total parenteral nutrition.
*The primary purpose of percutaneous intracardiac cathether line is for long-term antibiotic therapy without the complications of a peripheral line.
Source: Data from P Marino. The ICU Book. Philadelphia: Lea & Febiger, 1991.

- Damage to adjacent artery, nerve, or lymphatic duct
- Perforation of endotracheal tube cuff
- Pneumothorax or hemothorax
- Dysrhythmias from catheter tip

Physical Therapy Considerations for Central and Peripheral Lines

- The physical therapist should always ask for assistance when moving patients with invasive monitoring to avoid dislodging lines and catheters.

- To ensure accurate blood pressure measurement, the arterial line ("A-line") transducer should be at the level of the patient's heart. If the transducer is above or below the level of the heart, the patient's blood pressure reading will be falsely low or high, respectively. During functional mobility in the intensive care unit, the arterial line transducer can be attached to the patient's clothing with piece of tape at the level of the heart.

- When monitoring hemodynamic pressure during therapy sessions, the physical therapist should assess both the numeric value and the corresponding waveforms to be sure of accurate pressure readings. An accurate pressure reading displays a biphasic sinusoidal waveform.

Intracranial Pressure Monitoring

ICP, normally 4–15 mm Hg, may be measured in a variety of ways depending on how urgently ICP values are needed and the patient's neurologic or hemodynamic stability. Table IV-A.3 describes the different types of ICP monitors.

Physical Therapy Considerations for Intracranial Pressure Monitoring

- As with hemodynamic monitoring, be aware of both the ICP value and the corresponding waveform on the monitor. A normal ICP waveform has a triphasic sinusoidal waveform and should correspond to heart rate. The waveform may change shape with Cheyne-Stokes respirations or if cerebral ischemia occurs.

- For some ICP monitors such as the intraventricular catheter, the sensor and the transducer must be level. Check for signs posted at the bedside that state at what level the sensor and transducer should be (e.g., at the level of the ear).

Table IV-A.3. Intracranial Pressure Monitors

Monitoring Device	Location of Sensor	Considerations
Subarachnoid bolt	Subarachnoid or subdural space	For short-term use or if cerebral edema prevents the use of other devices Poor to fair reliability
Epidural/subdural sensor	Epidural or subdural space	Fair reliability
Intraventricular catheter (ventriculostomy)	Anterior horn of lateral ventricle (nondominant hemisphere if possible)	Can drain cerebrospinal fluid if needed Risk of hemorrhage Very reliable
Fiberoptic transducer–tipped catheter	Subarachnoid space, within the ventricles, or within the parenchyma	Very reliable

Source: Data from LA Thelan, LD Urden, JK Davie. Essentials of Critical Care Nursing. St Louis: Mosby–Year Book, 1992.

- Momentary elevations in ICP will normally occur. It is sustained elevation in ICP that is of concern and that should be reported to the nurse. Patients with elevated ICP are often positioned with the head of the bed at 30 degrees, which maximizes venous blood flow from the brain to help decrease ICP. Therefore, be aware that lowering the head of the bed may increase ICP. Other positions that increase ICP are the Trendelenburg position and lateral neck and extreme hip flexion. Additional conditions that increase ICP are the Valsalva maneuver, noxious stimuli, pain, and coughing. If ICP increases during bronchopulmonary hygiene treatment (in the mechanically ventilated patient) because of elevated partial pressure of arterial carbon dioxide ($PaCO_2$), manually hyperventilate the patient with an Ambu bag at a rapid rate until the ICP returns to the baseline level.

References

1. Aelhert B. ACLS Quick Review Study Guide. St. Louis: Mosby, 1994.
2. Thelan LA, Urden LD, Davie JK. Essentials of Critical Care Nursing. St. Louis: Mosby–Year Book, 1992.

IV-B

Tubes

Sean M. Collins

This appendix provides a basic explanation of commonly encountered tubes in the acute care setting.

Tubes are used primarily for feeding and drainage. The following descriptions explain these two actions:

1. A feeding system is initiated when patients, because of medical or surgical reasons, cannot sufficiently take oral feedings and are at risk for caloric and nutritional depletion.

2. Drainage tubes drain from gastrointestinal and genitourinary systems and spaces of the body (e.g., peritoneal space, surgical sites). They are used in an attempt to return normal drainage to an area when patients are unable to drain normal gastrointestinal or genitourinary contents or abnormal fluids that may accumulate because of medical conditions, surgical conditions (e.g., surgical-site edema), or both. Insufficient drainage of substances can be toxic to the body.

Feeding and Drainage Tubes

Commonly used tubes, their locations, and purposes are described in Table IV-B.1.

Table IV-B.1. Common Types of Tubes, Their Locations, and Purposes

Type of Tube	Location	Purpose
Nasogastric (NGT)	Nose to stomach	Enteral feeding Gastric drainage
Gastrostomy (G-tube)	Surgically placed in the stomach	Enteral feeding Gastric drainage
Jejunostomy (J-tube)	Surgically placed in the jejunum	Enteral feeding Small intestine drainage
Rectal catheter	Rectum	Rectal drainage
Urinary catheter	Bladder	Bladder drainage Foley catheter into bladder Texas or condom catheter can be applied externally on males
Suprapubic tube	Bladder, surgically inserted proxi- mal to prostate	Bladder drainage in case of abnormal hypertrophy of prostate
Jackson-Pratt drain (J-P drain)	Surgical site	Drainage of local edema and bleeding
Hemovac	Surgical site	Drainage of local edema and bleeding

Physical Therapy Considerations for Patients With Tubes

• Patients on nasogastric, gastrostomy, and jejunostomy tube drainage may be on suction, which can usually be removed before mobilizing the patient. Temporarily removing the suction should be confirmed with the nurse.

• Enteral feedings should be temporarily turned off before and during bronchopulmonary hygiene treatments. They can also be temporarily disconnected for mobility treatments after confirming with the nurse.

• Drainage tubes may rely on gravity for drainage and, therefore, should always be placed below the area being drained.

• After insertion of a gastric tube and before physical therapy intervention, the tube's position should be confirmed by means of a chest x-ray.

IV-C

Chest Tubes

Michele Panik

A chest tube promotes normal intrapleural pressures and mechanics by (1) removing air, fluid, or both from the pleural space and (2) preventing re-entry of air, fluid, or both into the pleural space. A chest tube drainage system consists of tubing that is inserted into the pleural space and connected to a drainage container. The drainage container has three components [1]: (1) drainage collection chamber, (2) water seal chamber with a one-way valve that prevents air or fluid re-entry, and (3) suction chamber, which decreases excess pressure in the pleural space.

The drainage system can be left to water seal or attached to regulated suction.

Indications for Chest Tube Placement

The following are indications for chest tube placement:

- After surgical opening of the pleural space
- Pleural effusion
- Pneumothorax, hemothorax, chylothorax, or empyema

Location of Chest Tube Placement

The location of the chest tube placement depends on whether air or fluid is being removed. If air is being removed, a chest tube is placed in the second, third, or fourth intercostal space(s) because air normally rises in the pleural space. If fluid is being drained, the chest tube is placed in the sixth, seventh, or eighth intercostal space(s) because fluid moves to the dependent portion of the pleural space.

Complications of Chest Tube Placement

The following are complications of chest tube placement [2]:

- Pain, bleeding, atelectasis, or subcutaneous emphysema at or near the chest tube site

- Tracheal or mediastinal shift

- An air leak (the escape of air) in the drainage system, at the chest tube site, or within the patient (Air leaks are observed as abnormal bubbling in the drainage container on coughing [3].)

Chest Tube Management

To ensure proper chest tube function, the drainage system should be below the level of chest tube insertion, and pulling, pinching, or kinking of the tubing should be avoided. The occlusive dressing over the chest tube site should remain intact. Avoid tipping the drainage system over. If this occurs, return the drainage unit to the upright position and notify the nurse. If the chest tube itself becomes dislodged, stop activity and notify a nurse immediately. If possible, place the patient in an upright sitting position [4]. Monitor the patient's breath sounds, respiratory rate and pattern, and vital signs for signs and symptoms of possible tension pneumothorax. The nurse will apply a temporary dressing over the chest tube site after the patient has performed a Valsalva maneuver.

Physical Therapy Considerations for Patients with Chest Tubes

- The presence of a chest tube should not in and of itself limit activity; in fact, position changes and mobility can facilitate drainage. A chest tube may be momentarily discontinued from wall suction to move the chest tube drainage system or temporarily discontinued (with permission from the physician) to facilitate out of bed activity. If the suction must remain on, extra tubing can be added or a portable suction device can be used for longer distance ambulation. Be sure to monitor for changes in breath sounds before and after activity.

- Modify hand placement during bronchopulmonary hygiene or assisted mobility so as not to press directly on the chest tube site.

- There is a risk of pneumothorax development during chest tube removal, thus a chest x-ray is normally taken after chest tube removal. Check the chest x-ray report for the presence, location, and size of pneumothorax before the next physical therapy treatment.

References

1. Carroll PF. The ins and outs of chest drainage systems. Nursing 86;16:26.
2. Mergart S. S.T.O.P. and assess chest tubes the easy way. Nursing 94;24:52.
3. Carroll PF. What's new in chest tube management. RN 1991:54;34.
4. Colizza DF. Actionstat: dislodged chest tube. Nursing 1995;25:33.

V

Postsurgical Physical Therapy Considerations

Michele Panik

The postsurgical recovery period is characterized as a time of physiologic alteration as a result of the operative procedure and the effects of anesthesia [1]. The physical therapist should be aware of the common postoperative complications (and the protocols and procedures to address them) in order to treat the patient as safely as possible, prioritize physical therapy impairments, and modify treatment parameters.

I. The major systemic effects of general anesthesia are the following:

   A. Neurologic effects. Anesthetic agents decrease cortical and autonomic function.

   B. Cardiovascular effects. Anesthetic agents create the potential for arrhythmia, decreased blood pressure, myocardial contractility, and peripheral vascular resistance [2].

   C. Respiratory effects [3, 4]

      1. Anesthesia has multiple effects on the lung, including decreased or altered
         a. Arterial oxygenation
         b. Response to hypercarbia or hypoxia
         c. Vasomotor tone and airway reflex
         d. Respiratory pattern

    e. Minute ventilation
    f. Functional residual capacity
    g. Mucociliary function
    h. Surfactant

2. The shape and motion of the chest are altered secondary to decreased muscle tone, which causes the following [1]:
    a. Decreased anteroposterior diameter
    b. Increased lateral diameter
    c. Increased cephalad position of the diaphragm

3. Other factors that affect respiratory function and increase the risk of postoperative pulmonary complications (e.g., atelectasis, pneumonia, lung collapse) include the following:
    a. Baseline pulmonary disease
    b. Incisional pain, especially if there is a thoracic or abdominal incision
    c. Smoking history
    d. Obesity
    e. Increased age
    f. The need for large intravenous fluid administration intraoperatively
    g. Prolonged operative time

II. During the postsurgical phase, the patient is monitored for the proper function or return of function of all of the major body systems. Common postoperative complications include the following:

  A. Neurologic complications

    1. Delayed arousal, agitation, or altered consciousness
    2. Cerebral edema, seizure, stroke
    3. Peripheral muscle weakness or altered sensation

  B. Cardiovascular and hematologic complications

    1. Hyper- or hypotension
    2. Dysrhythmia
    3. Myocardial infarction
    4. Coagulopathy
    5. Deep vein thrombosis
    6. Pulmonary embolism

    C. Respiratory complications
1. Respiratory depression
2. Airway obstruction
3. Hypoxia or hypercapnia
4. Aspiration
5. Pulmonary edema
6. Pneumothorax

    D. Renal complications
1. Acute renal failure
2. Decreased urine output
3. Fluid/electrolyte imbalance

    E. Other complications
1. Hypothermia
2. Pain
3. Infection or sepsis
4. Nausea or vomiting
5. Hyperglycemia

III. The development of these conditions in the immediate or secondary postsurgical phase determines further medical-surgical management and treatment parameters. A review of the anesthesia and surgical notes and doctor's order book can provide information about the patient's hemodynamic and general surgical status, unexpected anesthetic effects or surgical findings, operative time, vital sign parameters (including intracranial pressure ranges if applicable), electrocardiographic changes, degree of blood loss (and thus the need for blood products or IV fluid intraoperatively), positioning restrictions, activity level, and weight-bearing status (if applicable).

References

1. Litwack K. Immediate Postoperative Care: A Problem-Oriented Approach. In JS Vender, BD Spiess (eds), Post-Anesthesia Care. Philadelphia: Saunders, 1992;1.
2. Wilson RS. Anesthesia for Thoracic Surgery. In AE Baue, AS Geha, GL Hammond, et al. (eds), Glenn's Thoracic and Cardiovascular Surgery (6th ed). Stamford, CT: Appleton & Lange, 1996;23.

3. Conrad SA, Jayr C, Peper EA. Thoracic Trauma, Surgery, and Perioperative Management. In DB George, RW Light, MA Matthay, RA Matthay (eds), Chest Medicine: Essentials of Pulmonary and Critical Care Medicine (3rd ed). Baltimore: Williams & Wilkins, 1995;629.
4. Benumof JL. Anesthesia for Thoracic Surgery (2nd ed). Philadelphia: Saunders, 1995;94.

VI

Pain Management

Jaime C. Paz

In the acute care setting, physical therapists encounter patients who are experiencing pain for a variety of reasons, most commonly from surgical intervention. This appendix provides information on pain assessment and management that can facilitate the therapist's ability to provide care for a patient.

Assessment

The subjective complaint of pain is difficult to objectify in the clinical setting. Each assessment requires individualization while maintaining consistency among patients. Table IV.1 describes some of the more commonly used pain assessment tools in the acute care setting that complement a complete physical and diagnostic evaluation of the patient's pain [1].

Management

This section focuses on postoperative pain management; however, some of the methods described in Tables VI.2 to VI.5 can be used for pain management of patients with medical or oncologic diagnoses.

Table IV.1. Pain Assessment Tools

Tool	Description
Verbal descriptor scales	The patient describes pain by choosing from a list of adjectives representing gradations of pain intensity.
Numeric rating scale	The patient picks a number from 0 to 10 to rate his or her pain, with 0 indicating no pain, and 10 indicating the worst pain imaginable.
Visual analog scale	The patient marks his or her pain intensity on a 10-cm line, with one end labeled no pain, and the other end labeled worst pain imaginable.
Pain diary	A daily log is kept by the patient denoting pain severity, by using the numeric rating scale, during daily activities, such as walking, chores, and sitting. Medication and alcohol use, along with emotional responses, are also helpful pieces of information to record.

Source: Data from KP Kittelberger, AA LeBel, D Borsook. Assessment of Pain. In D Borsook, AA LeBel, B McPeek (eds), The Massachusetts General Hospital Handbook of Pain Management. Boston: Little, Brown, 1996;27.

Communication among therapists, nurses, physicians, and patients on the effectiveness of pain management is essential to maximize the patient's comfort.

Physical Therapy Considerations for Pain Assessment

- The physical therapist should recognize when the patient is weaning from pain medication (e.g., going from intravenous to oral administration), as the patient may complain of increased pain with a concurrent reduced activity tolerance.

- The physical therapist should be consistent with pain assessment. He or she should use the same pain assessment tool from day to day when evaluating pain before, during, or after physical therapy intervention.

- Often the best way to communicate the adequacy of a patient's pain management to the nurses or physicians is in terms of the patient's ability to complete a given task or activity (e.g., The patient is effectively coughing and clearing secretions).

Table VI.2. Nonsteroidal Anti-Inflammatory Drugs

Description
  Accomplishes analgesia by inhibiting prostaglandin synthesis, which
    leads to anti-inflammatory effects (Prostaglandin is a potent pain-
    producing chemical.)
  A useful alternative or adjunct to opioid therapy

Indications
  Used as the sole therapy for mild to moderate postoperative pain
  Used in combination with opioids for moderate postoperative pain,
    especially when weaning from stronger medications
  Useful in children younger than 6 months of age
  Contraindicated in patients undergoing anticoagulation therapy, with
    peptic ulcer disease, or with gastritis

Side effects
  Platelet dysfunction and gastritis

Generic name (brand name)
  Acetaminophen (Tylenol)
  Aspirin
  Ibuprofen (Motrin, Advil)
  Ketorolac (Toradol)
  Naproxen (Naprosyn)
  Trisalicylate (Trilisate)

Source: Data from JC Ballantyne, D Borsook. Postoperative Pain. In D Borsook, AA
LeBel, B McPeek (eds), The Massachusetts General Hospital Handbook of Pain Management. Boston: Little, Brown, 1996;247.

Physical Therapy Interventions to Maximize
the Patient's Comfort

- The physical therapist should be aware of the patient's pain
  medication schedule and the duration of the effectiveness of different pain medications when scheduling treatment sessions. (Phar-
  macist, nurse, physician, and medication reference books are good
  resources.)

- The physical therapist should also use a pillow, blanket, or his
  or her hands to splint or support a painful area, such as an

Table VI.3. Systemic Opioids

Description
  Block transmission of pain from the spinal cord to the cerebrum
  Can be administered orally, intravenously, intramuscularly, subcutaneously, and intrathecally
Indications
  Moderate to severe postoperative pain
Side effects and considerations
  Mood changes and sedation
  Respiratory and cough depression
  Pupillary constriction
  Decreased gastrointestinal motility and nausea and vomiting
  Pruritus (itching)
  Urinary retention
Generic name (brand name)
  Buprenorphine (Buprenex)
  Butorphanol (Stadol)
  Codeine
  Hydromorphone (Dilaudid)
  Meperidine (Demerol)
  Methadone (Dolophine)
  Morphine (slow release: MS Contin, Roxanol)
  Naloxone
  Oxycodone (Tylox, Percocet, Percodan)
  Propoxyphene (Darvon)

Source: Data from JC Ballantyne, D Borsook. Postoperative Pain. In D Borsook, AA LeBel, B McPeek (eds), The Massachusetts General Hospital Handbook of Pain Management. Boston: Little, Brown, 1996;249; and HL Fields (ed). Pain. New York: McGraw-Hill, 1987;253.

abdominal or thoracic incision or rib fractures, when the patient coughs.

• The physical therapist can use a corset, binder, or brace to support a painful area during functional mobility treatments.

• The physical therapist should instruct the patient not to hold his or her breath during mobility because doing so increases pain.

Table VI.4. Epidural Catheters

Description
  Placement of a catheter in the epidural space for the purpose of infusing
    pain medication, frequently a mixture including fentanyl and bupivacaine
  Fentanyl is a potent morphine-like substance, and bupivacaine is a
    fentanyl carrier.
  Prevents transmission of pain signals to the cerebrum at the spinal level
Indications
  Thoracic, upper abdominal, and lower abdominal surgeries, especially in
    patients with significant pulmonary disease
  Lower limb surgery, especially when early mobilization is important
  Lower extremity vascular procedures, when sympathetic blocks are used
Side effects and considerations
  Sedation and respiratory depression with morphine
  Decreased gastrointestinal motility
  Lower extremity weakness
Medications used according to age
  Younger than 1 year of age: 0.1% bupivacaine without fentanyl
  1–7 years of age: 0.1% bupivacaine with 3 μg/ml fentanyl
  Older than 7 years of age: 0.1% bupivacaine with 10 μg/ml fentanyl

Source: Data from JC Ballantyne, D Borsook. Postoperative Pain. In D Borsook, AA
LeBel, B McPeek (eds), The Massachusetts General Hospital Handbook of Pain Management. Boston: Little, Brown, 1996;252.

Table VI.5. Patient-Controlled Analgesia

Description
  A microprocessor pump that controls infusion of pain medicine, usually
    through an intravenous line
  Dosage, dosage intervals, maximum dosage per set time, and background
    (basal) infusion rate can be programmed
  Patient provided with a button that allows for self-dosing of pain medica-
    tion as needed
Indications
  Used for moderate to severe postoperative pain in patients who are capa-
    ble of properly using the pump
Side effects
  Similar to those of opioids (see the side effects listed in Table VI.3)
Considerations
  Preoperative education of the patient on the use of patient-controlled
    analgesia

Table VI.5. *Continued*

Ensuring that only the patient doses himself or herself

Medications used

Morphine is the drug of choice

Dilaudid or meperidine (when morphine is contraindicated or when it has failed)

Source: Data from JC Ballantyne, D Borsook. Postoperative Pain. In D Borsook, AA LeBel, B McPeek (eds), The Massachusetts General Hospital Handbook of Pain Management. Boston: Little, Brown, 1996;254.

References

1. Kittelberger KP, LeBel AA, Borsook D. Assessment of Pain. In D Borsook, AA LeBel, B McPeek (eds), The Massachusetts General Hospital Handbook of Pain Management. Boston: Little, Brown, 1996;26.

VII

Lower-Extremity Amputation

Jaime C. Paz

Introduction

This appendix describes lower extremity (LE) amputations in terms of common etiologies, types, and physical therapy evaluation and treatment considerations. Upper-extremity amputations occur less commonly and therefore are not discussed here.

Etiology

The majority of LE amputations are acquired from complications of peripheral vascular disease (64% of the cases) and nonhealing diabetic ulcers that lead to gangrene (21%). The least common cause of LE amputations are congenital, occurring only 1% of the time [1].

Types

The various locations of LE amputations are shown in Figure VII.1 and are described in Table VII.1.

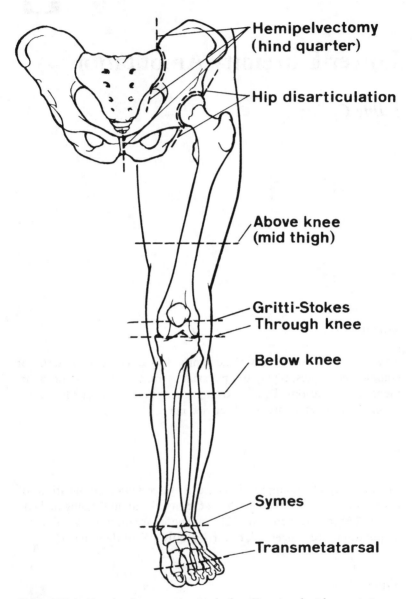

Figure VII.1. *Levels of amputation in the leg. (Reprinted with permission from A Thomson, A Skinner, J Piercy. Tidy's Physiotherapy [12th ed]. Oxford: Butterworth–Heinemann, 1991;261.)*

Table VII.1. Types of Lower-Extremity Amputations

Type	Comments
Toe	Initial weight-bearing postoperatively ranges from non–weight-bearing to partial weight-bearing (according to the physician's orders). Long-term need for adaptive shoes is generally not required.
Transmetatarsal	An adaptive shoe is required, with a rocker-bottom attachment on the sole to help facilitate push-off in gait. The initial weight-bearing status should be clarified with the physician.
Syme's (through the ankle mortise)	Syme's amputation is generally performed with traumatic and infectious cases. No prosthesis is needed.
Below knee	This is the ideal site for amputation, but healing is poor with vascular cases. Residual limb length ranges from 12.5 cm to 15.0 cm from the knee joint.
Through-knee disarticulation	This procedure leaves a strong residual limb with no residual muscle imbalance. It is rarely performed because cosmesis is poor, and prosthetic training is difficult.
Gritti-Stokes (femoral condyles)	This procedure heals well but is rarely performed because the prosthesis is unsightly.
Above knee	The above-knee procedure allows good healing but involves higher metabolic requirements to ambulate with a prosthesis.
Hip disarticulation (femoral head from acetabulum)	Hip disarticulation is indicated in cases of trauma or malignancy but not in cases of vascular disease. The pelvis remains intact.
Hemipelvectomy (hindquarter: entire lower limb and half of pelvis is removed)	Hemipelvectomy is indicated in cases of malignancy. A muscle flap covers the internal organs.

Source: Data from A Thompson, A Skinner, J Piercy (eds). Tidy's Physiotherapy (12th ed). Oxford: Butterworth–Heinemann, 1992;260.

Table VII.2. Physical Therapy Problems and Treatment Suggestions

Problem	Treatment Suggestion
Potential for skin breakdown	The physical therapist should provide instructions about the importance of frequent position changes to the patient and nursing staff and implement out-of-bed activities as soon as possible.
Potential for joint contracture	The physical therapist should provide patient education on residual limb positions and elevation.
	The physical therapist should provide the nursing staff with suggestions for pillow placements or provide splint boards as indicated.
	The physical therapist should begin active range of motion exercises and provide passive stretching as indicated.
Potential for residual limb edema and malformation	Physical therapy techniques range from ace wraps to preparatory prosthesis, according to the patient's needs and the facility's protocols (as clarified with the physician).
	The physical therapist should use elevation of the residual limb with emphasis on contracture prevention.
Potential for decreased functional mobility	Techniques should range from bed mobility training to transfer training to ambulation or wheelchair mobility.

Source: Data from LA Karacoloff, FJ Schneider. Lower Extremity Amputation: A Guide to Functional Outcomes in Physical Therapy Management. Rockville, MD: Aspen, 1985.

Physical Therapy Intervention for Patients with Lower-Extremity Amputation

The focus of physical therapy intervention in the acute care setting is on preprosthetic assessment and training. Prosthetic training, if appropriate, will most likely occur in the subacute or home setting. The primary components to assess in the acute care setting are (1) onset and type of amputation, (2) premorbid lifestyle, (3) discharge plans, (4) skin integrity and sensation, and (5) functional mobilit [2]. Table VII.2 outlines potential physical therapy problems and treatment suggestions for the patient status post LE amputation.

References

1. Thompson A, Skinner A, Piercy J. Tidy's Physiotherapy (12th ed). Oxford: Butterworth–Heinemann, 1992;260.
2. Karacoloff LA, Schneider FJ. Lower Extremity Amputation: A Guide to Functional Outcomes in Physical Therapy Management. Rockville, MD: Aspen, 1985.

VIII

Postural Drainage Positions

Michele Panik

The use of postural drainage as an adjunct to other techniques for the mobilization of pulmonary secretions can be highly effective. Figures VIII.1 to VIII.11 are diagrams of the various postural drainage positions. The physical therapist should note that there are clinical contraindications for postural drainage and considerations that may require position modification to maximize patient comfort or tolerance.

The following are contraindications and considerations for postural drainage [1, 2]:

- Bronchopleural fistula
- Unstable cardiac dysrhythmia
- Congestive heart failure
- Elevated intracranial pressure
- Significant hemoptysis
- Orthopnea
- Pleural effusion (large)
- Pneumothorax (unstable)
- Pulmonary edema
- Pulmonary embolism

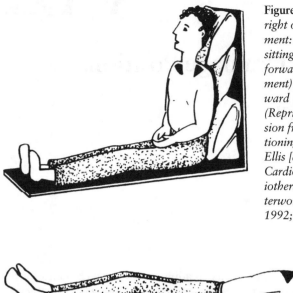

Figure VIII.1. *Lobe: right or left upper. Segment: apical. Position: sitting upright, slightly forward (posterior segment) or slightly backward (anterior segment). (Reprinted with permission from J Alison. Positioning. In J Alison, E Ellis [eds], Key Issues in Cardiorespiratory Physiotherapy. Oxford: Butterworth–Heinemann, 1992;181.)*

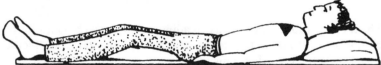

Figure VIII.2. *Lobe: right or left upper. Segment: anterior. Position: supine, bed flat, shoulders unsupported by pillow. (Reprinted with permission from J Alison. Positioning. In J Alison, E Ellis [eds], Key Issues in Cardiorespiratory Physiotherapy. Oxford: Butterworth–Heinemann, 1992;182.)*

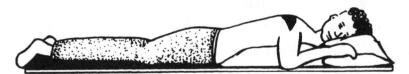

Figure VIII.3. *Lobe: right upper. Segment: posterior. Position: one-quarter turn from prone on left side, bed flat. (Reprinted with permission from J Alison. Positioning. In J Alison, E Ellis [eds], Key Issues in Cardiorespiratory Physiotherapy. Oxford: Butterworth–Heinemann, 1992;182.)*

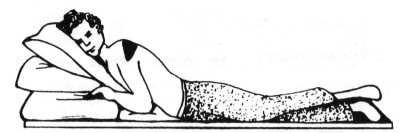

Figure VIII.4. *Lobe: left upper. Segment: posterior. Position: one-quarter turn from prone on right side, trunk supported by pillows to raise trunk 30 degrees or bed in 30 degrees reverse Trendelenburg. (Reprinted with permission from J Alison. Positioning. In J Alison, E Ellis [eds], Key Issues in Cardiorespiratory Physiotherapy. Oxford: Butterworth–Heinemann, 1992;183.)*

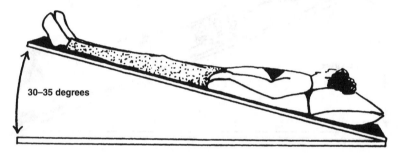

Figure VIII.5. *Lobe: left upper. Segment: lingular. Position: one-quarter turn from supine on right side, bed in 30 degrees Trendelenburg. (Reprinted with permission from J Alison. Positioning. In J Alison, E Ellis [eds], Key Issues in Cardiorespiratory Physiotherapy. Oxford: Butterworth–Heinemann, 1992;183.)*

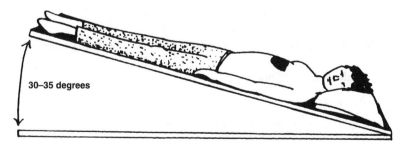

Figure VIII-6. *Lobe: right middle. Segment: lateral and medial. Position: one-quarter turn from supine on left side, bed in 30 degrees Trendelenburg. (Reprinted with permission from J Alison. Positioning. In J Alison, E Ellis [eds], Key Issues in Cardiorespiratory Physiotherapy. Oxford: Butterworth–Heinemann, 1992;184.)*

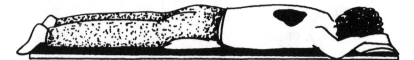

Figure VIII.7. *Lobe: right and left lower. Segment: apical. Position: Prone, bed flat, pillow under hips. (Reprinted with permission from J Alison. Positioning. In J Alison, E Ellis [eds], Key Issues in Cardiorespiratory Physiotherapy. Oxford: Butterworth–Heinemann, 1992;184.)*

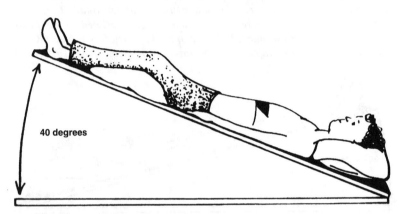

Figure VIII.8. *Lobe: right and left lower. Segment: anterior basal. Position: Supine, bed in 45 degrees Trendelenburg. (Reprinted with permission from J Alison. Positioning. In J Alison, E Ellis [eds], Key Issues in Cardiorespiratory Physiotherapy. Oxford: Butterworth–Heinemann, 1992;185.)*

The following are considerations for postural drainage [1, 2]:

- Abdominal distention
- Anxiety
- Extremes of hypotension or hypertension
- Position or range-of-motion restrictions
- Myocardial infarction (recent)
- Trauma

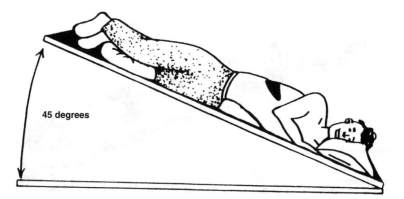

Figure VIII.9. *Lobe: right lower. Segment: lateral basal. Position: full left side-lying, bed in 45 degrees Trendelenburg, pillow under hips. (Reprinted with permission from J Alison. Positioning. In J Alison, E Ellis [eds], Key Issues in Cardiorespiratory Physiotherapy. Oxford: Butterworth–Heinemann, 1992;186.)*

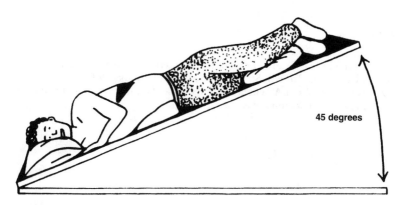

Figure VIII.10. *Lobe: right and left lower. Segment: medial basal (right) and lateral basal (left). Position: full right side-lying, bed in 45 degrees Trendelenburg, pillow under hips. (Reprinted with permission from J Alison. Positioning. In J Alison, E Ellis [eds], Key Issues in Cardiorespiratory Physiotherapy. Oxford: Butterworth–Heinemann, 1992;187.)*

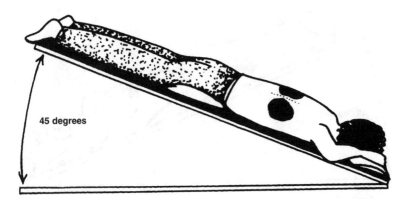

Figure VIII.11. *Lobe: right and left lower. Segment: posterior basal. Position: Prone, bed in 45 degrees Trendelenburg, pillow under hips. (Reprinted with permission from J Alison. Positioning. In J Alison, E Ellis [eds], Key Issues in Cardiorespiratory Physiotherapy. Oxford: Butterworth–Heinemann, 1992;188.)*

References

1. Frownfelter D, Dean E. Principles and Practice of Cardiopulmonary Physical Therapy (3rd ed). St. Louis: Mosby–Year Book, 1996;330.
2. Kisner C, Colby LA. Therapeutic Exercise: Foundations and Techniques (2nd ed). Philadelphia: FA Davis, 1990;577.

IX

Six-Minute Walk Test

Jaime C. Paz

Introduction

The 6-minute walk test is a symptom-limited measure of functional capacity in which a patient walks as far as possible on a premeasured course for a duration of 6 minutes. This test evolved from the 12-minute walk test, originally designed to assess disability levels in patients with chronic bronchitis. The 6-minute walk test was found to provide similar measures of exercise tolerance and therefore adopted by clinicians for its convenience (i.e., taking 6 minutes to perform a test rather than 12 minutes). Vital signs are measured before, periodically during, and after the test [1, 2].

Indications

Indications for the 6-minute walk test are as follows:

1.   As an objective measure of endurance before and after physical therapy intervention

2.   As a screening tool for functional deficits (e.g., gait or balance abnormalities) or limitations to activity

3.   As a tool to assist in the development of an exercise prescription (e.g., intensity, frequency, duration)

4. As a pre- and postoperative assessment tool (e.g., lung transplant or pneumoplasty)

Equipment

The equipment necessary to perform the 6-minute walk test are a stopwatch, pulse oximetry cart, portable blood pressure cuff, electrocardiograph machine (optional if a cardiac diagnosis is unlikely), rating of perceived exertion scale, visual analog pain scale, measuring wheel, and a recording sheet. Placing all this equipment on a cart or having assistance will provide convenience when conducting the test.

Procedure

The procedure for the 6-minute walk test is as follows:

1. The patient is instructed to walk as far as possible for 6 minutes within a designated test area of a premeasured distance (to facilitate distance calculation) and to report if he or she experiences shortness of breath, muscular pain, dizziness, or anginal symptoms, at which time the test will be terminated.

2. The patient is also instructed to rest whenever necessary during the 6 minutes but is asked to continue as soon as he or she is able.

3. The patient is discouraged from talking or asking questions during the test.

4. The tester tells the patient when 6 minutes has elapsed.

5. After the patient demonstrates comprehension of the procedure, resting vital signs can be taken.

6. Timing begins when the tester says "start" or "go."

7. During the test, the tester should walk alongside the patient and offer appropriate guarding as needed. (Walking behind or ahead of the patient influences his or her pace.)

8. Vital signs should be taken one to two times during the test and immediately at the end of 6 minutes.

9.   Chairs stationed at the ends of a hallway are useful in case the patient needs to sit and rest during or after the test.

10.   The distance covered during the 6 minutes should be measured with the measuring wheel.

11.   If the patient is unable to complete the full 6 minutes, the distance covered on termination is measured. The patient should also be asked for the reason for termination if different from those mentioned above (e.g., body pain, fatigue).

Interpretation of the Results

Many studies have examined the usefulness of the 6-minute walk test in specific patient populations (e.g., chronic lung disease, congestive heart failure, total hip replacement) and have found it useful in predicting oxygen consumption and determining the efficacy of surgical intervention on functional mobility [1–4]. No standards, however, have been established for the average distance a "normal" or nondiseased individual should walk in 6 minutes. Therefore, the test is most useful to physical therapists as a means of prescribing exercise intensity and measuring progress.

Exercise Prescription

The exercise intensity for a conditioning program (e.g., walking) can be determined from the 6-minute walk test by using the heart rate, rating of perceived exertion, respiratory rate, or visual analog scale (VAS) results attained at the end of the test. Each patient varies, and a comprehensive assessment of all systems should be performed in conjunction with the 6-minute walk test to safely prescribe an exercise program. The following are examples of exercise prescriptions.

Heart Rate Limitation

The heart rate measured at the end of the test can be used as a symptom-limited maximum parameter, if the patient is not short of breath, has a heart rate response (from start to finish) that shows a linear increase, and reports that he or she could not continue. Percentages (65–80%) of the heart rate can be used to prescribe intensity for an aerobic conditioning program.

Respiratory Rate or Rating of Perceived Exertion Limitation

The respiratory rate or the rating of perceived exertion measured at the end of the test can be used as the symptom-limited maximum parameter if, at the end of the test, the patient reports dyspnea as the limiting factor and the patient's heart rate response is below what is estimated to be a symptom-limited maximum parameter.* For example, if the patient's respiratory rate is 36 breaths per minute at the end of the test, the exercise intensity can be prescribed to allow exercise to continue at a respiratory rate below 36 (e.g., intensity = 36 × [0.65 – 0.80] = 23 – 29 breaths per minute). Note that patients on cardiac beta blockers have blunted heart rate responses; therefore, the above example may not be applicable.

Body Pain Limitation

The VAS report at the end of the test can be used as the symptom-limited maximum parameter if, at the end of the test (either at 6 minutes or any time before), the patient reports body pain as the limiting factor and the patient's vital signs are adaptive during exercise and below predicted symptom-limited maximum. Exercise can then be conducted as the patient's pain is monitored with the VAS, so that the end point of pain tolerance is not reached. To optimize activity tolerance, the patient's pain should be thoroughly assessed and treated.

References

1. McGavin CR, Gupta SP, McHardy GJR. Twelve-minute walking test for assessing disability in chronic bronchitis. BMJ 1976;1:822.
2. Butland RJ, Pang J, Gross ER. et al. Two-, six- and twelve-minute walking tests in respiratory disease. BMJ 1982;284:1607.
3. Cahalin LP, Mathier MA, Semigran MJ, et al. The six-minute walk test predicts peak oxygen uptake and survival in patients with advanced heart failure. Chest 1996;110:310.
4. Laupacis A, Bourne R, Rorabeck C, et al. The effect of elective total hip replacement on health-related quality of life. J Bone Joint Surg [Am] 1993;75:1619.

---

*A symptom-limited maximum is usually estimated at 75% if the age-predicted heart rate (i.e., [220 – age] × 0.75).

Physical Therapy Considerations for Patients Who Complain of Chest Pain

Michele Panik

This appendix can be used to help the physical therapist differentiate between cardiogenic and noncardiogenic pain. It also provides a description of unstable cardiogenic chest pain. Physical therapy considerations of noncardiogenic chest pain are discussed in individual chapters.

Chest pain can occur as a result of a variety of etiologies, described in Table X.1. Each etiology can have distinctive associated signs and symptoms, also listed in this table. If it appears that the patient's chest pain is cardiac in origin (angina), the therapist must then determine if the chest pain is stable or unstable.

Unstable angina is generally characterized by the following [1]:

- Chest pain that occurs with increasing frequency

- Onset of pain that is provoked at rest or with minimal exertion

- Chest pain that is not relieved by nitroglycerin

During an episode of unstable angina, an electrocardiograph may reveal ST segment elevation or depression with or without T-wave inversion that reverses when anginal pain decreases [1]. Additional clinical findings may include the following:

- Hypotension or hypertension

Table X.1. Possible Etiologies and Associated Signs and Symptoms of Chest Pain

Origin	Possible Etiology	Associated Signs and Symptoms
Cardiac	Coronary artery disease Myocardial infarction Mitral valve prolapse	Abnormal blood pressure, heart rate, and rhythm, or heart sounds
Pulmonary	Pneumonia Pulmonary embolism Tuberculosis	Abnormal breath sounds and respiratory rate, cough, hemoptysis
Pleuropericardial	Pleuritis Pneumothorax Mediastinitis Pericarditis	Pain with respiration, pleural rub, pericardial rub
Gastrointestinal	Hiatal hernia Esophagitis Esophageal reflux Acute pancreatitis	Nausea, vomiting, burping, and abdominal pain
Musculoskeletal	Muscle strain Repetitive coughing Rib fracture(s)	Reproduction of pain with range of motion or palpation, and pain with respiration

Source: Data from NH Holmes, M Foley, PH Thompson. Professional Guide to Signs and Symptoms (3rd ed). Springhouse, PA: Springhouse, 1997;153; and RL Wilkins, SJ Krider, RL Sheldon. Clinical Assessment in Respiratory Care (3rd ed). St. Louis: Mosby–Year Book, 1995;28.

- Tachycardia or bradycardia

- Irregular pulse

If the patient presents with one or more of these unstable anginal findings, the therapist should stop or defer treatment and immediately contact a nurse or physician.

References

1. Chandra NC. Angina Pectoris. In LR Barker, JR Burton, PD Ziere (eds), Principles of Ambulatory Medicine (4th ed). Baltimore: Williams & Wilkins, 1995;691.

Index

Note: Page numbers followed by f indicate figures;
page numbers followed by t indicate tables.

Cladribine, in cancer management, side effects of, 340t

Claudication, *versus* pseudoclaudication, 367t

Clofibrate, in cardiac disease management, 88t

Closed fracture, described, 165

Clotting, overactive, pharmacologic agents for, 396t

CMV infection. *See* Cytomegalovirus (CMV) infection

CNS. *See* Central nervous system

Coagulation
profiles of, 21
tests of, 363t
in hematologic system assessment, 359, 363t
zones of, 403f

Coarctation of aorta, secondary hypertension due to, 372t

Cognition
as factor in wound healing, 424
testing of, in mental status examination, 256, 258t

Colectomy, in gastrointestinal disorder management, 476

Colestipol, in cardiac disease management, 88t

Colitis, ulcerative, 469–470

Colles' fracture, 182, 183f

Colon, cancer of
risk factors for, 306t
surgical interventions for, 321t

Colonization, defined, 520

Colonoscopy
in cancer evaluation, 309t
in gastrointestinal system assessment, 451t

Colony-stimulating factor, in cancer management, side effects of, 344t

Color, in wound assessment, 426–427

Colostomy, in gastrointestinal disorder management, 476–477

Coma, hepatic encephalopathy and, 472–473

Comminuted fracture, described, 166

Communicable, defined, 520

Compartment syndrome, 375
casts and, 197

Complete blood count (CBC)
in cardiac system assessment, 20–21
in hematologic system assessment, 359, 360t–361t, 362f
values and interpretation of, 360t–361t

Compression fracture, described, 166

Computed tomography (CT)
in cancer evaluation, 309t
in gastrointestinal system assessment, 453t
in genitourinary system assessment, 493
in musculoskeletal system assessment, 164
in neurologic examination, 271–272
in vascular disorder assessment, 357t

Conduction disturbance, pathophysiology of, 34

Congenital vascular malformations (CVMs), 378

Congestive heart failure (CHF), 39, 42, 43t–45t
causes of, 39, 42
described, 39
management of, pharmacologic agents in, 49
patients hospitalized with, activity guidelines for, 44t–45t
signs and symptoms of, 43t

Consciousness, level of, in mental status examination, 255–256, 255t

Continent urinary diversion, in genitourinary disorder management, 516

Continuous arteriovenous hemofiltration (CAVH), for renal failure, 509–510, 509f

Continuous positive airway pressure (CPAP), 606–607

Contraceptives, oral, secondary hypertension due to, 372t

Contrast angiography, in vascular disorder assessment, 353, 357

Contusion, lung, 137